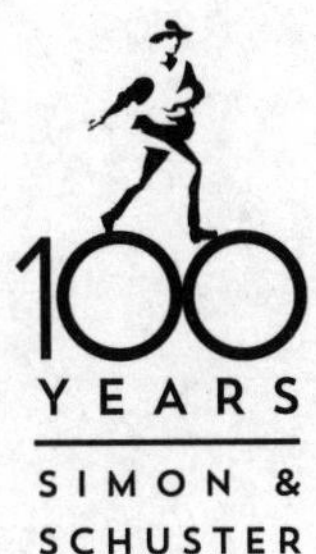
100
YEARS
SIMON &
SCHUSTER

Also by Donald G. McNeil Jr.

Zika: The Emerging Epidemic

The WISDOM of PLAGUES

LESSONS FROM **25 YEARS** OF COVERING PANDEMICS

Donald G. McNeil Jr.

SIMON & SCHUSTER

New York London Toronto Sydney New Delhi

1230 Avenue of the Americas
New York, NY 10020

First Simon & Schuster hardcover edition January 2024

SIMON & SCHUSTER and colophon are registered trademarks of Simon & Schuster, Inc.

Simon & Schuster: Celebrating 100 Years of Publishing in 2024

For information about special discounts for bulk purchases, please contact Simon & Schuster Special Sales at 1-866-506-1949 or business@simonandschuster.com.

The Simon & Schuster Speakers Bureau can bring authors to your live event. For more information or to book an event, contact the Simon & Schuster Speakers Bureau at 1-866-248-3049 or visit our website at www.simonspeakers.com.

Interior design by Wendy Blum

Manufactured in the United States of America

1 3 5 7 9 10 8 6 4 2

Library of Congress Cataloging-in-Publication Data

Names: McNeil, Donald G., Jr., author.
Title: The wisdom of plagues : lessons from 25 years of covering pandemics / Donald G. McNeil Jr.
Description: First Simon & Schuster hardcover edition. | New York : Simon & Schuster, 2024. | Includes bibliographical references and index.
Identifiers: LCCN 2023018091 (print) | LCCN 2023018092 (ebook) | ISBN 9781668001394 (hardcover) | ISBN 9781668001400 (paperback) | ISBN 9781668001417 (ebook)
Subjects: LCSH: Epidemiology. | Pandemics. | Public health surveillance. | Public health—United States. | CYAC: COVID-19 (Disease)
Classification: LCC RA652 .M36 2024 (print) | LCC RA652 (ebook) | DDC 614.4—dc23/eng/20230925
LC record available at https://lccn.loc.gov/2023018091
LC ebook record available at https://lccn.loc.gov/2023018092

ISBN 978-1-6680-0139-4
ISBN 978-1-6680-0141-7 (ebook)

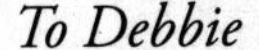

To Debbie

You superpowers spend billions on preparing for war and on fighting terrorism . . . and pennies on disease. That makes no sense. You can negotiate with your enemies to avoid war. You can change the behavior that makes you a terrorist target. But you cannot negotiate with a virus. And viruses kill more people than those ever will.

—Dr. Michael J. Ryan, World Health Organization coordinator of epidemic response, to the author, circa 2000

CONTENTS

Part One: Initial Reflections on Pandemics

Part Two: The Tangled Roots of Pandemics

Part Three: The Human Factors That Spread Pandemics

The WISDOM of PLAGUES

Part One

INITIAL REFLECTIONS ON PANDEMICS

Chapter One

COVID AS A NERVOUS CONDITION

It began innocuously.

On December 31, 2019, I saw a notice on the disease-alert service ProMED-Mail about unexplained pneumonia cases linked to a seafood market in Wuhan, China. I remember thinking, Huh—that sounds like the way SARS began: mystery pneumonia in a Chinese city, no more information. But I was busy with a story for *The New York Times* about the bad flu season then shaping up in the United States. Also, some ProMED alerts turn out to be false alarms. I filed it away mentally as something to keep an eye on.

In the earliest days, as more news came out of China, it didn't seem too serious. We speculated and made jokes about it. One colleague in China asked on an email chain if it could be a fish virus, since it was from a seafood market. I said I doubted it; I'd never heard of humans catching a fish virus, and besides, it caused pneumonia—and fish didn't have lungs. "Aquaman has lungs *and* gills," a foreign desk editor injected.

On January 8, China announced that, in 15 of the 59 pneumonia cases, it had detected a coronavirus that had never been seen before. I helped our Beijing and Hong Kong bureaus write that story. There were conflicting reports about how many of the known cases were connected to the market, which by then we knew also sold meat and wild game. There were also conflicting reports about whether there was any human-to-human transmission.

I suggested to my colleague Sui-Lee Wee that she keep an ear out for reports of "sustained" human-to-human transmission. Some limited human transmission was to be expected, since it had occurred in both SARS and MERS. Those coronaviruses—Severe Acute Respiratory Syndrome, which emerged in southern China in 2003, and Middle East Respiratory Syndrome, which emerged in Saudi Arabia in 2012—were highly lethal but ultimately containable because they did not transmit easily. Sustained transmission would be a much bigger threat.

We didn't know it at the time, but a week earlier, as soon as the first reports of pneumonia arose, Wuhan's mayor, Zhou Xianwang, had ordered a cover-up. An ambitious politician, he had a local party congress scheduled for mid-January that would advance his career. He was also planning a January 19 potluck dinner for 40,000 families that he hoped would put him in the *Guinness World Records* book. Police officers visited the doctors who had first reported the mysterious infections and told them to keep quiet or else face arrest. The market was shuttered on January 1. The sellers dispersed, their meat and live animals went elsewhere or into the trash, and the venue was hosed down. Even if that was a sensible decision for safety's sake, it amounted to trampling a crime scene, obscuring the origins of the pandemic to come.

On January 16, the CDC—the U.S. Centers for Disease Control and Prevention, based in Atlanta—said it would screen passengers arriving from Wuhan. However, it did only temperature checks, and we did not yet know that asymptomatic transmission existed. Unbeknownst to anyone, an infected passenger had arrived in Seattle on January 15.

On January 17, I went on vacation—a long-planned trout-fishing trip to Argentina. In retrospect, I clearly guessed wrong about how long it would take the virus to exit China. My editor in science news later told me that a foreign desk editor said: "He's on vacation? If he worked for us, he wouldn't be." (On the other hand, the paper was constantly pressuring us to take our vacation days because it disliked paying out our unused ones, as our union contract required.)

When I can't stay asleep—which is most nights—I listen to the BBC World Service, hoping it will lull me back under. In Argentina, I lay awake for long stretches listening to news from China. The old friends I was fishing with said, "You came to breakfast looking more worried each day."

In mid-January, Beijing sent an investigative team to Wuhan headed by eighty-three-year-old Dr. Zhong Nanshan, a hero of the 2003 SARS outbreak and nicknamed "China's Dr. Fauci." On January 20, Dr. Zhong said on national TV that there was clearly human-to-human transmission, including to medical personnel, and that Wuhan should be avoided. (He also said it was not as contagious as SARS, which later proved very wrong.) Three days later, Beijing shut down all travel to and from the city and the surrounding Hubei Province. At the time, there were only 500 confirmed cases and 17 deaths. The enormity of that decision would not become clear until later.

That same day, as I was leaving Argentina, the World Health Organization convened an expert panel to debate whether China's outbreak was a PHEIC, a "public health emergency of international concern." (I have heard PHEIC pronounced as "fake," "fike," "pike," and even "pick." As far as I can tell, there is no official pronunciation.) It concluded that it was not. My editor called to ask what I thought. I said that, given what we knew, the WHO decision made sense—on technical grounds. It was clearly a growing emergency inside China, but only a handful of cases and no deaths had occurred outside, so it wasn't really yet an emergency "of international concern." The expert committee, we learned later, was sharply split, and China had lobbied hard against declaring an emergency.

One week later, on January 30, even with fewer than 100 confirmed cases outside China, the WHO did declare one. The writing was on the wall.

Inside China, on January 27, Mayor Zhou apologized on national

TV for reacting too slowly. He offered to resign but was allowed to keep his job. (I found that strange, since some mayors had been summarily dismissed during the SARS epidemic and Hubei's officials were replaced. But Mr. Zhou is a prominent member of China's large Tujia ethnic group and perhaps Beijing was reluctant to humiliate him.)

On the evening of the 30th, China reported having nearly 10,000 cases with about 200 deaths. On the subway, mulling over the day's news, I realized with shock what that meant: this was not the return of SARS. A virus that could rocket from 500 cases to 10,000 in one week and that had had a fatality rate of 2 percent was very close to what the world had seen in 1918. That pandemic—the Spanish flu—had lasted two years, infected most of the world's population, and killed over 50 million.

I came in to work the next day very jittery. "This is it," I told my editor. "This is the Big One. This is going to be 1918 all over again."

She balked: "You have to talk to a *lot* of scientists before we can say that in *The New York Times*." I called a dozen of my regular sources—doctors who had played major roles in fighting smallpox, AIDS, Ebola, and other epidemics. They were divided: eight said yes, two said no, two were undecided. But one of the eight yeses was Dr. Anthony S. Fauci, whom I caught just as he was walking into the White House for a meeting about the outbreak. That helped convince my editor I wasn't crazy.

On February 2, the *Times* published my piece saying many experts felt a pandemic was inevitable.

By then there were 17,000 cases and 360 deaths and the virus was in 23 countries. Even so, I faced a mountain of disbelief. The article did not make page 1 or even get a "reefer"—a front-page one-sentence reference; it ran on page 12. The front page did have a well-written analysis of China's reflexive secrecy about disease, along with stories about impeaching President Donald Trump, Brexit, bullying inside Victoria's Secret, and the Super Bowl.

Only a few Americans were alarmed, but clearly some were. I went out to buy some masks and gloves and found none left at every pharmacy

I tried. I wrote an article about the possibility of shortages as the disease spread. When I called the CDC for comment, they seemed only mildly concerned; a midlevel official told me she had asked the big pharmacy chains to hold back supplies. When I called the chains, however, they professed to know nothing about any such request and were selling everything they could.

On January 31, after President Trump issued his executive order barring entry to noncitizens leaving China, I was asked to sit in on a meeting about what it would do to China-U.S. trade. After about half an hour of editors discussing story ideas, I interrupted to say, with some exasperation, "You don't understand. This isn't going to stop at China. Japan has cases. South Korea has cases. It's on the move." A deputy business editor looked at me condescendingly. "Are you saying flights to other countries will stop?" he asked. "Yes," I said. "This is going to affect the whole world." He made a blatant scoffing noise in my face and turned away.

Soon I found myself getting into email arguments, especially with foreign desk editors, and occasionally being reprimanded for my tone. That desk—whose correspondents in Beijing, Shanghai, and Hong Kong were regularly harassed and denied visas by the government—seemed to assume that everything emanating from Beijing was a lie. On February 12, when the case numbers in Wuhan doubled overnight, they assumed the books were cooked. I explained that, with tests for the virus in short supply, the government had permitted doctors to confirm diagnoses on the basis of X-rays alone, so case numbers had to jump. When China forced people into quarantine, the desk saw it as outrageous and believed rumors that the sick and the healthy were being quarantined together; I argued that mixing the two would make no sense, so I doubted there was any such policy. But isolating just the infected, harsh as it was, I said, could dramatically slow the spread.

All February, too much reporting focused on one passenger ship, the *Diamond Princess*, because it was full of Americans. Then a single passenger from the *Westerdam*—a second cruise ship that had been ordered away from port after port until it was finally allowed to disgorge its passengers in Cambodia—tested positive as she passed through Malaysia on her way home. The foreign desk dispatched half a dozen reporters to chase down *Westerdam* passengers, assuming they constituted a viral wave headed for America. I argued that, since the ship's captain said there had been no outbreak aboard, and since only one passenger had tested positive—and at a lab that did not meet WHO standards—it must have been a false positive. I wasn't believed; the reporters were kept chasing passengers. The CDC later confirmed my supposition that she'd never been infected. (In those days, the idea that a medical test could give a wrong answer was unfamiliar—except to medical professionals and science reporters.)

To be fair, at that time, most of the nation had trouble believing the threat was real. New York's mayor rebuffed suggestions that the St. Patrick's Day parade be canceled. A player for the Utah Jazz mocked reporters' questions about ending the basketball season by wiping his hands on all their microphones.

The stock market was initially slow to react. Then on February 24, the Dow Jones Industrial Average dropped 1,000 points, the first lurch in what would ultimately be a 30 percent drop. President Trump responded with a tweet: "The Coronavirus is very much under control in the USA. We are in contact with everyone and all relevant countries. CDC & World Health have been working hard and very smart. Stock market starting to look very good to me!"

The next day, in a phone call with reporters, Dr. Nancy Messonnier, the CDC's chief of respiratory diseases, effectively contradicted him, saying a major outbreak in the United States was "not so much a question of if this will happen anymore, but rather a question of exactly when this will happen, and how many people in this country will have severe illness." She suggested that Americans "start thinking about" how they would cope if their schools and businesses closed, gatherings were canceled, and travel was limited.

The markets tumbled further, enraging the president.

On February 27, prompted by Dr. Messonnier's words and the shaky markets, Michael Barbaro invited me onto his podcast, *The Daily*. He began by asking how many epidemics I had covered and how bad I thought this one could be.

I answered that I always spent a lot of time thinking about whether what I wrote was too alarmist—or perhaps not alarmist enough. Although this sounded alarmist, I said, the new epidemic looked to me like an echo of the Spanish flu. China's study of the first 45,000 cases had found a fatality rate of 2.3 percent—similar to estimates for 1918. We would not all die, of course, but 2 percent mortality meant we would all know someone who died. I mentioned a friend whose grandmother had died in 1918.

We talked about how spooky I found the reports from China. Despite the availability of lifesaving measures that had not existed a century ago—piped oxygen, ventilators, antiviral drugs, steroids for lung inflammation, antibiotics for bacterial pneumonia—large numbers of people were still dying. We talked about our own domestic shortage of ventilators. We talked about the Wuhan lockdown during Chinese New Year, which I compared to locking down Chicago at Christmastime. Most experts felt that making a vaccine would take more than a year, since the record was four years, set by mumps vaccine in 1967. I doubted that any of the drugs then being tested in China would prove effective. (If one had really been a miracle cure, I said, word would have already leaked out.) Therefore, I said, we might have to enforce our own China-style shutdown to stop the virus when it arrived. But I worried that we couldn't because Americans don't like to be told what to do, and many would resist.

Michael asked me what I was doing personally to stay safe. I told him I had bought a box of masks—I'd finally found some—but felt guilty because hospital workers needed them more. I worried about supply chains drying up, so I had ordered more of my blood pressure medicine. Also, I always had a month's worth of food in my basement "because that's the kind of guy I am." (I had stocked up after Hurricane Sandy in 2012.)

Later many *Daily* listeners, especially younger ones, told me that episode was what first made them take the threat seriously. Some Trump supporters, on the other hand, still accuse me of spreading panic, spooking the stock market, and triggering runs on grocery stores.

I was also meeting skepticism in my personal life. I played in a weekly softball game and a squash round-robin, and one of the squash players said he had heard me on *The Daily* but wasn't convinced. "I've got tickets for Greece in July," he said, "and I'm going." "I don't think your trip will happen," I said. "You should get your deposit back." "No," he insisted. "I *am going.* I don't care what you say." "OK, so don't get it back," I said with a shrug. "But I wouldn't be in a hurry to pay the rest."

One of my coworkers, a security guard, stopped me in the lobby to ask, "This disease doesn't affect black people, right?" "What?" I replied. "Where did you get that idea?" "Because it's not in Africa," he said. "That's because there aren't many flights there from China," I said. "It'll get to Africa. Don't kid yourself—you're not immune. Be careful."

In the paint store where my girlfriend worked as a color consultant, one of her coworkers assured her that he was safe because he never ate Chinese food or drank Corona beer. He wasn't joking.

Even one of my oldest friends at the paper was skeptical. He was an obituaries editor. I sent him an email saying his life would probably soon get very hectic because lots of Americans would die. But sports events would probably be canceled, so some great sportswriters would be idle. Why not, I asked, recruit them as obit writers?

He answered with a quasi-science-based argument: China had suffered fewer than 5,000 deaths, and the United States had only a third of China's population, so we should have only 1,500 or so. Of 1,500 random deaths across America, it wasn't likely that many would merit *New York Times* obituaries, so he wasn't worried.

"We're not going to have just 1,500 dead," I wrote back. "We're not China. We're not going to be able to control this." He wasn't convinced. (Ultimately, the whole staff and many freelancers wrote hundreds of mini obituaries under the rubric "Those We've Lost.")

The first time I got nervous for myself, however, was not until early March, when the CDC, after a disastrous two-month delay, finally rolled out large numbers of PCR tests—polymerase chain reaction tests that can detect the tiniest amounts of a virus's genes in a nasal swab. Up till then, New York's testing had been spotty. We knew about a big outbreak in a Westchester County synagogue and one at a New Jersey family dinner that killed four relatives. Now, suddenly, positives were pinging up all around me: a work colleague already hospitalized with pneumonia, another colleague's husband, a parent in a friend's child's school, five patients in the hospital where my girlfriend was a volunteer. I wrote a long email to my extended family, my friends, and all the squash and softball players I knew. New York was probably hot with virus right now, it said. Any subway pole or door handle could be contaminated. Any restaurant or party or meeting might be a superspreader event. So please be careful.

Most thanked me. Some thought I was being ridiculous.

On March 9, the *Times* began encouraging us to stop coming into the office. I kept going in until the 11th, to do one last *Daily* episode in the recording studio. By then my nights were only three hours long—I would basically drink myself to sleep at 11 p.m. with four glasses of wine at dinner. Nightmares would jolt me awake at 2 a.m., and I'd feel compelled to get up and keep reporting. I scanned Hong Kong and European news sites for what had happened the previous day, trying to guess how their crises would play out in the United States. I felt like Cassandra, the prophetess condemned to see the future but never be believed.

I could see Troy burning—in our case, thousands of Americans dying—so I couldn't stop, hoping something I said or wrote might blunt the blow.

By the third week of March, some of the crazy-sounding stuff I'd been spouting came true. The St. Patrick's Day parade was canceled; so was the basketball season. Schools closed, as did bars, restaurants, movie theaters, and Broadway. Most of us were asked to stay indoors and work remotely. We were divided into "essential" and "nonessential" workers. Masks were nowhere to be found, so YouTube videos appeared showing how to cut one from an old T-shirt or wrap your boxer briefs around your head. Hand sanitizer disappeared, so prisoners were ordered to make it. Stores saw shoving matches over toilet paper. We started washing down our groceries with bleach.

Day by day, the city's intensive care units filled up. Ventilators and personal protective equipment (PPE) ran short. Exhausted nurses were forced to protect themselves with garbage bags and wear the same masks day after day.

Soon New Yorkers began dying—first in drips, then in gouts, then in cataracts. Some nursing homes lost dozens of residents. Seniors and people with cardiac problems or diabetes died. So did frontline personnel: nurses, doctors, paramedics, police officers, transit workers, grocery clerks.

Mount Sinai Hospital became so crowded that tents were erected in Central Park to take the overflow. Hospitals forbade visitors, so thousands of New Yorkers died alone or said goodbye on cell phones. Hospitals stacked bodies in refrigerated trucks. Funeral homes ran short of caskets; Jewish burial societies ran out of shrouds. A photographer flew a drone over Hart Island, the city's pauper cemetery, and captured a deep mass grave with coffins stacked inside it.

At seven o'clock each night, we unglued ourselves from the news and stepped onto our stoops or leaned out windows to bang on pots and cheer for the emergency workers. In my girlfriend's U-shaped apartment building, we got to know the neighbors by waving at each other as we clapped. If a police car or ambulance turned into the driveway, we cheered until the crew got out and waved.

Everyone in the country was deeply frustrated and suffering—from the loss of jobs, from loneliness or grief, from the fear of death. By contrast, I felt more fulfilled than I ever had before, even as I worked harder than I ever had in my life. It was as if I had trained for twenty-five years for a story like this, and it had dropped in my lap just as I was contemplating retirement. I hadn't wished for it, but it made me useful, which was exhilarating.

The nature of my job also changed. Like all reporters, I was used to covering the past: something happens—a fire, a murder, an election, a coup—and you write it up. Suddenly the masthead, the paper's top editors, were assigning me to cover the future. Each month I would interview dozens of experts—epidemiologists, virologists, vaccinologists, medical historians, economists—and write long multichapter pieces synthesizing their thoughts and trying to envision what would happen next.

As the deaths mounted, my work got darker. My April 18 piece titled "The Coronavirus in America: The Year Ahead" was so grim that the photo editor illustrated it in black and white. The photos showed the entrance to one of the Mount Sinai tents, rows of refrigerated trucks on Randall's Island, an almost-empty Staten Island Ferry, a patient in an ambulance, a nurse checking her PPE, and a charity giving food boxes to families with children.

"It was impossible," I wrote, "to avoid gloomy forecasts for the next year. The scenario that Mr. Trump has been unrolling at his daily press briefings—that the lockdowns will end soon, that a protective pill is almost at hand, that football stadiums and restaurants will soon be full—is a fantasy, most experts said.

"'We face a doleful future,' said Dr. Harvey V. Fineberg, a former president of the National Academy of Medicine."

In retrospect, the story got much right—and much wrong. It took not months but years for society to return to normal. Our social restrictions went on and on, but they were "lockdown lite" and barely enforced. Americans quietly went on dates, held clandestine parties, drove anywhere they wanted. We flattened the curve of hospital admissions but never came close to stopping the virus. China kept its cities clamped tight until each had zero cases for two weeks; we never had fewer than 30,000 a day. Our work lives were so devastated that the government had to pour in billions to keep the economy afloat. Notions that once would have been deemed un-American became realities: Evictions and bank foreclosures were banned. Mortgage and tax payments were delayed. Millions who had recently had good jobs got unemployment checks.

Vaccines arrived far faster than the experts I had interviewed predicted. Convalescent plasma did not work as well as they hoped. Monoclonal antibodies did work, but never gained wide acceptance. "Immune passports" never became routine except in New York State, and even there mostly for entering restaurants. Young people did not deliberately infect themselves in order to rush back to normal life; normal life wasn't allowed.

To explain how the future would probably work, I cited Tomas Pueyo's seminal Medium essay "The Hammer and the Dance." First the "hammer" of lockdown would slow the spread, then we could briefly "dance" out to see how much freedom we could enjoy before deaths ticked up and the hammer fell again. Sadly, we never became organized enough to rationally cycle in and out of lockdowns like that. I also noted a prediction Mr. Pueyo made: the virus would initially kill Democrats because it was spreading in cities, but it would eventually reach rural states where Americans were older, heavier, farther from hospitals, and mostly Republican. He was proven right—but for a different reason, which neither of us foresaw: a year later, when the miraculously effective vaccines arrived, millions of conservatives would reject them. By late 2021, Americans living in counties that had voted for Trump in 2020 were three times as likely to die of Covid as those in counties that had voted for Joe Biden.

At the time I wrote that "Year Ahead" piece, New York had been closed down for less than a month and only 34,000 Americans had died. Nonetheless, it was considered so grim, and so contradictory to the president's rosy predictions, that orders came down from the masthead to make it more optimistic. When I resisted, saying that none of my sources were anything but gloomy, my editor simply inserted cheerful sentences like "Some felt that American ingenuity, once fully engaged, might well produce advances to ease the burdens." He insisted it end on an upbeat note. We finally agreed on "If a vaccine saves lives, many Americans may become less suspicious of conventional medicine and more accepting of science in general—including climate change, experts said. The blue skies that have shone above American cities during this lockdown era could even become permanent."

That was the first time in my career I had been ordered to change the mood of a story.

On *The Daily*, by contrast, Michael Barbaro let me describe how my sources actually felt and point out that reopening the country in May or June would lead to disaster. "If we all tried to come out at once," I said, "everything would look cool for about three weeks. And a week or two after that, the emergency rooms would start to fill again, and people would start to die again."

Now that seems obvious. At the time, however, the notion that you could fine-tune the number of dead with the strictness of your public health measures was not instinctively understood.

The first wave was a disaster because we had spent all January and February in a headless-chicken phase. We had had plenty of warning. But we reacted slowly because of disbelief, especially at the very top. Then we had no tests. Without them, we had no idea where the virus was. If we had, we might have shut down New York sooner. Even a week might have saved thousands of lives. If we'd known how rare the virus was elsewhere, we might have let much of the country stay open, then closed it hotspot by hotspot, not all at once. We might have slowed travel out of the hotspots, closed some school districts but not others, moved medical personnel and goods to where they were most needed, and so on. Everything might have been different. Common sense might have prevailed, instead of frustration and anger.

What no one—me, my sources, my editors, or *The Daily* producers—perceived back then was how polarized the country would become. In April there still was a feeling that we were all facing a calamity together; even President Trump had seen the projections of 240,000 deaths by midsummer and agreed to the pause he called "15 Days to Slow the Spread." No one yet imagined that the virus would be declared a Democratic hoax perpetrated to weaken his reelection chances by triggering a recession. No one imagined that so many Americans would reject masks and then vaccines even as their friends and family members died—and then insist they had died of other causes. No one yet imagined that the country would numbly accept the levels of death it ultimately did. When the toll hit 100,000 dead, the *Times* devoted its entire front page to their names. Two years later, when the toll was more than ten times as high, we were so battered that we could barely keep the right number in our heads.

Grim as my early piece was, the national insanity and the exhausted acceptance that would ultimately descend on us were still beyond contemplation.

Chapter Two

HOW I GOT HERE

I spent about twenty-five years covering global health for *The New York Times*.

My accidental introduction into the beat—and my education—began in 1998, when I visited an orphanage in Johannesburg, South Africa, the Cotlands Baby Sanctuary. The toddlers headed toward me, their arms out to be picked up and hugged. One chubby little guy with a runny nose wrapped himself around my calf as the teacher showed me the kitchen and the playrooms.

I felt terrible because I was at Cotlands for a reason. Except for a few with swollen glands, the children all looked fine—happy and healthy.

I finally detached the little guy and went out into the hall with the head nurse. I knew the answer to my next question—but I didn't want to ask it.

I nodded back toward the room full of kids. "They're all . . . going to die?" I whispered.

The nurse, Kathy Volkwyn, a white Afrikaner, almost burst into tears. "Yes," she said. "These babies are probably all going to die."

That Cotlands class was for the HIV-positive children, born to mothers who were themselves infected. All were African or mixed-race. Some of their mothers had already died; all the rest were doomed to.

In Africa in those days, adults with HIV usually lived five or six years after being infected. But babies who picked up the virus in the womb almost always succumbed sooner. Few of these kids would make it even to age four.

By that time, triple-therapy antiretroviral cocktails had been saving the lives of HIV-infected Americans for almost three years. AIDS in America was changing from an inevitably fatal plague into a manageable chronic infection. A triple-therapy pioneer, Dr. David Ho, had been *Time* magazine's 1996 Man of the Year. But there was no medicine for these kids.

"We have a hard time raising enough money to pay for milk and nappies," Reva Goldsmith, Cotlands's assistant director, told me. "We can barely pay for Ciprobay for their ear infections."

Back then, triple-therapy cocktails cost up to $15,000 a year. The companies that made them had zero interest in lowering their prices for Africans. Also, there were no pediatric formulations, nothing a child could swallow. The customers they wanted were gay men with health insurance in America, Europe, Japan, and Australia.

Nearly all other modern drugs were equally out of reach. Enough Ciprobay—ciprofloxacin, then a relatively new antibiotic made by Bayer, the aspirin company—to treat an ear infection cost about $40 in South Africa. There were generic versions made in India and elsewhere, but South African law, written to please the country's powerful pharmaceutical lobby, made importing them illegal.

I was just beginning to understand why.

I was not then a health reporter; I was a Johannesburg-based foreign correspondent covering southern Africa. I was on this particular story because, a few weeks earlier, a commercial attaché at the U.S. embassy in Pretoria had asked to meet me. He suggested I write about something the U.S. government—this was during Bill Clinton's presidency—strongly opposed. And that he personally considered outrageous.

The South African Parliament, he said, was on the verge of passing a bill that would make it possible for the national health minister to nullify any patent that pharmaceutical companies had registered in South Africa. If it became law and the minister thought a drug was too pricey, he or she could claim patent abuse and assign the right to provide the drug to someone else—even an Indian company.

My first reaction was identical to his: I thought the idea was outrageous. I'd been brought up reading biographies of the Wright brothers, Thomas Edison, and George Washington Carver, and I admired inventors. I thought it was terrible that someone could take a product inspired by genius, copy it, and sell it for less.

Also, in those days, the pharmaceutical industry was still basking in the afterglow of its post–World War II miracles. A torrent of new antibiotics had driven back tuberculosis, scarlet fever, and syphilis. Vaccines had beaten childhood scourges. Drugs that could cure cancer were being invented. Psychoactive drugs were helping victims of depression and schizophrenia lead normal lives instead of being institutionalized. The Pill had given women control over their sexuality. There was even talk of a magic pill that would one day help men get erections.

At the time, most Americans had very favorable views of the industry. It also wielded such power in Washington that, when President Clinton made his "African Renaissance" tour of the continent in 1998, he threatened to impose trade sanctions on South Africa if the patents bill became law.

But the more reporting I did—and especially after I talked to drug-access activists at Doctors Without Borders—the clearer it became to me that the real villains of the piece were the pharma companies. Rather than seeking to cure the greatest number of victims, they focused only on protecting their patent monopolies so they could keep charging the enormous markups to which they had become addicted. In public, they emphasized how much they plowed back into research. But the truth was that vast amounts were spent on lobbying, patent battles, and on wining and dining doctors. (Until 1997, it was illegal to advertise drugs to consumers on television, so they had long been spared that huge expense.)

In South Africa, the pharmaceutical lobby ran ads against the bill.

The most memorable one featured a crying baby. "Health Warning!" it read. "Remain Silent and the Unsafe Control of Medicine Could Cost You Forever." The new law, the ads said, would let unscrupulous operators import "counterfeit, fake, expired and harmful medicines." Generics, they suggested, were shoddy goods made by "pirates."

The companies coordinated their pressure tactics. Merck, Smith-Kline-Beecham, Bristol-Myers Squibb, Pharmacia & Upjohn, and Eli Lilly all either closed their South African factories or said they would drop expansion plans if the law passed.

The trade association's chief executive went even further: she publicly threatened to cut off all new medicines.

In an interview, I asked her if she was serious in saying that South Africans would be denied access—at any price—to the novel drugs then being developed for AIDS, cancer, and other diseases. She said yes.

"Are you literally," I asked, "threatening to let thousands of your fellow South Africans die if you don't get your way?"

She hemmed a bit, and then answered: "In so many words, yes. It's very clear—when countries start tampering with patent rights, the new innovations aren't released there."

I was shocked.

"Do you think that's a winning tactic?"

"Health is a very emotive topic," she answered. "When one party is totally unreasonable, the other becomes totally unreasonable. It becomes tit-for-tat. It's playground tactics, I'm afraid."

Even with such a blatant blackmail threat on the record, my first story about the law had a tone that was still ambivalent. What South Africa wanted to do seemed so radical. It certainly seemed radical to the business editor who handled it. Neither he nor I realized at the time that South Africa was merely granting itself the same absolute powers over patents that many governments—including the United States—already held.

That led me to reporting more stories on Africans dying because they couldn't afford medicine.

The majors were not keeping prices high only on antiretroviral drugs. For example, an antifungal sold in the United States for $25 a pill to cure vaginal infections and toenail fungus also cured thrush, an oral fungus that afflicted people with advanced AIDS. In a thrush-filled throat, one clinician said, a sip of water was "like swallowing razor blades." Another drug that eliminated women's facial hair could also cure sleeping sickness—which, despite its somniferous name, ravages victims like rabies before it kills them. But the companies wanted to make just pills or creams, not the intravenous versions needed to fight thrush and sleeping sickness. And they were uninterested in lowering their prices.

In the past, the U.S. government had not hesitated to employ its own tough patent love. In 1917, when the military wanted hundreds of airplanes for the war, it compelled all the manufacturers, including the Wright brothers' company, to "pool" all the patents they held on components like rudders and ailerons and accept a 1.25 percent royalty—a few hundred dollars per plane. The alternative, Franklin D. Roosevelt, then secretary of the navy, told them, was to see all their patents revoked.

In 2001, when anthrax-filled letters mailed in the wake of the September 11 terrorist attacks killed five Americans, the George W. Bush administration wanted to greatly expand the national stockpile of ciprofloxacin—which cures anthrax as well as ear infections. To force Bayer to lower its prices from about $5 a pill to less than $1, it threatened to ignore Bayer's patent and buy generics instead.

Some African countries definitely did have problems with substandard drugs from India, but I asked my Doctors Without Borders contacts which Indian companies had the best reputations. They named three.

I sought interviews and in 2000 went to India for the first time. Only one, Cipla Ltd., really welcomed my inquiries, so I profiled the company and its chairman, Yusuf K. Hamied. He was a Cambridge University–trained chemist and the son of a fierce Indian nationalist whom Gandhi himself had encouraged to start a pharmaceutical company to break the stranglehold that British pharma firms held on the country. Cipla ran spotless modern factories on budgets minuscule by Western standards. It made active ingredients for Western companies, so its factories had passed inspections by the U.S. Food and Drug Administration (FDA) and its European and Japanese counterparts. Dr. Hamied proudly showed me the inspection reports.

He made the $25 antifungal pills for 20 cents each and was turning a modest profit. Everything he did was legal under Indian patent law, and he was furious at being called a pirate.

On December 1, 2000—World AIDS Day—my profile of Cipla and its chairman made the front page of the *Times*.

Three months later, another drug-access activist told me that Cipla was willing to make a triple-therapy cocktail for $350 a year—less than a dollar a day. I called Dr. Hamied to confirm that, reaching him at midnight at a London dinner party. He said yes, that if he could get enough guaranteed orders to justify the cost of switching over his factories, he would offer that price to Doctors Without Borders and any African nation that could pay for them.

By then many outlets had done pieces about Africans dying because of Big Pharma greed. The story had become far bigger than it had been three years earlier when I had gone to Cotlands.

The drug companies, blind with hubris, had sued not just South Africa to overturn the patents law, but even its president, Nelson Mandela, who was regarded as a living saint. It was a public relations disaster.

More and more activists were joining the crusade, including Act Up Philadelphia, James Love of the Consumer Project on Technology, Bill Haddad of the Generic Pharmaceutical Industry Association, the advocacy group Health GAP, the Yale Law School Global Health Justice Partnership, Oxfam, and others. One HIV-positive South African activist had become famous for putting his own life on the line: Zackie Achmat refused to take antiretrovirals until all his countrymen had access to them. In late 2000, he had been arrested for smuggling generic fluconazole, the thrush-curing drug, in from Thailand. (He eventually took antiretrovirals in 2002 after

Mr. Mandela appealed to him as death was closing in and the South African courts were on the verge of forcing the government to provide the drugs in public hospitals.)

As vice president, Al Gore had made his own trip to South Africa, where he reinforced the administration's displeasure. When he ran for the presidency in 2000, American AIDS activists had begun interrupting his rallies with big banners reading "Gore's Greed Kills Africans." Puzzled campaign correspondents asked what they meant and began covering the issue. Since political reporters get far more readers than science reporters do, the story had grown that much bigger.

"Dr. Hamied," I said, "after tomorrow, your life is going to be different."

In part because my last story about him had made the front page, this one did also. His offer dropped like a bomb into the battle over global drug pricing.

Once it was accepted, which took months of negotiation, his generic competitors also piled into the market. Other countries in Africa, Asia, and Latin America began writing patent laws like South Africa's.

Since most poor countries had no equivalent of the FDA, the WHO created a division to assess the safety and efficacy of drugs.

Slowly, the price of AIDS cocktails fell from $15,000 to below $350 a year.

Those low prices allowed the George W. Bush administration to create the President's Emergency Plan for AIDS Relief (PEPFAR) in 2003 and later the President's Malaria Initiative. Kofi Annan, the UN secretary-general, led the creation of the Global Fund to Fight AIDS, Tuberculosis and Malaria. A rare bipartisan alliance in Congress between foreign policy liberals and Christian conservatives with links to African missionary hospitals supported all those efforts.

The foundation that President Clinton started in retirement began acting as a "market maker," bringing donors, developing countries, and all kinds of pharmaceutical companies to the table to work out cost-cutting deals.

Cipla's success—at one point it was supplying 70 percent of Africa's AIDS drugs, including pediatric formulations—made Dr. Hamied rich. Over the next twenty years, he gave so generously to Cambridge, his alma mater, that it renamed its chemistry department after him.

Now it's the norm for Big Pharma companies to offer "tiered pricing," including midlevel prices to middle-income countries and rock-bottom ones to the poorest. They take many precautions, of course. For example, they may change the name, the shape, and the color of a pill and its packaging to prevent leakage back into lucrative Western markets. They even compete to outrank each other on the Access to Medicine Index, which measures how much effort they make to help the world's poor: how much they cut prices, what patents they sublicense to generics makers, what neglected diseases they research, and so on.

Since those days, because of affordable drug prices and the generosity of donors—especially American donors—it's been estimated that the Global Fund, PEPFAR, and the Malaria Initiative have saved at least 30 million lives.

As I watched and reported, the world was changing its attitude toward the dying poor.

I changed, too. In 2002, at the end of seven years overseas, I was called back to New York. I was at loose ends. The last stint I had worked in New York was in culture news, covering Broadway—not as a critic, but writing about the theater business and its gossip. The executive editor asked me if I wanted to go back to the culture department. I said no. I didn't say so, but by then it seemed like something out of a half-forgotten previous life, and silly. (I realize this insults Broadway lovers, and I'm sorry—but it's how I felt after years in Africa.) He suggested science news. That sounded like a challenge, so I said yes. The science editor, Cornelia Dean, said she needed a health writer. I said I'd be happy to do that, but she had two MDs on her staff, Larry Altman and Libby Rosenthal, who were much better qualified than I was. They covered mostly the chronic diseases that Americans died of, such as cancer and heart disease, though Larry was also a pioneer in covering AIDS in America. I asked if I could instead specialize in global health, diseases of the poor. Cory first said, "We don't have a mandate for that"—there was no such beat. I argued that more than a billion people faced death from infectious diseases. We covered their deaths from wars or floods or famines—or even "bus plunges," a staple of short items in those days. So why not the ills they also faced? She said she'd make it an experiment—which became the rest of my career.

Chapter Three

WHAT I LEARNED ON THE WAY

I should also explain something else that changed in me over twenty-five years, because it deeply colored how I see pandemics, including—perhaps especially—Covid.

On February 28, 2020, I wrote a news analysis that, three years later, I am still occasionally attacked for. Mostly by the far right, but not always. It was under the headline "To Take On the Coronavirus, Go Medieval on It." It was prompted by two events that had happened in quick succession.

China had cracked down on Wuhan with startling ferocity. Eight million people had been frozen in place. Residents were ordered to stay inside, unable to even walk their dogs. Every three days, one family member could come out to shop for food. Some who broke the rules were pushed back in and saw their doors welded shut. Migrant workers with nowhere to go slept in parking garages.

A week later, on January 31, President Trump made a decision that had previously been almost unthinkable. Declaring the virus a public health threat to the United States, he barred entry to all foreign nationals who had recently been in China.

I was stunned. Tactics like closing borders and erecting a cordon sanitaire around a province were long out of favor in public health circles.

Penning citizens up inside poisoned cities to either die or stagger out weeks later as survivors was a fourteenth-century measure adopted to counter the Black Death.

For decades, the WHO had vigorously opposed border closures during Ebola outbreaks in Africa, arguing that they created stigma and halted trade, including vital medical supplies. It also opposed internal travel restrictions because they threw people out of work.

But both Chinese president Xi Jinping and Donald Trump had ignored modern liberal public health orthodoxy. For the first time in decades, I wrote that "the world has chosen to confront a new and terrifying virus with the iron fist instead of the latex glove."

Officially, the WHO was still leery of such ideas. But I'd been having long conversations with Dr. Bruce Aylward, whom I'd known for years. He had headed the small WHO fact-finding team that visited Wuhan in late January. It was becoming clear, he said, that the tactics were actually working.

What Americans did not understand—and still do not—was that China was not simply imposing a lockdown to create paralysis for its own sake. Freezing everyone in place was the precondition to taking the real steps to eliminate the virus. First, the flow of patients into overwhelmed local hospitals had to stop—death rates in the first two weeks were close to 5 percent. The city erected dozens of fever clinics, sometimes just tents in hospital parking lots, where PCR tests and CT scans could be done in a few hours. Every apartment building had to take residents' temperatures and report all who were ill. Everyone testing positive, even without symptoms, had to enter one of many "fangcang shelter hospitals"—quarantine wards set up in empty public buildings, hotels, schools, or gyms. Contact-tracers interviewed everyone who tested positive and then tried to hunt down everyone they had spent time with in the last few days—a mammoth task since, in a city with crowded markets, schools, and office and apartment buildings, each case could have dozens of contacts. Local hospitals were staffed by more than 30,000 doctors and nurses drafted from other cities.

Almost no one except emergency workers and couriers delivering groceries or medical supplies was allowed on the streets. Beijing's goal was to crush the outbreak so harshly that the return to normal would be rapid, reviving its temporarily paralyzed economy as fast as possible.

"If China can do this," said Michael T. Osterholm, the prescient epidemiologist who headed the University of Minnesota's Center for Infectious Disease Research and Policy, "it will be something amazing—like catching the wind in a butterfly net. No one's ever stopped a disease as transmissible as flu before."

It worked. A full year before vaccines existed, China's epidemic vanished. By April 2020, when the new-case count reached zero, fewer than 4,000 Chinese had died. The country reopened, but now with its cordon sanitaire moved out to its borders, blocking out the world. Almost no one got permission to enter, and those who did were locked in quarantine hotels for two weeks. Their doors were opened once a day to hand in a bag of food and remove a bag of garbage. Before coming out, they had to test negative twice, twenty-four hours apart.

The WHO eventually conceded that China's harsh measures had probably saved more than a million lives.

My news analysis said Trump was probably the only president who would have opted to shut the borders. It was in his xenophobic nature. Years earlier, he had opined that the heroic American doctors who got infected with Ebola while fighting it in West Africa should not be brought home for treatment but left overseas to die. He had been elected on a promise to build a border wall paid for by Mexico. As soon as he was in office, he had declared a ban on all immigrants from Muslim countries. His instincts were ugly. But harsh measures imposed early enough could save lives.

(In retrospect, of course, we now know that the virus had already been seeded in this country multiple times by February 28. We also know that China's viral suppression could not hold forever—but it did hold for almost three years.)

In my article, to illustrate how a government using iron-fisted tactics could save thousands of lives, I described something I had covered years before: Cuba's response to its AIDS epidemic.

In the 1980s, HIV reached Cuba and the United States almost simultaneously. Fidel Castro immediately saw the threat. Two years before President Ronald Reagan even uttered the word "AIDS," Castro predicted to his tropical disease specialists in the Pedro Khouri Institute that AIDS would be the "epidemic of the century." He charged them with stopping it.

Their methods, adopted with his approval, were coercive. As soon as kits were available, testing became mandatory for all Cubans returning from the multiple military missions he supported in Africa. Then it became mandatory for anyone who had been abroad, and then for anyone whose doctor suspected they were gay or even heterosexually promiscuous. (Cuban doctors are de facto public health officers with more power over their patients than American doctors have; every Cuban was expected to visit his doctor at least once a year.) Ultimately, testing became obligatory for all adults, even grandmothers who had never traveled. When I visited in 2012, Cuba's population of 11 million had been tested 43 million times.

Everyone testing positive was required to name all their sexual contacts, who would be tested in turn. Although Cuban law could not jail anyone who refused, heavy pressure was brought to bear. Anyone who balked at telling a nurse had to see a doctor. If they refused again, they saw the district psychologist. If they still held back, a committee from Cubans Living with HIV would drop by their home and ask them to cooperate for the sake of the nation's health. As a last resort, the local Committee for the Defense of the Revolution—neighbors who acted as government spies and enforcers—would come over to remind the uncooperative that their housing and their food coupons were granted at the pleasure of the state.

The pressure worked. Dr. Arachu Castro (no relation), a Harvard doctor who worked in Cuba, told me she knew of only one woman who had refused every request, insisting she had never had sex with anyone but her husband, who was HIV-negative. The doctors finally gave up, she said. "We called her the Immaculate Infection."

Far more controversial was what happened next: in those days, everyone infected was forced to move into a quarantine camp. It was then assumed to be a life sentence because most people lived only six months or so. (As in the United States, that was often true early on because sufferers were diagnosed only when they were emaciated and near death.) If you could get a pass for a brief family visit, an escort went along to make sure you did not have sex.

The camps were gilded prisons but, despite rumors spread by anti-Castro forces, were not hellholes. The nicer ones had bungalows, gardens, theater troupes, medical care, and more food than people living outside often had, especially after the Soviet Union disintegrated and Cuba's heavily subsidized economy collapsed. Some desperate homeless youths in Havana actually injected themselves with blood from other patients in order to get in, Dr. Jorge Pérez Ávila, the country's chief HIV doctor for many years, told me. (Two former camp residents confirmed that. "They died fast," one said.)

Initially, only a minority of camp residents were gay. Most were former soldiers, engineers, nurses, teachers, and others who had worked in Africa and were infected through heterosexual sex or medical needle accidents. Inside, couples met and married. Those who were gay sometimes faced less discrimination than they had outside in macho rural Cuba. In the revolution's early days in the 1960s, homosexuals had been fired from jobs, beaten, and sentenced to hard labor. (Late in life, Castro said he regretted his homophobia.)

The amount of sex that had taken place in the camps became evident in 2015, when scientists identified a new dangerous crossover HIV strain thought to have emerged in them. While the American epidemic was almost all of one Zairian strain, Cuban infections included strains from Angola, Ethiopia, and other countries where Cubans fought.

In the 1990s, most of the camps closed. Initially, about 40 percent of residents chose to stay, Dr. Pérez said. After triple therapy arrived, most left. In 2012, I was allowed to visit two of the three last remaining camps. The few residents in each said they were there voluntarily. They were from poor families and had more space, food, and medical care than they would have outside.

"At home, we have seven in my family's apartment," said Carlos Emilio García, an HIV-infected nurse who both lived in and worked at the Santiago de las Vegas sanitorium just outside Havana. "Here, well, you can see what I have." The camp was on the grounds of Los Cocos, an estate that once belonged to a relative of Fulgencio Batista, the dictator ousted by the revolution. Its buildings were run-down, but the grounds were lush, with towering palm trees, broad lawns, and fountains. Mr. García had his own bungalow with a kitchen, a TV, an air conditioner, and a garden for flowers or vegetables. He got his state salary, and a cafeteria served basic meals. "I'd like to let my nephews move in with me," he said. "But it's against the rules."

By contrast, in the United States, the Reagan administration's reaction as AIDS deaths mounted was indifference. His Christian conservative supporters saw the disease as divine vengeance on homosexuals and drug users. They also opposed teaching teenagers about homosexuality, safe sex, or needle exchange, so interventions that might have slowed the epidemic were not even discussed. When I interviewed students in Cuba, one said she had been shown how to put a condom on a model penis when she was twelve. One of her classmates rolled his eyes, saying, "Sometimes they do so much sex education you get tired of it."

At the same time, in cities like New York and San Francisco, the gay rights movement was gaining strength. The focus was emphatically on protecting the privacy and civil rights of the infected above all. Not only was testing not compulsory, but it was even illegal in some states to offer a test without first doing a separate counseling session behind closed doors, which scared off many men.

From a human rights point of view, this was correct, of course. In those days, any American who was HIV-positive would be denied both health insurance and life insurance. Even asking for a test would be tantamount to admitting being gay, which could lead to dismissal from many jobs, ostracism by coworkers, and bans from some fields, such as teaching. It would lead to a dishonorable discharge from the military. In many conservative and religious families, it would lead to ejection from the family fold.

Also, during the fifteen years before antiretroviral treatment was invented, having a positive test amounted to a death sentence. Many gay men simply chose to not know. They crossed their fingers and hoped they weren't infected—or infecting anyone else.

But from a public health point of view, making privacy and individual rights paramount was an utter disaster. The men who did not know, the men who chose to not know, the men who knew and lied, infected other men by the thousands.

In the 1980s, as the United States protected civil liberties at all costs, health officials confidently predicted a vaccine and a cure within three years. It would all be over soon, they promised. The latex glove would save us. Cuba, by contrast, chose the iron fist.

Forty years later, there still is no vaccine and no cure. It took fifteen years to develop drugs that could suppress the virus but not cure it. The first regimens had such harsh or disfiguring side effects that many men avoided them. It took thirty years to come up with something resembling a vaccine: a PrEP pill that protects if taken daily. It took almost forty years to come up with longer-lasting injected versions.

The result? During those forty years, more than 700,000 Americans died of AIDS. Fewer than 5,000 Cubans did. Cuba's per capita infection rate is still a fraction of that of the U.S. It's down on a par with Finland and Singapore—and that's true even though the virus probably arrived in Cuba earlier, and even though Cuba is, to some extent, a sex tourism destination. (It has an underground but thriving sex industry, employing *jineteras* and *jineteros*—"jockeys.")

Cuba has roughly the same population as the New York City

metropolitan area. In the epidemic's first thirty years, fewer than 2,500 Cubans died of AIDS. Over 78,000 New Yorkers did.

My feelings about all of this are complex and make me highly unpopular in some circles. After I cited that example in my essay, I received a furious email from Gregg Gonsalves, a Yale epidemiologist and gay rights activist whom I greatly respect. How dare I, he wrote, speak approvingly of such brutal measures against gay men? How would I have felt if my colleague Jeff Schmalz had been frog-marched out of *The New York Times* and forced into a concentration camp?

Jeff was a *Times* reporter who died of AIDS at age thirty-nine after chronicling his own diagnosis and decline. He had collapsed from a seizure in the newsroom when the virus reached his brain. His autobiographical essay "Covering AIDS and Living It," a landmark in AIDS journalism, appeared in the *Times* less than a year before his death. He died in 1993, a mere two years before triple therapy became available.

I answered Gregg that I felt torn over that very question. Jeff and I had been friends. Not close friends, but work pals. We were the same age and in the mid-1970s had both come to the *Times* as copy boys—him while attending Columbia, me soon after graduating from the University of California, Berkeley. We had both worked on the city desk, him as an editor, me as a reporter, and we occasionally went out for drinks or dinner in Times Square. (It was a more dangerous place then: a mugger once slashed Jeff's head with a razor when he left after finishing a night shift.) He was then still in the closet—everyone gay at the *Times* was because the executive editor, Abe Rosenthal, was openly homophobic and even ordered the city desk to ignore the annual Gay Pride Parade. Jeff never explicitly told me he was gay but he made enough gender-vague jokes about "liking young blonds" and such to intimate it—presumably because he trusted me.

Since Jeff died in 1993, I told Gregg, he had almost undoubtedly been infected not in the first wave, but sometime in the mid to late 1980s. Had the United States responded as toughly as Cuba had, I said, Jeff might be alive today.

So how do you choose? When you're one of the lucky living, it's easy to shriek about your right to personal freedom—whether it's to dodge a test, refuse a vaccine, not wear a motorcycle helmet, or insist on carrying a gun.

But who speaks for the dead? Was America right to let more than 600,000 gay men die in order to protect the privacy of a few thousand—or perhaps even a few hundred—infected in the first wave?

When does a government finally say "No—this public health order must be obeyed"? When is it right to restrict the liberty of a few citizens to save the lives of the many? And how much and for how long?

There is no easy answer. In this book, I will describe much of what I learned—and what changed in me—between that moment in the Cotlands orphanage in 1998 and the present. Those babies instilled a sense of empathy for the utter helplessness of victims. I hope I still have it. But now that's tempered by a feeling that we must somehow balance the civil rights of victims against the lives they in turn put at risk.

After decades of watching epidemics and seeing how a few countries beat them while most failed to, I've come to feel that the Western focus on personal liberty above all else can kill.

Nothing in our Constitution enshrines my inalienable right to give you a fatal disease.

But we often act as if it does—as if no one else's life but ours matters.

Like all Americans, I adore life, liberty, and the pursuit of happiness. But I place life first. The dead enjoy neither liberty nor happiness. Once they're gone, no one speaks for them to say, "I didn't have to die." Over the years, I've come to feel that speaking for them is part of my job.

I expect my views will provoke some anger.

A few years ago, I said to a friend, "The longer I cover disease, the more of a public health fascist I become."

"For God's sake, Donald," he replied, "don't ever say that. That is so politically incorrect. Don't ever write it down."

No doubt good advice. I have a history of getting in trouble by speaking my mind.

However, I do think the long, awful trauma of Covid has moved some Americans closer to my way of thinking. This was the saddest epidemic I've ever covered. Other nations showed us how to control it. We ignored them. We produced the cure—vaccines that were truly miraculous in their combination of safety and efficacy. Tens of millions of Americans rejected them. Ordering anyone to take them, they argued, was fascism.

Many Americans seem to have grown up believing that their rights are paramount, that they trump any national interest. In my brief moments of optimism in the pandemic's early days, I hoped we would coalesce as a country to beat the virus, as my parents' generation had to fight World War II. Instead, we divided into warring camps. The flags read "Don't Tread on Me," but all I heard was the infuriated screams of the spoiled nine-year-old I once was: "I won't do it, and you can't make me."

Of course, my parents often *could* make me, and I wondered what America my fellow citizens had grown up in. When I was young, the government could snatch me out of college, force me into the military, inject me with whatever vaccine they liked, and send me to Vietnam to kill or be killed. My only recourse would have been prison or abandoning my citizenship. (I was spared by a high draft number, but friends had less luck.)

I don't miss those days. But I'm shocked at what's left—a sense that we have no obligation to protect each other, or even each other's children and parents. An insistence on following our own whims, "doing our own research," regardless of the cost.

Covid coarsened something in us as a nation. It wasn't just the virus. It was the way we reacted, the way we were coached to react—the indifference to each other's lives, the utter disdain for sensible advice, the demands that science be infallible or shut up. In the wake of the pandemic, I see evidence of that coarsening everywhere: in the January 6, 2021, insurrection, of course, but also in the speeding on the highways, in the turnstile jumping and loud music on the subways, in rising violent crime rates, in plunging vaccination rates. That coarsening cracks our national skin. It makes us more vulnerable to infection.

New pandemics lurk just over the horizon. Once they arrive, they blunder into a fusillade of responses driven by medicine, commerce, politics, diplomacy, bigotry, news judgment, and a dozen other factors. Mistakes are made—including major ones, the equivalent of bungled military assaults that throw away thousands of lives for nothing.

I've watched many such battles in many countries. Sometimes human brilliance shines through. Sometimes greed and stupidity prevail. There are moments of great generosity, both in money and in the sweat and tears of doctors and nurses. And moments of utter selfishness and national frustration as the deaths needlessly drag on.

The question I've always asked myself is: What saves the most lives? This book, I hope, will be a hard look at some answers.

Part Two

THE TANGLED ROOTS OF PANDEMICS

Chapter Four

WHAT IF WE'D HANDLED COVID DIFFERENTLY?

What are the consequences of how the United States handled Covid-19?

As I write this, in the late spring of 2023, the pandemic is officially over. The American government and the WHO have ended their health emergencies. The websites tracking infections and deaths have shut down. About 1.1 million Americans have officially died of Covid. Total excess mortality for the pandemic is yet to be finally tabulated, but has been estimated to be as high as 1.7 million. That includes all extra deaths during the three years the pandemic lasted, whether from Covid, cancer, heart disease, suicide, drug overdose, car accident, or any other reason.

If we had taken the threat seriously from the outset, and had reacted more intelligently, how many lives might have been saved?

Various analyses have attempted to measure this. They've come up with a range of results, but the numbers are always distressingly large. A study in the *Journal of the American Medical Association* by researchers from Brown University and the University of Pennsylvania found that the United States, adjusted for its greater population size, had up to 466,000 more deaths than 20 "peer nations."

But it measured only the Delta and Omicron waves *after* vaccines became available. It ignored the 2020 spring wave in New York, the summer wave in the Deep South, and the terrible winter of 2020–21, when 3,300 Americans died each day—a peak we never reached again.

A study from Brown, Harvard, and Microsoft's AI for Health unit found that 318,000 deaths could have been prevented if all adults had been vaccinated. But it looked only at data from January 2021 to April 2022, again ignoring the early days and measuring only the impact of vaccine.

I think a simpler and more reasonable method is to compare our final outcome to those of our closest peers that reacted from the very beginning in ways that we could have replicated—but did not. To me, Germany and Canada are the best candidates.

They roughly match us in per capita income and public health expertise. They also roughly match us in risk factors like obesity and old age. (More of our population is overweight, but because we have a steady flow of young immigrants, less of ours is over sixty-five.) Our cultural norms are similar. We all have open debate and histories of political protest, sometimes violent. Americans, Germans, and Canadians were not previously in the habit of wearing masks.

All three countries got mRNA vaccines soon after they were available. All three ultimately faced serious demonstrations against lockdowns, masks, and vaccine mandates. Canada's capital, Ottawa, was paralyzed for weeks by angry truckers. But by early 2023, as the pandemic wound down, we in the United States had suffered almost twice the per capita death rate of Germany and almost three times that of Canada.

In a population the size of ours—330 million—that means we could have lost only 560,000 Americans instead of 1.1 million if we had handled ourselves well enough to land somewhere between Germany and Canada.

What cost those 540,000 Americans their lives was poor leadership.

In my eyes, that was the single biggest difference between them and us. German chancellor Angela Merkel and Canadian prime minister Justin Trudeau took the threat seriously from day one and worked hard to get their populations to accept social distancing, business closures, and masks. Their lockdowns were far more restrictive—and effective—than ours. A year later, when vaccines arrived, they strongly backed them. In the United States, we had denialism, finger-pointing, and polarization, much of it coming from the top.

By the pandemic's end, the per capita death rates in East Asian countries were a mere fraction of those in Western Europe and North America. This was true not just in China—even after its January 2023 wave of deaths—but in Japan, South Korea, Taiwan, Singapore, Vietnam, Thailand, and more. Compared to them, we never had a chance. I'm not going to speculate about the "national characters" of Asian countries versus Western ones—that quickly degenerates into racist nonsense. The numbers are what they are. Low death rates prevailed across both autocracies and democracies. Death rates were also very low in Australia, New Zealand, and Iceland—and apparently across much of Africa, although many governments there lack the capacity to compile accurate national statistics. (Low death rates may or may not have prevailed in India, Indonesia, and some other populous countries; serious doubts have been raised about the numbers those governments released.)

In Asia, much of this was a legacy of SARS and bird flu. In 2003, SARS struck hard there, and since the 1990s there have been small but lethal outbreaks of H5N1 avian flu in humans. When China revealed that its outbreak of mysterious pneumonia in Wuhan was caused by a new coronavirus, Asian countries instantly grasped the threat. Some already had battle plans and activated them.

Soon after China released the virus's genetic sequence on January 11, 2020, many Asian countries raced to produce their own PCR tests and started hunting for cases. Thailand reported its first confirmed case on January 13, Japan on the 16th, South Korea on the 20th, and Singapore and Vietnam on the 23rd.

When epidemics start, reaction time makes all the difference. If a virus is introduced by just five visitors and doubles every five days, it is far easier to control it in the first month, when those 5 cases become 320, than it is in the second, when those 320 cases become 41,000. This is even more true when the virus is capable of unpredictable superspreader events in which one person infects 10 or even 100 others.

Wuhan clearly had hundreds infected before China even identified the cause. Other Asian countries did not need to be nearly as aggressive because they had more warning. But many did move forcefully anyway. Most canceled all flights from China and required anyone who had recently arrived, especially from the Wuhan area, to spend two weeks in quarantine—not at home but in a hotel or quarantine center. Release from quarantine generally required two negative tests twenty-four hours apart. In countries that did allow foreigners in, new arrivals usually had to turn over their cell phone numbers or download apps that automatically sent their locations to the police. If the phone left the quarantine hotel, the app dialed the police. If the phone even remained stationary too long—suggesting the owner had slipped out without it—it also dialed the police. Violating quarantine could result in fines of thousands of dollars.

Thanks largely to the experience of SARS two decades earlier, mask use in Asia was almost universal and not controversial. That slowed early transmission.

Asian governments quickly trained large cadres of contact-tracers. In Wuhan alone, 9,000 contact-tracers were working by mid-February. It was not until June that New York City had even 3,000. That program—intended to be a model for the United States—quickly fell into chaos. Few New Yorkers cooperated, and it was ultimately judged a failure.

Across much of Asia, anyone who tested positive was immediately isolated away from home. (Early studies suggested that at least 75 percent of all transmission was within families.) Those in isolation were asked to name everyone they had been in contact with. Those contacts were traced and tested, and often their contacts were as well.

As a result, most Asian countries suffered very little in the first spring 2020 wave. By May 27, 2020, when the death toll in the United States had reached 100,000, Japan had suffered only 857 deaths, South Korea a mere 269. China, struck with no warning at all, had fewer than 5,000.

Europe and North America had more time to prepare than Asia did. We could have been more ready.

Germany reported its first case on January 27, 2020, after a young woman from Shanghai whose parents had visited her from Wuhan flew to Stockdorf, near Munich, to visit the auto parts company that employed her. (Her case briefly became famous as the first example of asymptomatic transmission; it later turned out she was not truly asymptomatic. She had felt fatigued in Germany but assumed it was just jet lag; on the flight home, she began running a fever and was more seriously ill.) That German cluster was contained within two weeks and never exceeded 16 cases. That was possible partly because a laboratory at Berlin's Charity Hospital had produced a PCR test by January 16; it became the WHO's standard and was mass-produced. Also, the auto parts company quickly shut down its Stockdorf plant to contain the outbreak. Because it used electronic calendars it was relatively easy to trace everyone who had met the employee from China.

Germany did not have a second cluster until February 25, at a winter carnival in Heinsberg. By then the government had rolled out a public information campaign and had a national response plan. Nonetheless, the Heinsberg cluster soon grew too big to contain, so the rapid contact-tracing and isolation that was effective in Asia and in Stockdorf became impossible. In mid-March, Germany closed its borders and shut down all schools from kindergarten to university. Six states imposed curfews; others prohibited contact with anyone outside one's household. By the end of April, all the states had mandated mask-wearing in stores and on public transit. Germany subsequently went through roughly the same pattern of viral waves that the United States did—including outbreaks in meatpacking plants. Chancellor Merkel, who had been a chemistry researcher before entering politics, took a cautious approach to reopening and to permitting summer travel despite complaints from the premiers of some German states. When the 2020–21 winter wave of infections set in before vaccines were available, Germany imposed two further partial lockdowns to slow the spread.

Like the United States, Germany saw protests against its shutdowns and mask mandates. It even had a fatal shooting by a gas station customer turned away by an attendant for not wearing a mask. Like the United States, Germany has powerful far-right groups, conspiracy theorists, and an anti-vaccine movement.

By the time the United States had 100,000 deaths, Germany had only 8,260. (It has about a quarter of America's population, so that was the per capita equivalent of about 33,000 dead.)

Italy, just south of Germany, detected its first cases in late February, about the same time that Germany did. Judging by how many Covid deaths ultimately occurred in northern cities like Bergamo and Lodi, it is likely that Italy's outbreak had begun earlier than Germany's but went undetected because Italy initially tested no one unless they had been to China. Once the folly of that became clear, it still offered tests only to people who were hospitalized. Also, local authorities there strongly resisted closing restaurants, churches, soccer matches, and such, so there was a long delay until an initial weak lockdown was imposed. Then, as deaths kept mounting, the lockdowns were broadened and tightened until, for a time, Italians could not stray far from their homes without a letter to show to the police explaining why. By April, Italy had six times Germany's death rate.

By the time the United States had 100,000 deaths, Italy had about 33,000. Given that Italy's population is less than a fifth of the U.S., that was the equivalent of 182,000 dead. Nonetheless, the United States would later go on to surpass Italy, ending the pandemic with about 10 percent more deaths per million residents.

Canada also had its first known case in late January; it was in a Toronto resident who had visited Wuhan. But that cluster died out, and Canada had no confirmed community transmission until March 5. It closed its borders and ordered everyone who had arrived earlier to isolate for ten days. Later, when the most populous provinces had surges, the government imposed strict lockdowns and curfews until caseloads dropped. In areas with few cases, like the Atlantic Provinces, the lockdowns were rarer and briefer.

The first case in the United States was found on January 20 in a thirty-five-year-old man who had flown into the Seattle-Tacoma airport five days earlier after visiting family in Wuhan. By the time the CDC lab in Atlanta confirmed his test results, he had been sick for several days and was initially told to go home and isolate himself. Assuming no one else with the virus was in Seattle that early in the epidemic, he somehow started a chain of infection that was never contained. By mid-February, it had reached a nursing home where it infected 129 residents and staff, killing 23 of them.

By February, the virus had been introduced into the New York area several times. The first confirmed case was found on March 1 in a woman who had returned from Iran. But genetic testing later revealed that multiple strains had arrived from Europe, possibly starting as early as late January. (In Europe, the virus had picked up a mutation that distinguished it from the Wuhan strain.)

But because it took the CDC until mid-March to distribute a working test to state labs and because the FDA forbade private companies from making them, only about 100 tests a day were done across the whole country in February while other nations did tens of thousands daily. Infighting within the Trump administration over who would lead the White House pandemic task force left a leadership vacuum. During our first two months, we were flying blind.

Once vaccines became available, Canada quickly approved four of them. In October 2021, it imposed vaccine mandates on all federal workers and those in public transportation. It barred domestic air, rail, and ship travel to anyone who was unvaccinated and created vaccine passports to show who had gotten the shots. When the border with the United States reopened, no one unvaccinated was allowed through—including Canadian truckers. As a result, vaccination rates rose much higher in Canada, at 82 percent versus 64 percent here.

Ultimately, Canada had the same patterns of cases and deaths the United States did, but in a much more muted way. It also had peaks in spring 2020, winter 2020–21, in the Delta wave of October 2021, and the

Omicron wave of January 2022. But when American peak deaths hovered near 3,000 a day, Canada's were about 150—one-twentieth as high while its population is one-eighth as big. Canadian hospitals were never as overwhelmed as American ones were.

The United States produced the world's best vaccines, but they became a pawn in election year politics. Even though President Trump could have gloried in much-deserved credit for ordering them, he instead accused vaccine makers of delaying their clinical trials to hurt his reelection chances. He never endorsed them to his followers. For months, he even kept secret the fact that he and his wife had been vaccinated in January 2021, as soon as they could have been.

In Canada and Germany, with strong backing from the top, vaccine uptake was far higher. By January 2022, at the peak of the Omicron wave, it had become clear that three doses, not two, were needed to prevent hospitalization and death. Only 25 percent of Americans got the third "booster" dose. By contrast, 40 percent of Canadians and 50 percent of Germans did. That third shot made a huge difference in relative death rates.

The toll of 1.1 million dead amounts to a fatality rate of almost 3,500 Americans per 1 million population. The United States did considerably worse than all its Western European peers, worse even than Poland or Brazil.

By contrast, Germany's per capita death rate was about 2,000 per million and Canada's less than 1,400. If our death rate had ended up halfway between theirs, at about 1,700 per million, we would have lost about 540,000 fewer dead.

Who speaks for them?

This is not to argue that autocratic leadership cannot backfire—especially if it becomes arrogant and inflexible. In China, Xi Jinping's draconian "zero Covid" policy was brutally efficient and saved both lives and China's economy. By the end of the pandemic, in the spring of 2023, Taiwan's fatality rate was less than 800 per million population, South Korea's was below 700. Japan, despite its aged population, was below 600.

By contrast, as 2022 drew to a close, China's 5,300 dead amounted to a mere 4 deaths per million. Its economy had reopened when its national caseload reached zero in April 2020—after just seventy-six days of lockdown—and it had functioned at near-full strength for two years while the rest of the world struggled with on-and-off closures. The effectiveness of President Xi's iron-fisted policies had helped him retain his grip on power for a historic third term in October 2022, making him the most powerful ruler since Mao Zedong.

As we all now know, however, the supremely transmissible Omicron variant that emerged in 2022 finally broke the back of Mr. Xi's strategy. No matter how quickly factories, universities, neighborhoods, or cities were closed, the virus kept spreading. The repeated closures in attempts to stop it threw people out of work. Citizens used to being obedient in return for being cared for by the state suddenly found themselves going hungry. By mid-November, multiple cities were in revolt. Rioting crowds tore down the metal fences penning them in and fought police with the stanchions. In unprecedented shows of defiance, they gathered in public squares and called for the fall of both President Xi and the Communist Party.

Mr. Xi's arrogance and bullheadedness had backed him into a corner. Even after it was clear that the Omicron variant was milder, Chinese propaganda portrayed all Covid as deadly. His scientists had made only mediocre vaccines, and he had refused to buy better ones from Pfizer or Moderna. China, he insisted, would develop its own mRNA vaccines. Then it failed to do so. Uptake of the two domestic vaccines, CoronaVac and Sinopharm, was high among workers who could be forced to get them, but low among vulnerable seniors, who heard rumors of harsh side effects. In early December 2022, Mr. Xi tried to ease out of his "zero Covid policy." Instead it collapsed completely. Infection rates shot up so fast that emergency rooms all over the country filled with elderly patients. Despite the Communist Party's attempt to suppress the bad news, videos leaked out showing hundreds of patients lying unattended in hospital corridors. Reports emerged of doctors and nurses falling ill and oxygen supplies running out. Long lines of hearses were photographed outside crematoriums. Funeral workers reported processing ten times as many bodies as they normally did. Some epidemiologists predicted that China would see between 1 million and 2.1 million deaths. But there was no way to know: in December, China simply stopped reporting cases and deaths.

To judge from leaked news reports, the deadly explosion ended relatively quickly. By some estimates, the wildly contagious Omicron variant infected 80 percent or more of China's population in January alone. In mid-February, the Communist Party leadership declared a "major, decisive victory" and said the China CDC had recorded only about 83,000 deaths since December. That was ridiculed as an obvious cover-up of the true toll. The government had ordered doctors to report only deaths of hospitalized patients who had test-confirmed Covid and succumbed to pneumonia. (Chinese cities also stopped publishing cremation data.) Various outside epidemiologists used different methods to estimate deaths; one model was based on Lunar New Year travel data, one on reports about a brief 2022 outbreak in Shanghai, one extrapolated from American death rates. (*The New York Times* took a novel approach: it tracked published obituaries of prominent elderly Chinese scientists and found that they spiked eight times higher than normal.) Overall, studies estimated that between 1 million and 1.5 million had died. The high end of the most extreme estimate was 2.3 million.

Even 2.3 million dead would still be a fatality rate of only 1,630 per million, about tied with Switzerland and and just above Canada and Israel. One million dead would be 700 per million, in the neighborhood of Taiwan and South Korea. Either result would be an impressive success, but the party was clearly not content with that and chose to instead create a fictional narrative.

Mr. Xi's policy shifts had effects on the world economy that no one had predicted. China's initial airtight lockdown lasted only from January to April of 2020. Exports from its factories were cut off—but only briefly. The most immediate impact was that the world was left desperate for masks, gowns, gloves, and medical equipment. After April, China got back in gear in time to supply both that and the "lockdown buying spree" that Americans went on because they were bored at home, collecting government checks and spending nothing on travel. Then the United States economy slowed because of computer chip shortages, clogged ports, and other obstacles. In 2022, China fell out of sync as the rest of the world slowly recovered: Omicron defeated its most extreme prevention measures; "zero Covid" shuttered some factories again. Finally, China restarted its economy only by sacrificing a generation of the elderly—essentially the same choice the United States had made over the previous three years by imposing only "lockdown lite." The difference was that our elders died off more slowly but in greater numbers.

In 2020, South Korea, Taiwan, and New Zealand and other Asian countries all imposed lockdowns nearly as tight as China's. But they eased them in 2021 as soon as vaccines rolled out. And, crucially, they convinced most of their populations to accept vaccination. As a consequence, they suffered few deaths *and* relatively little economic damage. (Of course, the major advantage several of those countries had was isolation—Taiwan and New Zealand are islands and South Korea is effectively one since there is no travel across its land border.)

The takeaway lesson seems obvious: if your goal is to avert both deaths and economic collapse, you have to constantly temper and rebalance your responses. The iron fist can save lives, but it's not an end in itself. It's a way to buy time until you can do something smarter, such as roll out a vaccine or find a cure. In the meantime, you must educate your populace, gain their trust, and get as much support as you can for measures that will save lives—even if you ultimately have to impose them by fiat. Finding a way to balance lost freedoms against deaths averted is difficult—but necessary.

Chapter Five

WHAT IF WE'D HANDLED MONKEYPOX DIFFERENTLY?

As of this writing, in the late spring of 2023, the global monkeypox outbreak that struck in the spring of 2022 has largely—but not completely—disappeared.

For a generation of gay men in one hundred countries outside of Africa, of course, it was a major scare. Almost 86,000 caught it. The vast majority recovered. But thousands were hospitalized for pain management or to treat secondary infections, some were left with permanent scars—and about one hundred died. To what extent it will stay inside the gay male networks it started in remains to be seen.

At least two major strains are still circulating in Africa, still killing some victims. A highly lethal one pops up unpredictably in small clusters in central Africa, mostly in the rain forest regions of the Democratic Republic of the Congo. A less lethal but more transmissible one circulates in West African cities, particularly in Nigeria. It was a variant of that lesser strain that made its way around the world.

One would imagine that, having just survived a pandemic that had altered all of our lives, we would have reacted judiciously to the new one and suppressed it quickly. Particularly since we not only knew what the disease was but also already had two vaccines that could stop it.

Instead, our response was, to be charitable, disappointingly slow.

There was nothing like the top-down leadership failure that had crippled us from the outset of Covid. Denialism did not stop us from reacting. Medical experts, not politicians, directed the counterattack. Nothing divided us into warring tribes. We ultimately did drive the virus down to very low levels. Nonetheless, to my mind the whole effort was more flawed than it should have been. It worked mostly because of dumb luck.

It's not as if we had no warning. The few scientists who study monkeypox had been sounding alarms for years. In 2003, we had lived through a serious domestic outbreak, one that made me believe then that we would have another someday, although the 2022 one evolved in ways I never expected.

The 2003 one was caused by a shipment of African rodents, including Gambian pouched rats, rope squirrels, dormice, and porcupines imported by a Texas exotic pets dealer. The pouched rats were briefly stored in an Illinois pet warehouse near about 200 American prairie dogs, which were then sold to pet stores all over the eastern half of the country. The first sign of a problem was a three-year-old Wisconsin boy who developed a high fever and rash after being bitten by the family's new pet prairie dog. Alert state health officials made the correct diagnosis, which triggered a frantic search for the rest of the prairie dogs.

Before the outbreak was declared over two months later, 71 Americans had had either lab-confirmed or likely cases, and 94 of the prairie dogs that had been found and necropsied had the virus. There were some family clusters, suggesting human-to-human transmission had taken place. But because everyone with symptoms had also had at least fleeting contact with a prairie dog, the CDC concluded that there was no firm evidence that the virus could jump between people.

As a consequence of that outbreak, two important decisions were made. First, it became illegal to import African rodents. Unfortunately, a clandestine trade in exotic pets, from parrots to tortoises to chimpanzees, still persists. Second, a vaccine then in development in case smallpox was ever used in a bioterrorism attack was tested in monkeys against monkeypox. It worked, and stockpiles of that vaccine would prove essential in 2022.

Scientists assume monkeypox circulated in Africa for centuries and occasionally infected humans but was mistaken for smallpox, its more lethal relative in the orthopox family. Rodents, not monkeys, are its natural reservoir. It got the name because it was first discovered in a shipment of research monkeys at a Danish laboratory in 1958. Oddly, they were not African monkeys but crab-eating macaques from Singapore.

How those Asian monkeys got it remains a mystery. The disease's incubation period is just a week, and they had been delivered apparently healthy almost two months earlier. The investigators' best guess was that some monkeys had arrived with silent infections and it circulated among them until a few susceptible ones fell ill and displayed pox. In the next few years, there were outbreaks in Holland and several American labs, always in macaques or rhesus monkeys from India, Malaysia, or the Philippines. The first known human case was in a nine-month-old boy in what was then Zaire, now the Democratic Republic of the Congo, in 1970.

The global vaccination drive that eliminated smallpox in 1980 also suppressed monkeypox. After elimination, however, the use of smallpox vaccine was discontinued because it had some rare but occasionally deadly side effects. Starting in the 1990s, isolated clusters of monkeypox began cropping up in Africa, usually in children born after 1980. When the cause could be found, it was most often a bite or scratch from a rodent.

Then, in 2017, a sudden outbreak of 38 cases in southeast Nigeria suggested that the virus had mutated to adapt better to humans. A medical professor who investigated that outbreak, Dr. Dimie Ogoina, even suspected that male-to-male sexual contact was involved; he noticed that most of the victims were adult males and had anal, genital, or oral lesions. But when he tried to reveal that at a major international medical conference, he later told an NPR reporter, he was told to keep quiet.

Since then, the virus had circulated steadily but at low levels in Nigeria, including in cities, apparently transmitting between humans without any rodents involved. It also was diagnosed several times in Britain or the United States, in individuals who had recently visited Nigeria. We were warned.

As we all now know, in early May 2022, it suddenly burst out among gay men in Europe, initially in those who had patronized certain venues: the Darklands leather fetish festival in Antwerp, Belgium; the Maspalomas Gay Pride party in the Canary Islands; a techno rave party at the Berghain nightclub in Berlin; and the Paraíso sauna in Madrid.

From the very beginning, it seemed clear that the initial risk group was a small subgroup of gay men with an interest in leather fetishes and group sex. Darklands involves harnesses and bondage gear between dominants and submissives. (That year's motto was "Are You Ready to Go Deep?") The Paraíso, which has thirty darkened cubicles, a bar, and a sadomasochism cell with a bondage rack, is more of a sex club than a spa.

Under names like "party-n-play" and "chemsex," this sexual network was already well-known to medical clinics catering to gay men for having high levels of oral and anal syphilis and other STDs. Men who have sex with multiple partners a night often use a mix of alcohol, amphetamines, ketamine, Viagra, and other drugs to keep going. Some are wealthy enough to fly from one festival to another. The initial spread was clearly within a small but very high-risk network with transglobal links.

Starting on May 23, 2022, when there were fewer than 100 cases outside of Africa and only one confirmed case in the United States, I published a series of articles on Medium trying to raise the level of alarm. Because the virus had already been detected in multiple countries from England to Israel to Australia and because it had a two-week incubation period, I feared there could soon be thousands of cases.

The CDC's initial reaction struck me as phlegmatic and tone-deaf. Their chief concerns seemed to be to damp down alarm and to avoid stigmatizing gay men by avoiding any mention of the fact that almost all the new victims were male and gay. They described the disease as "mild and self-limiting" and confidently called it "containable." Many health journalists also seemed intent on reassuring their readers, "Don't worry, it's not Covid," and on avoiding stigmatization by repeating the CDC mantra, "Anybody can get monkeypox."

Some public health experts, including at the WHO, seemed to think the most urgent issue was not to stop the virus but to find a new name for it, on the grounds that *monkeypox* stigmatized Africans. That led to six months of public hearings and debate, after which the WHO officially renamed the virus *mpox*—and then said it would take a year to phase in the new name and that *monkeypox* would still function as a search term. Since the *m* clearly stood for *monkey*, I hardly saw how the change helped.

The first advice issued by the CDC was so off-target and evasive as to be laughable. It was aimed at travelers and suggested they avoid eating or touching rodents and monkeys, avoid contaminated bedding, and avoid anyone "with open sores." None of it was bad advice—but it was ludicrous. There cannot be many Americans who go abroad to eat rodents, but some do to attend leather sex festivals. The risk to those travelers was simply not mentioned. The warning also suggested wearing a mask—very odd advice for a virus transmitted by anal sex. That paragraph was quietly removed, and in early June, the whole page disappeared from the CDC website.

In the United States, more cases began cropping up, first among men who had attended the International Mr. Leather conference in Chicago, and then among many thousands more who celebrated at Gay Pride festivals in Montreal and then in New York.

To its credit, the CDC later created a new advice page. It was so startlingly graphic that it read as if a different agency had written it. It frankly addressed risky anonymous encounters, described the dangers of sex toys and fetish gear, and even used the words *cum* and *poop* to help men who might not recognize *seminal fluid* or *feces*. (Later versions of the page edited out those words, but helpfully followed up *anus* with *butthole*. One has to wonder what debates within the agency are like.)

The first tactic suggested by the WHO and adopted by the CDC was "ring vaccination," which requires tracing and vaccinating the whole "ring" of contacts around each infected person. Anyone familiar with HIV, including journalists like myself, instantly knew that was doomed to fail. Contact-tracing is difficult with any sexually transmitted disease because people resist admitting to marital infidelity, patronizing sex workers, bisexuality, or whatever other activity caused them to get infected. When the sex is between men who meet anonymously and sometimes wordlessly in dark cubicles, it's impossible. No one takes names and phone numbers at an orgy.

The only way to stop the spread, I argued, was:

> Why don't we offer the vaccine voluntarily to all gay men who contemplate having sex with strangers? We should probably also offer it to all sex workers of all genders. Why? Because if you have sex with anyone you don't know well enough to say, "Uh, before we begin, can I check your body for sores?" then you are already in the high-risk group for HIV, gonorrhea, syphilis, chlamydia, herpes and hepatitis. And it's looking like monkeypox is worming its way into those sexual networks.

June opened with a period of confusion about vaccines. There were two, and the newest, Jynneos, approved in 2019, was clearly the safest. Testing had shown it was even safe enough to give to someone with HIV or skin diseases, which the older vaccine, ACAM2000, was not. A press release from the Danish vaccine maker, Bavarian Nordic, said it had delivered 28 million doses to the U.S. government in the past, but some had expired. It didn't say how many. Even the CDC didn't know how many doses were in the U.S. Strategic National Stockpile. At a news conference, a CDC representative publicly guessed "more than 1,000." I called a spokeswoman for the stockpile to ask what the correct number was. She refused to say because the doses were, she said, "a biodefense asset." It was absurd—an example of the fog of war that every epidemic begins with.

Ultimately, the stockpile's administrators revealed that they had only

2,400 doses ready to inject. It was the equivalent of the U.S. Army facing an assault, calling up its tank battalions, and seeing them arrive with one tank. The government scrambled to get more but ran into multiple roadblocks. Bavarian Nordic had another 780,000 in Denmark, but in frozen bulk form, not in vials. It had not put them into vials because the Covid pandemic had delayed FDA plans to inspect the company's new "fill and finish" plant. Plans to make more vaccine existed—but no doses were due before 2023. Now more than 100 other countries were clamoring for the shots, and there were none to spare.

The national stockpile also contained 100 million doses of ACAM2000, the older smallpox vaccine. It had some serious side effects: In anyone with a depressed immune system—such as someone with undiagnosed HIV—it might lead to a full-body case of the weakened pox used in the vaccine, which could be lethal. If it was given to someone with severe eczema or psoriasis, the vaccination "blister" might become necrotic, cause nearby tissue to die, and even require amputating the arm. Also, there was about a 1-in-500 risk of myocarditis and pericarditis—inflammation of the heart and the tissue around it.

On the other hand, ACAM2000 was an improved version of the same smallpox vaccine I'd been given three times as a child with no ill effects—at nine months, at age eight, and at age thirteen. With careful screening, such as HIV tests and skin checks, it seemed to me to be safe enough to use in a crisis. Myocarditis could be treated with steroids. The CDC, I heard from sources inside, was having an internal debate over whether to roll it out. Ultimately, it decided not to, which was later portrayed by one angry gay activist as "the heterosexuals deciding what's safe enough for us."

It slowly dawned on health experts that ring vaccination would not work. First Canada, then Britain, and then on June 23, New York City began offering it to any man who said he'd had multiple male sex partners in the previous two weeks. But it had very few doses on hand and, as soon as word got out, they were virtually all snapped up by white men who followed the Twitter feeds of certain insiders. That included most of the doses offered at a Harlem clinic, which created anger about racial disparities. Five days later, the CDC adopted the same policy, and "ring vaccination" was dead.

Because there was so little vaccine, the FDA soon authorized the intradermal injection of one-fifth doses. The skin contains far more immune cells than muscle or fat do, so small doses there can still produce lots of antibodies. But sliding a needle between skin layers at a steep angle takes training that many injectors did not have.

Given the combination of high risk and a vaccine shortage, I argued, the best way to slow the outbreak would be to delay the Gay Pride events scheduled for that summer. The danger was not the parades, of course: it was sex at the after-parties. If, I suggested, the party sponsors would agree to hold off until autumn—and perhaps the government could reimburse them for losses they suffered by rescheduling—there would be enough time for tens of thousands of men to be vaccinated. By autumn there might even be a rapid test that could be used at the door to any party.

But Pride events are big moneymakers with corporate sponsors, so no major ones were canceled. In an echo of the argument used by gay bathhouse owners who had refused to close down in the face of AIDS forty years earlier, party organizers insisted their events should go ahead because they would be "educational" if they handed out fliers. One after another, those megaparties turned into superspreader events. Cases in New York surged after Pride Month celebrations in June. In San Francisco they surged after Electroluxx Pride and the post–Burning Man Afterglow Blacklight Discotheque. In Massachusetts, they surged after Provincetown Bear Week. It was not until Labor Day weekend that any state's officials had enough vaccine to justify calling a Pride event helpful rather than harmful: nearly 700 men were vaccinated at the Southern Decadence celebration in New Orleans.

I also argued that infected men should be offered temporary housing, along with food, medical care, and modest payments, to help them isolate for the four weeks they were infectious. Men I interviewed or heard interviewed in the early days were confused, scared, and lonely. They felt dirty and shunned for having the virus. One said the stigma was "worse than HIV." Some were in pain from marble-sized lesions in their rectums. Some had maddening itching. Some lived with roommates they feared infecting. Some wanted to go out with friends to relieve the boredom. Some initially could not find treatments like Tpoxx or even a doctor familiar with the disease. And a few had to sell sex to pay the rent and buy food. If all those men had been offered a way to isolate safely, in a central location among fellow sufferers going through the same crisis, and with access to medical professionals who knew the symptoms, both suffering and ongoing transmission could have been lessened.

Finally, on July 23, the WHO declared the spread of monkeypox a PHEIC, a public health emergency of international concern. It was not until August 2 that the Biden administration named a national monkeypox response coordinator, and then, two days later, declared a national health emergency.

That same week, we learned later, was the peak of the outbreak, with 450 cases detected each day. By June of 2023, one year after the outbreak reached the U.S., that number had tailed off to fewer than four cases a day. We appeared to have achieved victory. But to my mind, some worrying trends were emerging.

Case clusters had appeared, one in central France and one in Chicago, in which the majority of men had been fully vaccinated. It was already known that the vaccine was only partially effective, especially in people whose immune systems were compromised by HIV. Cases among the fully vaccinated suggested that efficacy also waned with time.

A British study of more than 2,700 cases found that more than half had been transmitted *before* the person suffering from the infection felt any symptoms.

In mid-May, the CDC warned that the virus might soon surge again. Although 1.2 million doses of Jynneos vaccine had been administered, the agency said, less than a quarter of all Americans considered at risk for the disease—gay and bisexual men and their sex partners—had been fully vaccinated.

Also worrying was the fact that, the longer the epidemic persisted, the greater was the proportion of new cases found in young gay black and Hispanic men, particularly in southern states. Because those men often do not have doctors or health insurance, they have historically been hard to reach with health messages and vaccines. Many from religious families are reluctant to even ask about taking steps to protect themselves because they fear being exposed as gay and shunned—in some cases, even by their own parents. Some lead double lives and have children. Also, black and Hispanic men in the U.S. are more likely to be sent to prison, where male-male sex is common but rarely openly discussed.

This meant the virus was shifting into a new, more hidden network. A CDC technical report released in November 2022 showed that each month, a greater fraction of all those who tested positive were unable or unwilling to reveal how they got infected. As of October, it was 80 percent. A CDC study released in January 2023 suggested that the number of cases in women—particularly in black women—was increasing. Most of them were transmitted by sex.

Even though the weekly case count fell to very low levels, I suspected that cases were going unreported. Doctors are also de facto segregated into networks; some have patient populations that are mostly white gay men; others mostly treat black women. Those doctors and their patients live in different neighborhoods and have different peer groups and different medical specialties. (Women with health insurance often have ob/gyns as their primary care physicians; gay men obviously do not.) Doctors are taught to "think horses, not zebras" when they hear hoofbeats—that is, they are trained to first suspect that their patients have common diseases, not exotic ones. Also, many doctors admit in surveys that they rarely discuss sex with their patients unless the patients initiate the conversation. If a patient presents with painful sores, a doctor who treats many gay male patients is likely to suspect monkeypox and test for it. A doctor who has never seen the pox and whose other patients don't have them is not. Eventually the sores usually go away, but in the meantime, they can cause a lot of suffering.

Another worrying trend appeared: a small but increasing number of cases were in children and adolescents. More than 80 percent of them were black or Hispanic. Most of the children under age twelve were infected through household contact like diapering or bathing, but the teenagers, male and female, were mostly infected through sex.

That fact put new pressure on public health leaders. When my father was young, the worst thing you could be called was a communist. When I was young, the worst thing you could be called was homosexual. Now the worst possible accusation is that you are a racist or a homophobe. Public officials are deathly afraid of being called either; it can destroy their careers. They shy away from even discussing problems like disease transmission by sex between men of color or sex involving minors. But if a problem can't be discussed, it can't be stopped.

Early in the outbreak, a struggle over how to address infections among gay men convulsed the New York City health department. A respected senior epidemiologist advocated asking them to temporarily have fewer sexual partners. He was reassigned to a lesser job by a new health commissioner who wanted the department's messages to be "sex-positive." The commissioner even authorized an advisory saying men with monkeypox could have sex safely if they avoided kissing and covered their sores with bandages. That was patently unsafe advice, since there was already preliminary evidence that there was asymptomatic transmission. Internal emails leaked to *The New York Times* showed that some officials inside the health department were outraged—as they were right to be.

I feel strongly that public health leaders must get over their squeamishness and fears of criticism. They must directly address whoever is at highest risk and counsel them on how to protect themselves.

Most such officials are MDs. They learned in medical school to project a caring bedside manner and to think first of their patient and his or her right to privacy. They want their patients to like them. Until Covid, it had been so long since we faced a truly threatening pandemic that we had become used to having kindly, comforting experts in charge. But a craving to be liked is, in many ways, antithetical to the ability to be a good public health leader. That vocation was once, like the military, quite a tough-minded one. Public health leaders were often vilified because they were forced to curtail the rights of an angry few to save the lives of the many. Good generals must be empathic, but they needn't be popular. They sometimes must order one unit to fight a suicidal rearguard action to protect the retreat of the larger force. Public health experts don't like making choices like that. But when they abjure them, they consign innocents to suffer or die.

Chapter Six

WHERE PANDEMICS CAME FROM, AND HOW THEY CHANGED US

Over the last 500 million years, the fates of most species on this planet were determined by massive geological or meteorological events: asteroid strikes, volcanic eruptions, atmospheric heating or glaciation, tectonic drift. Forces like those caused the five extinction events, each of which destroyed more than 75 percent of the species then in existence (the most recent being the Cretaceous-Paleogene extinction of 65 million years ago, which ended the reign of the dinosaurs and made room for smallish mammals like us). In the last few millennia, the handful of species that survived into the age of *Homo sapiens* have suffered mostly at our hands. While we humans lacked the power of volcanos, we had unique talents that wiped the woolly mammoth and the giant kangaroo from the land, the passenger pigeon from the sky, the Steller's sea cow from the oceans, and the dodo from remote islands. We used fire, dams, and bulldozers to make rain forests and river basins disappear.

Now that we have come to dominate the landscape—at least temporarily—a different kind of force is shaping the course of our own history: disease. Pandemics have had more impact than any earthquake or eruption, any new weapon or infantry tactic, any new religion or political system. And certainly—although we flatter ourselves that history is shaped by our hands—more than any single human.

We write biographies of emperors and despots, of philosophers and scientists, of living saints and victorious generals, but grubby little microbes have done more than any other force to win and lose wars, destroy economies and empires, and even wipe out whole peoples. Maybe someday an asteroid or a nuclear exchange will put paid to us as an endless winter did to the dinosaurs, but thus far in our history, only diseases have done damage to rival that. Even climate change, which threatens to force us to abandon coastal cities, leave once-fertile lands arid, and watch thousands die in weather-driven storms and fires, pales by comparison. Only one force wiped out 95 percent of the Americas and several times killed wide swaths of Eurasia: pathogens.

Wars, with their outsize personalities and heroic legends, get far more attention from historians. But until the invention of vaccines and antibiotics, diseases always felled more combatants during wartime than swords, arrows, bullets, or shrapnel and so did more to rewrite history.

The Plague of Athens in 430 BC struck in the second year of the Peloponnesian War. Athens was the cradle of democratic ideals while Sparta was a military state controlled by a ruling elite, so the course of Western democracy might have been quite different. Athens lost an estimated quarter of its population, but the Spartans besieging the city were so terrified of the slayer inside its walls that they withdrew.

Two plagues probably hastened the decline of the Roman Empire: rinderpest, a virus related to measles that attacks the guts of cloven-hoofed beasts, including cattle (in pastoral societies, losing your herds causes economic collapse and starvation); and the Plague of Justinian, roughly AD 541–543, caused by the same *Yersinia pestis* bacterium that later caused the Black Death, and which killed perhaps a quarter of the people in the Mediterranean basin. It so weakened Emperor Justinian's Constantinople-based dominions that he abandoned his plans to drive the Vandals and Goths from Rome and reunite the old empire. (Admittedly, plague wasn't his only setback. A pair of major volcanic eruptions, one in 536 in Iceland and another possibly in North America in 540, darkened the skies for years and caused crop failures from China to Ireland.)

In the 1300s, the Black Death killed a third of Europe and undetermined numbers of people in Asia and Africa. It was massively disruptive: Initially, fields went untilled and famine threatened. Then, with fewer mouths left to feed, agricultural land, the bulwark of the medieval system, lost value. Serfs drifted away from the estates to which they had been bound and swelled cities. Belief in God and the Church was shaken; religious fanaticism rose. In some historians' eyes, the plague triggered the end of the Middle Ages and laid open the path to the Renaissance and later the Protestant Reformation.

At least two diseases helped destroy Napoleon's invasion of Russia, which undertaking, if he had succeeded, would overshadow European history today. He crossed the River Niemen with the largest army ever assembled—estimates run from 422,000 to 680,000 men. In impoverished Poland, the Grand Armée met flea-borne typhus. *Rickettsia typhi* bacteria brought on fevers, nausea, rashes, and, ultimately, organ failure and death. As the French outmarched their mud-bogged supply wagons, the retreating Russians burned the farms and fields in their path to deny them forage. Hunger set in. Bacteria from the guts of men and horses spread dysentery in the streams they drank from. The Battle of Borodino, deep inside Russia, was the bloodiest ever fought until World War I. It opened the way to Moscow, but Napoleon by then had only 100,000 able-bodied men left. Before he could establish winter quarters, the Russians set fire to their own wooden capital. With his army facing starvation and lacking winter uniforms, Napoleon turned back. On the march home, freezing weather, Cossack cavalry, hunger, and disease took their toll and only an estimated 10,000 men made it back across the Niemen. France's domination of Europe ended.

A pandemic altered the resolution of World War I and, it can be argued, helped bring on World War II. By the time the Spanish flu struck the

European front in the fall of 1918, the military outcome of the Great War had largely been determined. Fresh American troops had helped stop the last German thrust at Paris. But the pandemic greatly amplified the war's already awful toll. President Woodrow Wilson, determined to win at any cost, ordered jammed troopships to set sail despite the risks that many aboard would get infected and die. In the closing weeks of the war, in the crowded conditions of military camps, in trains, ships, and in the trenches themselves, flu killed more soldiers than battle did.

In April 1919, after he arrived in Paris for treaty negotiations, Wilson himself fell seriously ill. Wilson's delirium is vividly described in historian John M. Barry's *The Great Influenza*: fevers reaching 103 degrees deranged him. He became convinced that French spies were everywhere. He obsessed over the cars used by the mission and made scenes over furniture he insisted had been stolen when it had not even been moved.

"We could but surmise that something queer was happening in his mind," his chief usher, Irwin Hoover, later recalled. "One thing was certain: he was never the same after this little spell of sickness."

Wilson had come to Versailles determined to stop France's prime minister, Georges Clemenceau, from imposing harsh conditions on the defeated Germans, and planning to push his own pet project, the League of Nations. But once the flu had sapped his stamina, he folded as the other Allies dismembered the former German empire, demanded reparations payments, and forbade Germany to rearm—grievances that Adolf Hitler exploited in his rise to power.

Even Covid-19 may have helped trigger a war. Although this is psychological speculation, many Russia specialists observing President Vladimir Putin suggested that his paranoia and refusal to heed advice had been exacerbated by two years of pandemic isolation. The Kremlin had released many pictures of bizarre tableaux: Putin meeting with dignitaries and even his own cabinet from the opposite ends of a thirty-foot-long table, suggesting he had a morbid fear of the virus. Isolation from his advisors may have doomed his disastrous 2022 invasion of Ukraine from the start.

He overestimated his own army, assumed it would win quickly and be welcomed as liberators, and massively underestimated Ukraine's will to resist and the resolve of NATO to oppose him.

How did all this misery and death get started?

As the last Ice Age ended about 11,000 years ago—a mere blink ago in the 4.5-billion-year history of the earth—we *Homo sapiens* hunter-gatherers shifted our behavior in a way that had consequences we could not foresee. We began taming animals, raising them in large numbers for food and crossbreeding them for assets like fatter meat or thicker wool. First sheep and goats, and then a host of others: cattle, swine, chickens, ducks, horses, camels, llamas, alpacas, guinea pigs, and so on. (Dogs were domesticated earlier, probably 14,000 to 29,000 years ago, but we raised them in small numbers as hunting assistants, guards, sled pullers, and companions, and only rarely for food.)

Before that era, we humans probably rarely came close to a sheep, goat, pig, cow, or camel unless we had brained it with a rock, impaled it on a spear, or broke its neck in a pit trap. It was probably alone, having been abandoned by its fellows, and dead soon after encountering us. If it harbored a disease, it was unlikely that our ancestors caught it.

Even if one ancestor did, it probably would not have spread far. We lived in small bands because most landscapes could support only limited numbers of hunter-gatherers. Interactions with other groups—for trade or the exchange of brides—were dangerous and therefore probably brief. If a deadly new disease popped up in one band, its members would likely all die of it or be recovered and noninfectious by the time they interacted with another band. Archeological studies suggest that ancient hunter-gatherers were a remarkably healthy bunch. They died of wounds, broken bones, or starvation, or perhaps as prey to wilier predators. But evidence of infectious diseases is rare.

With domestication, that changed. We began living amid flocks of creatures we owned from birth to slaughter. Their bacteria and viruses adapted to us. As fellow mammals, our cells were biologically similar enough to make that easy.

Raising crops and tending herds allowed us to stop wandering in pursuit of migratory animals and seasonal foods. We built cities, grouping thousands of us closely together. We stored our new abundance of food in granaries, attracting rats, mice, and other disease-spreading rodents. We dug cisterns for fresh water, pits for sewage, and dumps for our food waste. That helped mosquitoes, flies, and other disease-spreading insects adopt us as new hosts. They laid their eggs in our standing water, feces, and garbage. Human proximity itself encouraged the spread of epidemics: we sneezed in each other's faces, defecated in each other's drinking water, and slept with each other's spouses. We opened pathways for animal bacteria, viruses, worms, parasites, and fungi to spread among us.

Thanks to our lust for meat, we exited the Ice Age and entered the Pandemic Age.

In 1999, I got an up-close look at the man-meat boundary. I took a week-long trek to a pygmy village in the rain forest of eastern Cameroon to meet a hunter who specialized in killing chimpanzees and gorillas.

I had arranged it through Karl Amman, a Swiss photographer and conservation activist who was fighting the bushmeat trade. My goal was to show how the great apes were in danger of being hunted to extinction. Their decimation was not only in itself a loss to the planet but also a disaster for medical science. Dr. Beatrice H. Hahn, a virologist then at the University of Alabama at Birmingham, was trying to prove that a chimpanzee virus was the source of HIV. She feared the chimpanzees would be wiped out before she could finish her work. "These chimps are information we need," she told me. "Killing them for the pot is like burning a library full of books you haven't read yet."

It was a two-day drive from Yaoundé, Cameroon's capital, to the village in the Dja Faunal Reserve in the country's southeast. The Dja was supposed to be a national park and animal preserve, but it was full of hunting villages. They supplied meat to the many illegal logging camps scattered throughout the reserve, run by the companies that chopped down and trucked out the huge teak, pearwood, and sapele mahogany trees.

Once outside the capital, the drive was mostly unpaved roads, some graveled, some just dirt tracks cut through the forest by bulldozers. On the outskirts of every town was a police roadblock, usually just a nail-studded plank laid across the road to puncture the tires of any car that failed to stop. The officers would approach, ask my driver what his business was, see me in the back, and come around to my window to ask, in French: "Boss, can you spare a little beer money?" Two dollars got us thanks and a wave onward.

We slept the first night in a sort of hotel-bar-bordello catering to truckers and loggers. Dinner was meat stew and bottles of Beaufort beer, served out of a shipping container that was both the kitchen and the management office, and eaten on a plastic chair in a mud courtyard. My room, which cost a dollar a night, was a wooden box with a corrugated tin roof and a padlock. Inside was a wooden platform with a dirty foam mattress; forewarned, I had bought a sleeping "cocoon"—a bag of silk woven tightly enough to keep bedbugs out. It took me a minute to figure out the light, which was a naked bulb linked to an auto battery; to light it, you hooked together the bent ends of two dangling wires. After a visit to the outhouse, I secured the door by switching the padlock to the inside hasp. Soon it was pouring rain, so I was grateful for the tin roof.

With the roads muddier, it took much of the next day to reach the village. My guide-translator, Joseph Melloh, was a former gorilla hunter, and not at all sentimental about his fellow primates. "A gorilla is still meat," he said. "It has no soul." But he had agreed to help Mr. Amman with his efforts—including guiding journalists like me to hunting camps—because it paid better and because he saw the economic opportunity in his plans. Mr. Amman was lobbying the government and donors to create a reserve where chimps and gorillas could be habituated to humans and visited by tourists, as in East Africa. "Killing a gorilla means being paid just once for it," Mr. Melloh said. Making it a tourist draw meant being paid every day. "And," he added, "you don't have to carry the firewood to smoke it."

This village we were headed for, Mr. Melloh explained, was home to "his" pygmies. When I probed, he explained that he didn't own them, but they worked just for him. He provided tools, cooking pots, guns, ammunition, wire for snares, and other things from the faraway cities. They paid him in bushmeat. He took wives from among their women. I later learned this wasn't an uncommon relationship in parts of rural Africa. Centuries before, Bantu farmers migrating in from the west had displaced pygmy hunter-gatherers. They had chopped down and burned the trees to make fields and pastures. The farmers avoided the forests, fearing predators and snakes, but the woods were full of things they coveted. So many Bantu villages developed overlord relationships with nearby pygmy villages: in return for vegetables, grain, and beer from the farmers, pygmies would supply meat, skins, honey, nuts, and other forest products. Mr. Melloh said he did consider pygmies to be fellow humans—but not his equals.

When we arrived in the late afternoon, I was in luck. Dieu-Donné Bima Bima, an affable young man regarded as the village's best hunter, had just killed a whole gorilla family: a silverback, a mother, and their baby.

"I shot the big male as it charged me," he told me as we stood next to the fire outside his hut where he was smoking the bodies. "The baby was on the mother's back. When she turned around to look at me, the baby did, too." He did an imitation of a baby's scrunched face. "I shot her in the face, and the bullet went through it, too. Bouf! One bullet, two gorillas!"

I asked if he would hold up each bit of the smoking meat so I could photograph him. He first hoisted the silverback's hands and feet, and then picked up the baby, which he had split in half and butterflied. It looked so human, so like my own kids when they were infants, that I betrayed my distress by briefly clutching my chest. He laughed at me. "Why do you want to protect gorillas? They're just animals."

I spent that night in a mud hut too small for me to stand up in. My bed was a rack of split bamboo poles, with an enormous hairy tarantula clinging motionless to the wall near my head. I decided to just leave him alone and try not to think about him instead of poking him and finding out what he could do when threatened.

At 4:30 a.m., Mr. Melloh shook me awake, saying we had to leave immediately. Some men in the last village we had passed had seen me in the car, he said, and were coming to kidnap me. As we took off, he mentioned that this had happened once before: he and a South Africa TV cameraman had been caught by surprise and had to run through the forest with men chasing them until they could circle back, jump in their SUV, and gun out of there.

Every other village in the area also had meat for sale. Dead animals dangled on lengths of twine from sticks jammed in the ground: tiny forest antelopes called duikers, monkeys, pangolins, porcupines, and rodent-like things I couldn't name.

There were two sets of buyers, Mr. Melloh explained. The loggers wanted meat for their stews. It was cheaper to hunt it than to drive in refrigerated trucks full of pork or chicken. The others were the drivers of the logging trucks shuttling between the forest and the port cities, where the sawmills were. Almost every truck had a blood-caked burlap bag or two stashed behind the cab.

In Yaoundé, Mr. Amman showed me where that meat ended up. There was an open market only a few blocks from the presidential palace and the downtown Hilton. Laid out in rows were smoked and fresh monkey and duiker meat, bushpigs, snakes, and even rows of fruit bats ready to be made into soup.

At the tables selling ingredients for fetishes rather than food, the offerings were even more exotic: The skulls of monkeys, lizards, and birds. The bright red tails of endangered African gray parrots. Four-inch cylinders of sliced elephant trunk. Antelope horns. Dried snakes. What looked like the dried hands of a baboon. The sellers were friendly but wary; they would talk to me but not let me take photos.

A fetish vendor named Elie shared some of his medical knowledge. If you had a weak son, feeding him gorilla meat or scraping a gorilla bone into his bathwater would help him grow strong. Chimpanzee hands could cure stomach pains. Pressing a heated chimpanzee skull against a broken bone would heal it faster. The sliced elephant trunks would scare off bugs or birds that would eat a family's crops.

Behind the fetish tables, a group of rough-looking men guarded a pile of dark, hairy pieces of meat. The long bones, Mr. Amman said, meant they must be gorilla or chimpanzee limbs. Those men would not talk to us at all, and he said they had mobbed photographers who had tried to take pictures, grabbing their cameras. It was illegal to sell great apes, but the law was rarely enforced. There was even a rumor that the president had given the national soccer team's goalkeeper a gorilla skull to bury in front of the net to scare off other teams' penalty kicks.

But the bushmeat trade extended far beyond the capital. To get back to my home in South Africa, I had to fly via Paris. My takeoff in Cameroon was delayed and the plane sat on the runway for five hours in sweltering heat. When we disembarked in Paris, I got to the luggage carousel late. Circling around and around with my suitcase were two big cardboard boxes. Blood-tinged water was seeping out, running in streaks down into the machinery. Clearly, they contained frozen bushmeat that had thawed during our long wait on the tarmac. Now they might never be claimed, but presumably they had been destined for local African restaurants that, alongside their regular menus, had secret "specials" for guests who could be trusted to keep quiet. Mr. Amman said he knew of wealthy Africans who sneered at domestic beef and pork as "white man's meat" and paid far more for bushmeat from home. "I know a woman who has to take chimpanzee meat to her family whenever she goes home," he said. "You can order a gorilla for Christmas the same way I'd order a turkey."

(My smoked-gorilla photographs never appeared in the *Times*. In those days, the paper banned photographs of dead human bodies and the foreign editor vetoed mine as too graphic. However, when my article was shifted from his pages to the Sunday magazine, they ran with Karl Amman photos of dead gorillas. The magazine had its own rules.)

I went to Cameroon because of what the bushmeat trade means for endangered species. But it is also an invitation to a medical disaster. The butchering of any one of dozens of forest species could have brought the hunter into contact with an unknowable threat. They could harbor *anything*.

The small number of species we have domesticated have been in close contact with us for millennia. We have presumably caught most of the ills they had to share and have built up some immunity.

Measles, for example, probably came to us from cattle, who suffer from rinderpest, a lethal intestinal disease caused by a related morbillivirus. Ducks, geese, and their waterfowl relatives are the reservoirs for all influenza viruses. From all over the globe, they migrate north into the Arctic Circle each summer and swap flu genes in the evanescent tundra pools they share. As they fly south in the fall, they shed the new strains into the urban ponds used by their human-habituated relatives who have taken up permanent residence in parks, or in the fishponds and rice paddies where flocks of domesticated ducks with clipped wings are allowed to fatten up on snails.

Dogs may have given us whooping cough; kennel cough is caused by another bacterium from the *Bordetella* genus. Although we probably got malaria from apes—their parasites are the most similar to ours—birds may be the original reservoir. Almost all bird species can play host to malaria parasites without being sickened by them. (The best-known exception is penguins, which do die of bird malaria. Since there are no mosquitoes in Antarctica, they never had to evolve resistance.)

Coronaviruses like Covid-19, SARS, and MERS appear to have

originated in bats, but typically reach us through domesticated intermediaries such as camels or semi-wild animals bred for food or fur, like palm civets, raccoon dogs, or mink. The lyssavirus rabies, the filoviruses like Ebola and Marburg, and the henipaviruses Nipah and Hendra also circulate in bats. They usually reach us in bat bites or through contact with other animals like dogs, raccoons, pigs, or horses.

Pathogens' need to be passed on to new hosts makes them cunning. Those that are not easily shed in breath, feces, or insect saliva may find other routes. In some cases, they even reach the host's brain and modify its behavior in a useful way. Rabies makes docile animals aggressive and more likely to bite, which moves the virus to a new host. The parasites of *Toxoplasmosis gondii* may be the most fiendish of all. Felines are its natural hosts. It can be lethal to human fetuses, which is why pregnant women are warned to avoid cat litter boxes. It can infect many other animals but it must somehow return to the intestines of a feline to reproduce. Therefore, it has developed a devious strategy: It makes its host more likely to be eaten by a feline, whether a saber-toothed tiger or a house cat. In the brains of mice or rats, toxoplasmosis parasites somehow make them lose their fear of cats. Cat urine, which normally repels them, becomes attractive. Toxoplasmosis is also called "cat lady disease" because it is suspected of somehow making certain humans obsessively fond of cats. When the lady dies, it may be some time before her body is found—in a house full of starving felines. One can imagine . . .

Once a disease finds a new host, it can ricochet unpredictably through other species that the host interacts with, wild or domestic. For example, in the 1990s, the rangers in South Africa's Kruger National Park realized that their Cape buffalo herds were dying of tuberculosis, which is not normally endemic in them.

It's an ancient disease. The *Mycobacterium* genus it belongs to may have originated more than 150 million years ago, when the continents were squeezed together into Gondwanaland. Bone damage from it has been found in both Egyptian and Peruvian mummies, so it was in the

Americas long before Columbus arrived. Modern strains have an ancestor that circulated in East Africa between 35,000 and 15,000 years ago.

But the most virulent strains may have evolved in just the last 250 to 1,000 years. From the seventeenth to the nineteenth centuries, it was known as "Captain Among These Men of Death" and was a slow but relentless killer, especially in the crowded cities. Its features—pale, sunken cheeks and blood-flecked coughs—were romanticized in the deaths of Mimi in *La Bohème* and Satine in *Moulin Rouge*. Its closest relative is a cattle disease, *Mycobacterium bovis*. It's not entirely clear whether our cloven-hoofed companions had it first and gave it to us, or whether we gave it to them, adding insult to the injury of domestication.

In Kruger, the rangers soon decided that their buffalo had caught it from domestic cows. The park is the size of Switzerland, and its western border abuts the farms and ranches of Limpopo and Mpumalanga Provinces. It had electric fences to keep its big vegetarians, such as elephants and rhinoceroses, out of farmers' crops and its big carnivores, such as lions and leopards, away from farmers' herds and families. But the electricity sometimes broke down, so buffalo and cattle could get close enough to at least nuzzle each other through the wire. Mutual attractions between buffalo and domestic cattle were common, rangers said.

Once the fence was reinforced, the TB-eradication plan was to cull all the park buffalo, starting at the southern end, and then to repopulate with imported disease-free buffalo. The rangers created a buffer zone about twenty-five miles wide between the new southern herds and the older northern ones. Any buffalo wandering into the zone would be shot by helicopter or foot patrols. As more calves were born in the southern herds, the rangers slowly moved the kill zone northward.

Then the plan ran into unexpected complications. First, lions began getting tuberculosis, apparently from the buffalo. When a pride tries to drag down an adult buffalo, one lioness often leaps on the fearsome beast's head and clamps her jaws over its muzzle to cut off its air. The dying buffalo coughs its last breaths right down the lioness's throat—a perfect mode of transmission. Also, lions eat the tubercle-ridden lungs and other organs of their kills, another possible transmission mode. Also, the whole pride shares in any kill, with lions, lionesses, and cubs grouped with their heads closely together over the carcass, tearing away. Whenever rangers spotted an infected lion—fairly easy because they became emaciated and weak as the bacteria devoured their lungs—they would cull the entire pride. (Although lions are the king of beasts, they breed quickly and adapt to many landscapes, so any royal family can be replaced.)

Then some baboon troops also got tuberculosis, which was a mystery. Baboons have teeth bigger than leopards' and kill small antelopes and other game. But they aren't nearly powerful enough to hunt buffalo, and they are terrified of lions. Eventually, the rangers realized their own carelessness was to blame. The disease was first seen in the troops closest to park headquarters in Skukuza. The headquarters complex included a large necropsy room with tables big enough to accommodate lions and buffalo. Field veterinarians would open them up to see what had killed them. When the veterinarians went out to lunch, they sometimes left the big doors open for the breeze. Opportunistic baboons would dash in and grab organs right off the necropsy table.

That's how a disease can pass from species to species; in this case it might have been human in origin and ended up in one of our close relatives.

Primates are so nearly identical to us genetically that we can easily share each other's diseases. Most of us don't fraternize outside our own genus and species, but a few of us do intensively. Rain forest hunters, gorilla-trekking guides, zookeepers, and scientists who use "nonhuman primate" models are in regular contact with live animals, while researchers and vaccine makers are in contact with their cells.

AIDS came to us from great apes. SV-40, a simian virus that causes brain and bone cancer, contaminated early batches of polio vaccines that were grown in broths of rhesus macaque cells. Primate viruses infect us so readily that we even use them as vaccine vectors. A chimpanzee adenovirus is at the core of AstraZeneca's Covid vaccine. Primate viruses can invade our cells but almost none of us have encountered them and we therefore lack antibodies to them. Adenoviruses were chosen because they usually cause only mild colds.

Much more common is the dangerous role that mammals play as intermediate species or as mixing vessels for diseases that otherwise could not reach us.

It's often hard to pin down the origins of Ebola outbreaks, because they begin in remote forested areas and may have gone on for weeks before epidemiologists arrive to investigate. The huge 2014 outbreak in West Africa was, at least theoretically, traced to a tree full of bats where children played in the village of Meliandou, Guinea. But others are thought to have started when rural people scavenged the carcasses of apes that had died of the disease—which also kills them. Bats are the reservoir for the virus, but the apes may have picked it up from saliva left on fruit gnawed by bats.

Middle East Respiratory Syndrome, or MERS, a bat coronavirus found in the Arabian peninsula, reaches us via camels that may also have picked it up from bat-gnawed tree fruit. Pig farmers in Southeast Asia were the first known victims of Nipah disease. Their pigs, raised in the open, may have gotten it the same way.

The "mixing vessel" phenomenon is even more disconcerting. We keep our future meals penned so closely together in stockyards, hog barns, and chicken coops that the rapid spread of any new pathogen is inevitable. When two similar viruses infest the same population, swapping of whole gene segments can occur. That process, called recombination, is more likely to produce something unpredictable than the single-point mutations that occur when viruses make random mistakes while copying themselves. Something like this triggered the 2009 H1N1 pandemic. Although it was called a swine flu, it was actually a jumble of human, bird, and swine flu genes.

When influenza viruses enter cells, they fall to pieces, producing multiple gene segments that reassemble themselves. If more than one virus happens to infect a cell, segments from each one may end up sticking together and creating something totally new.

The novel 2009 flu contained a "cassette" of several genes that had circulated in North American pigs for a decade. That cassette contained North American pig flu genes, a bird flu gene, and a human flu gene. What was suddenly and unexpectedly added was a gene segment from a flu that had previously circulated only among Eurasian pigs.

There lay the mystery. Humans and birds fly unhindered all over the world, so avian and human flu genes can mix anywhere on the globe. But pigs, as they say, don't fly. Hogs are frequently moved across the Canadian, Mexican, and U.S. borders; in Asia and Europe, they can cross borders everywhere from China to the Netherlands. It is extremely unlikely, of course, that any one pig would travel from Beijing to Amsterdam, but a pig disease easily can. It is illegal, however, to export pigs from anywhere in Europe or Asia to the Americas, and vice versa. Even uncooked pork products or frozen sperm can carry diseases and are therefore forbidden. Pigs have many ills besides flu—African swine fever, blue-ear disease, porcine diarrhea virus, and so on. Most can't infect humans, but they can devastate pig farms, so the pork industries in each hemisphere make strenuous efforts to keep pigs from the other one out.

Also, because pigs thrive anywhere in the world, there is usually no profit in importing them, except for breeding purposes. In the rare cases where imports are permitted, they are supposed to be quarantined until they are clearly disease-free. During the 1980s fad for tiny Vietnamese potbellied pet pigs, it was reported that every one in the United States descended from a single breeding pair cleared after a long quarantine.

But the H1N1 strain first found in La Gloria, Mexico, had a Eurasian swine flu gene. How did it get there? Who had imported a Eurasian pig that happened to be suffering from the flu?

That, it turned out, was probably the wrong question to ask. Although it was impossible to prove, virologists said, the most likely explanation was that the gene arrived not in the snout of a pig, but in the sinuses of a human—and the flu might even have circulated in Asia before reaching Mexico.

Pigs can't fly but people can. Pig farmers, pig auctioneers, pig slaughterers, and others who work with pigs do occasionally catch swine flus. Someone from anywhere from China to France—or even an American child who had visited a petting zoo or farm overseas—could have come home with a runny nose that, unbeknownst to anyone, was caused by a swine flu. Which perhaps infected one pig that child played with or was passed to an adult who raised pigs, or whatever. That gene could have circulated widely in pigs, since it was not being tested for, and might have gone unnoticed for weeks or months until it happened to recombine with the more common cassette and produce the La Gloria outbreak.

Unless the world goes vegan, we will live under constant threat from the centerpiece of our diets: the meat dish. Of course, that isn't the way the world is trending. Global meat consumption now averages over 90 pounds per person per year and has doubled in the last thirty years. The average American eats more than 250 pounds a year.

Then, of course, there is another set of animals playing a role in the spread of disease. These animals view *us* as food, either wanting to share what we eat, or wishing to eat us—in very small portions that we hardly miss but that can have serious consequences.

Any list of those animals would include rats, mice, squirrels, chipmunks, pigeons, crows, bats, snails, grubs, mealworms, cockroaches, mosquitoes, sand flies, ticks, tsetse flies, house flies, deerflies, kissing bugs, wasps, fleas, ticks, head lice, body lice, skin mites, and a host of internal parasites like tapeworms, hookworms, liver flukes, and schistosomes.

An equally incomplete list of what they can transmit to us would include plague, malaria, rabies, yellow fever, dengue, chikungunya, West Nile, Zika, Lyme disease, babesiosis, Rocky Mountain tick fever, Crimean-Congo hemorrhagic fever, La Crosse virus, St. Louis and Japanese encephalitis, sleeping sickness, elephantiasis, leishmaniasis ("Baghdad boil"), hantaviruses, trachoma, leptospirosis, histoplasmosis, Chagas disease, rat lungworm disease, and on and on.

Most of these diseases are rare in wealthy countries with temperate climates. But we shouldn't smugly assume we're permanently safe. In 1793, a yellow fever epidemic killed 10 percent of the population of Philadelphia. Another in 1822 led thousands of New Yorkers to flee north to a bucolic hamlet called Greenwich Village. Far from the fetid swamps of lower Manhattan, they built rooming houses and even bank headquarters, and the city soon expanded north to fill the gap.

Even in the twentieth century, malaria was endemic in the southern United States. In the nineteenth century, during hot summers it could appear as far north as Boston. The *Aedes* mosquitoes that carry yellow fever and the *Anopheles* mosquitoes that carry malaria still inhabit our low-lying wet areas.

The more common threat now is West Nile. In summer, even northern cities like New York send spray trucks into the streets and spray helicopters over the marshes in Queens. Even in Times Square, the epitome of urbanism, I've watched city workers toss poison packets into corner storm drains to kill mosquito larvae.

The chief reason we rarely face insect-borne outbreaks anymore is not our climate but our prosperity. Our homes have windows, screens, tight-fitting doorjambs, fans, and air-conditioning. A mosquito can't fly in a quarter-mile-an-hour wind, and it desiccates and dies in an air-conditioned room. They crave darkness and humidity, which is why they often end up lurking in our showers.

Also, we have tests and treatments. For almost any disease, if you have a way to quickly diagnose and cure the infected, you can usually stifle an outbreak. After 1912, as other parts of the country prospered, malaria was confined mostly to the rural South. That's why the CDC is in Atlanta, not Washington. It began life as a malaria-control center.

Mosquito diseases still threaten. Dengue virus, which can cause a lethal hemorrhagic fever, was detected in Florida in 2009 after seventy-five years' absence. Local transmission of chikungunya was found in Florida and Texas in 2014 and 2015.

When I was a child, having a tick bite was merely an annoyance; the biggest worry was infection from scratching it with dirty fingernails. That all changed in 1975 when doctors realized that some children from Old Lyme, Connecticut, who had what appeared to be juvenile rheumatoid arthritis actually had a tick-borne illness. Now there may be more than 300,000 cases of Lyme disease in the country each year. Ticks have been found to transmit a range of bacteria and viral ills, including babesiosis, anaplasmosis, ehrlichiosis, relapsing fever, Powassan virus, Heartland virus, and Bourbon virus. Some of these can kill or cause permanent brain damage. Lone star tick saliva transmits a sugar molecule that causes alpha-gal syndrome; the molecule so resembles a meat protein that people who recover from the bite develop severe allergies to red meat.

In the continental United States, the ranges of disease-bearing ticks are increasing; warmer winters no longer kill most of them off. Also, our living habits favor them. After World War II, developers bought farmland or clear-cut forests to build suburbs. Since then, the land between those houses has reforested itself. In our woody but populous suburbs, we tolerate the deer and mice that play host to the ticks but don't tolerate the mountain lions, wolves, and hunters that would keep deer in check, and we can't foster enough coyotes, foxes, weasels, hawks, and owls to control the mice. New tick species are also making homes here. The Asian long-horned tick arrived in 2017; thus far it has not been shown to carry any pathogens here, but a disease it transmits in East Asia has a 15 percent fatality rate.

Because we have showers, we forget how many hours each day our ancestors spent grooming each other like chimps, going over each other's bodies to pick off ticks and other bloodsucking pests. For older animals, tick burden is a major threat. The old lions one sees on African safaris may not die in battle with younger rivals—they succumb ingloriously to a horde of external and internal parasites. Even the magnificent American moose is threatened by ticks. In areas where winters have become warmer, up to 70 percent of tagged moose calves are slowly bled to death by the ticks covering them: no matter how fast they eat, they cannot replace the protein drained away by their joyriders.

The roots of our pandemics are ultimately in animals—the big ones we eat, and the little ones that come along for the feast. The tinier the foe, the greater the impact it is likely to have on us. Malaria parasites are so small that more than 1,000 can fit in a mosquito's salivary glands. Those parasites can teem with bacteria, and every bacterium can be invaded by viruses. The list of threats is endless.

Chapter Seven

WHY NO PANDEMIC WILL BE OUR LAST

It is impossible to predict what the next pandemic will be. What will matter is how intelligently and how fast we respond. Whether we have prepared for something like it. And whether we get lucky—as we did with monkeypox by having a vaccine already made.

I was born in 1954 and, by my count, have survived five true pandemics and quite a few near misses.

The five comprised four flus and one coronavirus. The near misses were pathogens that circled all or significant portions of the globe but never achieved pandemic status because of some limiting factor, such as infection via insects or sex or vomit or any method less effective than coughing and sneezing, which are the light and heavy artillery of transmission. Among these I would count AIDS, Ebola, West Nile, Lyme, SARS, MERS, Zika, dengue, chikungunya, and monkeypox. Statistics tell me the same thing my gut does: they seem to be arriving faster and faster.

A 2008 study in *Nature* estimated that 335 diseases that could infect humans had emerged between the years 1940 and 2004. The tab came to about five new potential pandemics each year.

A 2016 report from the United Nations Environment Programme and the International Livestock Research Institute looking back several decades estimated that new pandemic threats emerged an average of three times a year.

A 2022 WHO analysis found that, in the years 2012 to 2022, there were 63 percent more outbreaks of zoonotic diseases in Africa—those jumping from animals to humans—than there had been in the previous decade.

The exact number doesn't matter. In every scenario, it's a lot.

Obviously, the number seems higher than was once apparent because the invention of genetic sequencing has made it possible to distinguish previously identical-looking ills from one another. But what that really revealed is that more threats exist than we thought.

The reports blamed the proliferation on many factors, including population growth, deforestation, bushmeat hunting, factory farming, live animal markets, jet travel, antibiotic overuse, and global warming.

The two influenza pandemics of my childhood were the 1957 Asian flu and the 1968 Hong Kong flu. By conservative estimates, each killed more than 1 million people in its initial year. Some recordings of live classical music performances are notorious for heavy coughing by the audiences. Two of the most famous are Sviatoslav Richter playing Mussorgsky in Bulgaria in 1958 and Vladimir Horowitz playing Rachmaninov in Carnegie Hall in 1968. Given the dates, I suspect those two pandemics were behind the unusual coughing.

In 1977, the mysterious Russian flu led to about 700,000 deaths. It almost entirely affected people less than twenty-six years old. In 2015, genetic sequencing revealed that it was almost identical to the H1N1 strain that had circulated before the Asian flu of 1957, which was an H2N2, replaced it. (The old H1N1 strain was a weakened seasonal descendant of the 1918 Spanish flu.) Since flu viruses constantly mutate, the only way it could have remained almost unchanged for twenty years, according to Trevor Bedford, a flu expert from the University of Washington, was for it to have been in a freezer all that time. Its reappearance in 1977 may not have been an accident, such as a lab leak. Some changes in the genome suggested deliberate attempts to attenuate, or weaken, it. It might have been an attempt to make a vaccine against the pre-1957 strain that went awry and got loose, either in the Soviet Union or in Mao's China. (Cases of the new virus were first detected in northern China; it was first reported to the WHO by the Soviets after it appeared in Siberia. Neither country admitted releasing it.)

The H1N1 2009 swine flu from Mexico was also a true pandemic, a novel mix of swine, human, and avian flu genes that spread globally. Luckily, it turned out to be relatively mild. Ten years after it ended, the CDC estimated that it had killed 150,000 to 575,000 people worldwide. It affected young people more than old; the assumption was that those born before 1957 still had some residual protection from flus they caught as children. (A concept in virology jokingly known as "the doctrine of original antigenic sin" holds that the first version of a virus you are infected by—usually as a child—imprints itself on your immune system so thoroughly that, for the rest of your life, you mount your best defense against that strain, and less-effective defenses against later variants.)

Covid-19 is a coronavirus rather than an influenza virus. It also was a true pandemic and more lethal than the four flus. To most experts, that came as a shock. For many years, whenever prominent virologists were asked on television or in public forums, "What disease do you worry about most? What's the most likely to be the Big One?" almost all answered "flu." Their fear was that something like the H5N1 or H7N9 bird flus that have so far killed only a few hundred humans would get into pigs, monkeys, minks, or some other mammal and pick up mutations that would help it attach to human nose and lung cells. Disaster would follow.

The only virologist I remember saying otherwise was Dr. W. Ian Lipkin, director of Columbia University's Center for Infection and Immunity. He was involved in the early days of both SARS and MERS, and he said he worried just as much about coronaviruses as he did about flus. In 2019, he was proven right. (Recently, I've noticed that virologists who are asked the same "What's the Next Big One?" question tend to hedge their bets, saying it might be an influenza, a coronavirus, a paramyxovirus, an adenovirus, or another. Since those families include hundreds of known viruses, they are unlikely to be wrong.)

The "near misses" I've lived through were not considered pandemics only because they didn't spread either as easily or as far as influenza or coronaviruses.

AIDS has killed 37 million people worldwide and still kills about 680,000 each year. For decades it was a sword dangling over the heads of all gay men, and it still ravages Africa. But because it is transmitted by semen, blood, and vaginal fluid, it spreads relatively slowly.

Ebola also spreads slowly because it requires physical contact with infected human fluids.

Monkeypox is a disease in transition. Most cases used to come from contact with rodents, and it was in only a few species. Now most spread is through close human-to-human contact, including sex, so its potential range has increased enormously; but, like AIDS and Ebola, it spreads slowly.

SARS and MERS are both novel coronaviruses that reached many countries. Because they are spread by respiratory droplets, they could have proved rapidly transmissible. Thus far, however, most clusters have involved only family members or medical caregivers. Transmission appears to require inhaling a much higher dose of the virus than Covid does. Such diseases can usually be held in check once health authorities recognize the threat, isolate the sick, and make caregivers take basic infection-control precautions like masks. But if either virus mutates to become more transmissible, all bets could be off.

Zika virus is not "novel" since it was discovered in Uganda's Zika Forest in 1947, but it was novel to the Western Hemisphere in 2015. Like Zika, dengue, chikungunya, and West Nile are spread by mosquitoes, which need heat and humidity. They're a danger only in the tropics and during hot, wet summers in the temperate zones.

Lyme disease is spread by ticks, which expand their ranges more slowly than mosquitoes do, but seem better at persisting once they breach a new zone. Lyme is odd in that it may be only an "apparent" pandemic. That is, it now appears to be an ancient disease that has been infecting us since the Ice Age, but that was only recognized in 1975 because a large cluster of arthritis cases in children in Connecticut raised alarms. That led to a hunt for the cause, which turned out to be the *Borrelia burgdorferi* spirochete, which led to the creation of a test. For years after it was identified, it was thought to be confined to the northeastern United States. Then it was found in Michigan and the Upper Midwest, and then in California and the South—but nowhere in the Mountain States in between, which seemed odd.

Since the mid-1980s, however, similar cases have been found in Europe from as far west as Ireland to as far east as Ukraine. Odd symptoms associated with tick bites, including bull's-eye rashes and arthritis, have been described by European doctors since the nineteenth century. Since 2011, cases have been found in South Korea and then in Japan. The spirochetes that cause it and the ticks that spread it vary by region, so its apparent spread may be a combination of factors: some movement by infected humans, some by infected ticks—and perhaps mostly just new tests identifying an old problem.

Given the many factors that affect how diseases spread, the one thing we can count on is that the next threat will *not* be the one we prepare for.

For example: New flu strains have typically emerged in rural Asia, where millions of poor farmers sleep under the same roofs in winter as their pigs, ducks, and chickens. But the 2009 flu emerged in La Gloria, a pig-farming town in Mexico's Veracruz state. It was transmitting inside the United States before we even knew it existed.

"We weren't focused on Mexico," Dr. Thomas R. Frieden, a former director of the CDC, said later. "All our resources are concentrated on detecting new flu strains in Asia."

In 2009, two prominent virologists attempted to predict which of dozens of insect-borne diseases were the most likely to be the next threat to the Americas. The two biggest dangers they named were Rift Valley fever and Japanese encephalitis. Instead, Zika appeared in Brazil in 2015 and by the following summer was in Miami. (To be fair, Zika had been on the virologists' list of potential threats but was not a leading candidate.)

In the jet age, viruses can travel thousands of miles in a few hours, carried by any one of the 12 million people who catch flights each day. Whether or not the hitchhiker spreads upon arrival, however, depends on many other almost totally unpredictable factors.

West Nile virus, for example, arrived in the United States in 1999. It has killed almost 2,500 Americans and left far more than that with brain damage. About 6 percent of those who are known to get it die, but it's likely that many silent cases are never diagnosed.

Scientists believe it arrived from Israel, since the closest genetic match was to an outbreak among geese there. Also, it was first detected in New York City's borough of Queens, home to John F. Kennedy International Airport. But it is unknown whether it arrived in the blood of a human, in a stowaway mosquito, or even possibly in a bird that was either blown thousands of miles off course by storms or trapped in an airplane's cargo hold. After it arrived, it took five years to spread across the country to the West Coast.

Simply arriving on these shores was not enough. It also had to get extraordinarily lucky. First, it had to land in an area that harbored a mosquito that could transmit it—that is, a species whose immune system allowed the virus to wriggle out of the half-digested blood meal in its abdomen and make its way into the salivary glands without being degraded. Happily for the virus, the *Culex pipiens* mosquito thrives in this country, particularly in the suburban and peri-urban residential areas where tens of millions of Americans have lived since the mid-twentieth century. (In an earlier era, when the urban-rural divide was sharper, West Nile might have died out: the asphalt jungle of most American cities is not hospitable to culex mosquitoes, and farm families lived too far apart to allow sustained spread.)

Next, it had to also find a helpful bird species. Although humans can die from the disease, they generally don't build up high enough viral loads in their blood to pass it on. That is, if a mosquito bites a human harboring West Nile, it doesn't get enough viral particles to trigger the disease in another human. (Yellow fever and malaria, by contrast, are definitely shuttled between humans by mosquitoes.) Birds, however, do build up high viral loads. But not just any bird will do: the virus kills some species too quickly. Dead exotic birds in the Bronx Zoo and dead crows in Queens helped tip veterinary authorities in New York to the fact that a new virus was circulating. Again, luckily for the virus, someone had introduced the European house sparrow, *Passer domesticus*, to the United States, probably two hundred years before. Sparrows build up high levels of virus but don't die from it.

In another happy coincidence for the virus, European house sparrows like living close to humans in cities and suburbs because they feed in our gardens. They nest, moreover, in close-knit bunches, so it was easy for a few mosquitoes to spread the virus to many birds. Sparrows, however, do not travel very far in their lives. Having arrived in New York City, the virus might have remained stuck in the metropolitan area, or east of the Appalachian Mountains. Again, in a happy circumstance for the virus, it also could proliferate in species like crows, blue jays, and robins, which are not migratory but range much farther than sparrows do in search of food. Even though some would die of it, those species may have been the ones that moved the virus steadily and incrementally a few states to the west each spring and summer until it reached the Pacific Ocean in 2004.

The virus also had to arrive at an opportune time weather-wise. Mosquitoes transmit viruses more efficiently at high temperatures. Luckily for the virus, global warming had begun to kick in, and the summers of 1999 to 2004 were hotter across the United States and Canada than the thirty previous summers had been.

Finally, the virus had to have no local competitors that would have rendered birds or humans immune to it. Luckily for West Nile, its cousin, St. Louis encephalitis—another flavivirus spread by the same mosquitoes and birds—had been slowly disappearing over the decades since it had produced an explosive outbreak of brain infections in St. Louis in 1933.

In short, West Nile found the perfect conditions to let it become an epidemic.

More candidates await. Some, like dengue ("breakbone fever") and chikungunya ("bending-up disease"), have become familiar because they circulate in tropical climes where many Americans vacation. Each infected vacationer is another chance for a virus to visit the continental United States. Once in a while, one might get lucky as West Nile did. Further afield are many others with currently unfamiliar names like O'nyong'nyong fever, Semliki Forest virus, Machupo and Mayaro viruses, Lassa fever, and Congo-Crimean hemorrhagic fever. Their arrival is not out of the question.

In the last few years, we've learned that some of our long-standing assumptions about pathogens are wrong. For example, we used to believe that, even though many pathogens mutate rapidly to make better attachments to cells, they always clung faithfully to their original modes of transmission. That is, a disease that was normally spread by coughing or by insect bite would never, for example, evolve so much that it could be spread by sex.

Ebola was the first to upend that shibboleth. For forty years, we assumed it was spread only by vomitus, feces, and blood. Then, in the 2014 West Africa outbreak, a few cases spread by sex were found. Then living, viable virus was found in the testes and even in the eyeballs of patients long after recovery. That was a shock. A change in transmission modes was the equivalent of us already knowing that the dog genome is so malleable that crossbreeding can produce either a Chihuahua or a Great Dane, and suddenly discovering that the genome could mutate enough to produce a dog that sprouts wings and flies away.

Soon Zika, which we thought was spread only by mosquitoes, turned out to also be transmissible by sex. Then monkeypox, a disease previously spread mostly by rodents, began rapidly spreading through the skin-to-skin contact inherent in sexual liaisons.

For centuries, the most devastating pandemics, such as plague, tuberculosis, and cholera, were caused by bacteria, which are complex living organisms, rather than by viruses, which are simple sets of genetic instructions. With the discovery of antibiotics, we assumed we had brought that era to a close and that we would never again face a bacterium like *Yersinia pestis*, the cause of the Plague of Justinian and the Black Death. But bacteria are constantly evolving resistance to our antibiotics. We may one day meet—or create, accidentally or otherwise—a bacterium that outflanks all our defenses.

We also assume that viruses, which evolve remarkably fast under pressure, tend to ultimately become more transmissible and less lethal. That follows the Darwinian principle of survival of the fittest. In theory, the variants that too rapidly pummel their hosts into their beds or their graves are rarely passed on, while the weaker ones that jolly their hosts into remaining upright and going to parties reach far more receptive noses and throats, and thus conquer with kindness. But Covid's Delta variant, which was equally lethal to its predecessors but more transmissible, showed us that rule is not written in stone. (Admittedly, Delta was later chased out by Omicron, a weaker variant, which reestablished the paradigm. But Omicron, too, could kill.)

Nothing is fixed. New threats are evolving all the time. We must be constantly on guard.

Part Three

THE HUMAN FACTORS THAT SPREAD PANDEMICS

Chapter Eight

THE NETWORKS THAT TRIGGER BLAME

Once a new disease has made itself known, a whole series of forces rise up to affect how it spreads and how many people it infects.

These forces are constant and yet inconsistent. That is, they often reappear, but not every time—because every disease is different. Some differ in merely practical ways—aerosol transmission is different from droplet transmission, for example. Some carry moral baggage. We silently pass a different judgment on someone who picks up a sexually transmitted illness than on someone bitten by a mosquito. We may even draw finer discriminatory lines, such as drawing different conclusions about someone who encounters a tick in his or her own backyard versus someone who travels to the Middle East to be bitten by a sand fly. Among those forces, I count response time, denialism, fatalism, bigotry, corruption, rumors, media coverage, political opportunism, hygiene theatrics, and profiteering.

A first principle is this: although most pathogens can infect any member of our species, they almost inevitably first appear in a smallish network of similar and related people.

This inevitably has two consequences:

First, the members of that network get blamed for the disease—even if they are merely its first unlucky victims.

Second, public health officials face a moral dilemma. The most opportune time to stop an epidemic is while it is still within that small network. But because those networks are often made up of one ethnic group or one marginalized group—such as gay men, the homeless, ultra-Orthodox Jews, or Amish farmers—health officials doing their jobs are liable to be accused of bigotry.

This issue rears its head in almost every outbreak. As I described earlier, when monkeypox appeared in New York City, some officials were so afraid of being seen as "not sex-positive" that they offered advice that could spread disease. To my mind, that's malpractice on a grand scale.

There is no question that stigmatization is deplorable. It is also inevitable. Perhaps the most famous example is syphilis.

The disease first appeared in Europe in the army of Charles VIII of France besieging Naples in 1495. The "Great Pox" was devastating. It started with fever and genital lesions, then sometimes progressed to a blanket of sores all over the body, leaving bone-deep pain and stinking abscesses. Once it reached the brain, it could slowly lead to dementia and death.

No one knew where it had come from, but Charles's army was composed of mercenaries, a few of whom had gone to the New World with Columbus. Scholars now believe they caught it from the natives of Hispaniola, the island where he first landed (in what is now the Dominican Republic). Later accounts by Spanish missionaries who learned local languages suggested that the symptoms had been known in the New World for centuries. Genetic analysis of the family of spirochetes that includes syphilis now confirms that it was a New World disease. It was the lone counterpunch the inhabitants of the Western Hemisphere were able to land before the diseases brought by Europeans nearly wiped them out.

Charles's army was trailed by "camp followers," including women who sold food, laundry services, medical care, entertainment, and, of course, sex to the troops. Since camp followers would follow whatever regiments had money to spend, diseases easily spread from one army to another.

The Great Pox was the most feared epidemic since the Black Death of 150 years earlier, and every country across Europe and Asia blamed it on their enemies.

The French called it "the Neapolitan curse." The English, Italians, and Germans called it the *morbus Gallicus*, or "French pox." The Dutch called it "the Spanish itch," the Russians called it "the Polish disease." Poles and Persians called it "the Turkish disease." Turks called it "the Christian disease." Tahitians, who got it from visiting sailors, called it "the British disease." Indians called it "the Portuguese disease." The Japanese called it "the Chinese pox," while other Asians called it "the Persian fire."

This tendency goes back into prehistory. Athenians blamed the Plague of Athens on the Spartans. Romans in Constantinople, capital of the eastern Roman Empire, blamed the Plague of Justinian on Egyptians.

Jews have been a focus for such accusations for centuries, often related to the fact that in many countries, by choice or because of bigotry, they lived apart from other ethnic groups. During the Black Death, more than two hundred Jewish communities in Western Europe were wiped out by murder, arson, and forced emigration.

In 2009, the Yeshiva University Museum in Manhattan mounted an exhibit about one item: a chest containing thousands of gold and silver coins. It had been unearthed during a construction project in what had long ago been the Jewish quarter of Erfurt, Germany. The last king depicted on the coins had reigned in 1349, the year the Black Death reached Erfurt. The city had been the scene of one of the worst massacres—more than a thousand Jews were killed. One of them, presumably, was the owner of the chest, who never dug it up.

Jews were blamed in part because of the perception that their neighborhoods were spared. The plague bacterium, *Yersinia pestis*, was carried around Western Europe from port to port by fleas that lived on ships' rats. When those rats disembarked and passed their fleas to their landbound cousins, plague radiated inland. Neighborhoods in those days were often built around wells, and Jewish neighborhoods were rarely the first hit—so Jews were accused of poisoning the wells of Christian areas. One theory as to why Jewish neighborhoods were not first is that grains attract rats and at Passover, Jews were obliged to rid their houses of all wheat, barley, oats, rye, and other grains. Plague tended to surge in the spring, the same time of year that Passover occurs, which may have helped foster that theory.

A more likely explanation, in my opinion, is that rats traveled between inland cities in farm wagons loaded with produce. Wagons don't move in winter snows, and farmers have little to sell in winter. In Western Europe, Jews were rarely farmers because they were usually not permitted to own land. On market days, the Christian farmers probably off-loaded their wagons first—or almost exclusively—in Christian neighborhoods. The rats on their wagons would have hopped off there, like their shipborne cousins. Markets in Jewish neighborhoods would presumably have focused on goods they produced, such as clothing, shoes, and tools, so the rats and fleas would not reach those areas until later.

In 1892, Jews were blamed for outbreaks of both cholera and typhus in New York City. In those cases, Jewish immigrants may actually have introduced the pathogens. The SS *Massilia*, a passenger ship carrying Jews from Odessa to New York, had a typhus outbreak aboard. Cholera outbreaks occurred that year in several European port cities, including Hamburg, where many ships embarked for America. But they were unknown because the mayors suppressed or denied reports of cholera diagnoses.

In 2019, New York suffered one of its worst measles outbreaks in decades. The cases in both New York City and its suburbs stayed almost entirely within the ultra-Orthodox Jewish community. Its catalyst was a large 2017 outbreak in Ukraine that climbed to over 70,000 cases. In that country, it was not limited to any one ethnic group. Many Ukrainian children were unvaccinated for various reasons: the government had rejected an inexpensive Indian vaccine but was unable to afford replacements. Trust in government was low, and the country was embroiled in a war with Russian-backed separatists.

In 2018, measles spread from Ukraine to Israel because of a religious tradition. Every year on Rosh Hashanah, tens of thousands of Hasidic men converge from all over the world at the grave of Rabbi Nachman of Breslov, founder of a branch of Hasidism. (The event, held in the Ukrainian city of Uman, is jokingly referred to as "Hasidism's Burning Man.")

From Israel the virus spread first to ultra-Orthodox communities in North London and then to New York. Most ultra-Orthodox Jews did vaccinate their children—prominent rabbis have for centuries argued that it is obligatory to protect one's children against disease. But the American anti-vaccine movement had been targeting Orthodox Jews, and some local rabbis opposed vaccination. At the start of the measles outbreak, New York City health officials estimated that 80 percent of the Hasidic children in Brooklyn were vaccinated. But measles is so transmissible that it can sustain an outbreak when immunity falls below 95 percent.

To contain it, the mayor and health commissioner threatened to fine parents $1,000 for each unvaccinated child and to close any school that could not prove that all its students were vaccinated. To fend off accusations of anti-Semitism (already being voiced in some quarters), the municipal order did not mention Jews or yeshivas. It targeted everyone who lived or worked in certain zip codes—which happened to roughly coincide with the ultra-Orthodox neighborhoods. The outbreak lasted more than a year and more than 1,200 were infected.

Unfortunately, the combination of vaccine rejection and the breakdown of health systems during the Covid pandemic had further consequences—and in the same ethnic network. In the summer of 2022, a twenty-year-old ultra-Orthodox man in upstate Rockland County, New York, who had not recently been overseas was paralyzed by polio. It was the first case of local transmission of the virus in the United States since an outbreak among the Amish in 1979. Sewage sampling found several strains of the virus circulating in Brooklyn and in four suburban counties with ultra-Orthodox populations, each of which matched strains circulating in similar neighborhoods in Israel and London. Health officials estimated that only about 60 percent of Rockland Country children below age three had had all their vaccines, and in some Hasidic neighborhoods, it was below 40 percent.

Any network can end up being blamed for disease. In 1900, a new wave of bubonic plague that had emerged in southern China in 1855 was finally detected on American territory, presumably arriving on ship traffic from China. Honolulu's Chinatown burned down when fires set to drive out rats got out of control. Within weeks, a death from the disease had occurred in San Francisco's Chinatown, which was immediately cordoned off by the police as health inspectors invaded rooming houses to search for cases. The cordon led to a long legal and political battle between city and federal officials, Chinatown's ruling council, and the companies and wealthy families who wanted their Chinese employees back at work. The controversy of course greatly fueled the anti-Asian prejudice already common in California.

Mexicans were targeted after the 2009 swine flu outbreak began there. In Chile, a Mexican soccer player was called a "leper" by a Chilean opponent; when he responded by spitting on his tormenter, the Chilean news media accused of him of germ warfare. A month later, Argentinians stoned buses entering from Chile, claiming they were spreading the virus. European countries soon warned their citizens against visiting Argentina—but not against visiting the United States, where the virus was far more widespread.

In the 1990s, New York City faced a wave of homeless people and drug abusers with antibiotic-resistant tuberculosis who would not take their medication. The city's director of tuberculosis control, Dr. Thomas R. Frieden, locked the most recalcitrant ones in a hospital on Roosevelt Island for months, forcing them to take multiple antibiotics until they were no longer infectious. Boston and Denver did the same. There were few objections because the homeless have no political clout. (Dr. Frieden later went on to be the city's health commissioner and then CDC director.)

However, it is important to note that transmission networks are not always composed of the poor or the marginalized. Viruses seek opportunities wherever they can.

In mid-2020, following the spring surge of Covid deaths, which was concentrated in a few urban areas, there was a long summer lull during which deaths dropped as low—relatively speaking—as 520 a day. In early autumn, cases began rising rapidly again. That reversal was largely triggered by the movement of a privileged strata of American society: college students. In many states, particularly in the Midwest and the border states of the American South, the first outbreaks were in university towns, especially in the "Greek" neighborhoods abutting universities. Childishly defiant fraternity brothers and sorority sisters disdained masking rules and ignored university bans on large parties. The virus spread from gown to town—from students to older, more vulnerable residents. A few months later, students heading back home for Thanksgiving and Christmas contributed to a double peak of case surges, each of which began after those two holidays. Covid's peak mortality was reached in early January 2021, when the country had an average of 3,300 deaths per day.

Another network that exemplifies white privilege—Alpine skiers—contributed to two separate waves of death during the Covid pandemic.

From Wuhan, the virus spread first to popular tourist areas in Asia, including beach destinations in Thailand. It then reached Iran, perhaps via a merchant from Qom who had visited China. Or perhaps via a Chinese Muslim visiting Qom, a Shia holy city. Its earliest substantial emergence in Europe was in northern Italy. It's not entirely clear why, though there are business connections between Wuhan and the Italian city of Bergamo, Italy's hardest-hit city, which sits on the edge of the Alps.

Once there, the virus spread first to ski towns in the Austrian Alps. From there it moved to Germany. Early cases in Iceland and Norway were traced to skiers who had visited Austria. Skiers may also have played an early role in its spread to France and Britain. Several of France's first cases were found in Les Contamines-Montjoie, a mountain ski town where a British businessman who flew in from Singapore infected pals with whom he shared a chalet.

In the United States, the largest outbreaks of the spring wave were heavily concentrated in a few cities, including New York, Seattle, San Francisco, New Orleans, Detroit, and Miami.

There were very few cases anywhere in the Mountain States—except in one unique setting: ski resorts. Skiers and workers in Sun Valley, Idaho; Vail, Colorado; and a dozen other Rocky Mountain ski towns fell sick. On a per capita basis, Sun Valley was a bigger hotspot than New York City; a greater percentage of its tiny population died.

Almost two years later, that pattern repeated itself. The Omicron variant was first described in the Johannesburg-Pretoria region of South Africa in late November 2021. Over the next weeks, it sparked major outbreaks in London, Oslo, and Copenhagen. By mid-December, it was spreading widely in New York City, and then throughout the Northeast, and to most of the South and along the Pittsburgh-Chicago "Rust Belt."

Once again, there were very few Omicron cases in the Mountain States—except in areas with ski resorts. On January 6, 2021, on *The New York Times* map of new cases, one county in every Rocky Mountain state was deep purple, indicating more than 250 confirmed Covid cases per 100,000 residents in the past week. In Idaho, it was Blaine County. In Utah, Summit County. In Wyoming, Teton County. In Colorado, Pitkin County. In Montana, Gallatin County, and in Oregon, Deschutes County. Those were the home counties of Sun Valley, Idaho; Park City, Utah; Jackson Hole, Wyoming; Aspen, Colorado; Big Sky, Montana; and Mount Bachelor, Oregon.

By then, Europe had recognized the danger that skiers presented. Resorts in the Italian Alps required all winter visitors to prove that they had been vaccinated, had recovered from Covid, or had just tested negative.

When diseases are not contained within the first network they circulate in, they soon jump to others.

Holiday travel forces members of unrelated networks to cross paths. Even when airplanes are rendered relatively safe by mask mandates and HEPA filters, travelers are pressed together in airport lines, elevators, restaurants, shuttle buses, bathrooms, and so on. When families gather for holiday celebrations, each person at the dinner table has left his respective network—a university, a military unit, a factory, an office, a shared house—and may either introduce the virus to the family or bring it back.

Almost every year, the December–January peak of flu season has a pronounced "double hump," rather than a single one. Epidemiologists say it is caused by Christmas vacation. Flu is typically spread into a family by its children, who pick it up in school or day care. Transmission markedly drops during the two weeks of vacation, then resumes when classes do.

Sometimes the network that accelerates the spread is global rather than local. In 2010, the first conference in a new field, "mass-gathering medicine," was convened. It took place in Saudi Arabia, in recognition of the fact that the Saudis were experts in mass-gathering medicine, and with reason. For centuries, the hajj, the annual Muslim pilgrimage to Mecca, was an important focal point for pandemics, and the Saudis had worked hard to minimize that.

The nineteenth century's cholera epidemics several times reached Mecca and spread from there to new countries. The hajj also played a role in Europe's last smallpox outbreak, which occurred in Yugoslavia in 1972. Although there was no smallpox in Mecca that year, a Muslim pilgrim from Kosovo returning by bus visited several shrines in Iraq, which had the virus. Because he was vaccinated, he suffered only a mild rash, but he became a carrier, apparently infecting a Kosovo teacher upon his return, perhaps through attendees at his welcome-home party. The teacher fell seriously ill and was transferred to a hospital in the capital, Belgrade. He was misdiagnosed as suffering from a bad reaction to penicillin and then died of internal hemorrhaging, a rare smallpox complication—but not before infecting several doctors and nurses.

Although Yugoslavia was behind the Iron Curtain, its Dalmatian Coast beaches were popular with Western European tourists. Not wanting to lose the hard currency those tourists spent, the government initially hid the outbreak. Ultimately, however, the spread of cases within Belgrade made that impossible—and scared off tourists. Reversing course, the administration of President Josip Broz Tito, whom many historians consider a dictator, began an intense crackdown that resembled the one China would impose almost fifty years later. Kosovo's borders were closed. All public events, meetings, and weddings were banned. Empty tourist hotels were converted into quarantine centers. Mandatory vaccination was imposed; 15,000 were quarantined and their contacts traced. Ultimately 18 million Yugoslavs were vaccinated or revaccinated, ending the outbreak after 175 cases and 35 deaths.

In 2020, fearing a repeat of earlier disasters, the Saudi government canceled the hajj, which was scheduled for July. Only one thousand pilgrims—all of them local—were allowed to enter Mecca that year.

But another religious mass gathering boosted Covid.

India's Hindu festival of Kumbh Mela is far larger than the hajj, although it occurs in twelve-year cycles and lasts four months, not just a week. The 2013 Kumbh Mela drew 100 million worshippers to Allahabad to bathe in the Ganges River, which is the festival's main event. That year's festival passed with nothing more serious than outbreaks of diarrhea and upper respiratory infections, but that has not always been the case. The 1783 and 1891 Kumbh Melas were both interrupted by massive cholera outbreaks; in the first, more than 20,000 pilgrims were said to have died.

The 2021 Kumbh Mela was held in Haridwar, where the Ganges exits the Himalayas and runs across the flat Deccan Plateau. It began in April just as India's Covid-19 epidemic appeared to be waning. In the weeks before, confirmed cases in India had dropped to less than 12,000 a day, down from a peak of 100,000 in September 2020. Prime Minister Narendra Modi, a Hindu nationalist, rebuffed appeals to cancel the festival, and 9 million pilgrims attended. Tests on many who returned ill suggested that the disease had been widespread in Haridwar. Several important holy men died of the virus. In the following month, cases in India shot up to 400,000 a day. Some virologists believe the Kumbh Mela gathering spawned the lethal and more-transmissible Delta variant of Covid-19, which spread around the world.

In 2008, World Youth Day, a gathering for young Roman Catholics, drew 223,000 pilgrims from 170 countries to Sydney, Australia. It was held in mid-July, the height of the Southern Hemisphere's winter flu season. More than 100,000 young people stayed in gymnasiums, community centers, churches, and the city's former Olympic Village, often sleeping on mats in rows on the floor. The final mass, presided over by Pope Benedict XVI, was attended by more than 400,000 pilgrims and locals.

Flu was widespread, and genetic sequencing showed that World Youth Day had been a giant mixing bowl. Investigators found strains from Europe and Malaysia that had never been seen in Australia before. Some had mutations making them resistant to the anti-flu drug Tamiflu, another wrinkle that Australians had never encountered. And, of course, some pilgrims took those home.

Depending on how a disease spreads, only some networks can sustain transmission. In others, it dies out.

AIDS is a prime example. How it spread from a few apes in the Congo Basin into a worldwide pandemic—but only in some populations—is described in detail by the Canadian epidemiologist and medical historian Dr. Jacques Pépin in his 2011 book, *The Origin of AIDS*.

The ancestor virus for HIV was SIV_{cpz}—a simian immunodeficiency virus circulating in chimpanzees. That virus was itself a blend of two variants of a virus that had circulated for at least 32,000 years in two separate African monkey species—red-capped mangabeys and mustached guenons. At some point, the two viruses mixed—possibly in one chimpanzee that had eaten both an infected mangabey and an infected guenon. (Chimps hunt monkeys, chasing them through the treetops and swatting them to the ground. A chimp may have gotten infected through mouth cuts caused by the sharp ends of crunched bones.)

In Africa, there are four groups of human HIV, each one representing a separate jump from chimpanzees—presumably to hunters who cut themselves while butchering chimp carcasses. One, group M, accounts for 99 percent of all human cases, and molecular dating suggests it reached us in the early 1920s.

It hadn't happened earlier, Dr. Pépin argues, because it's extremely difficult for a man to kill a chimpanzee without a gun, and Europeans didn't introduce large numbers of guns into equatorial Africa until the early 1900s.

In the mid-twentieth century, the virus began spreading. Heterosexual sex, however, is far too inefficient at transmitting HIV for it to have been the path the virus took from a handful of hunters in remote villages to thousands of urbanites. Heterosexual sex is inherently safer because the vaginal walls are hardier than the fragile skin of the penis and rectum. Studies in Africa have found many "sero-discordant" couples in which the virus is not transmitted from one to the other even after years of unprotected sex.

Dr. Pépin offers evidence that the blame for the initial rapid spread should be placed on the massive campaigns against yaws, leprosy, and other diseases conducted by the British, French, Belgian, and other colonial authorities, in which hundreds of villagers would be lined up for injections. Those campaigns were made possible by the invention of factory-made syringes in the 1930s and injectable antibiotics in the 1940s. (Previously, syringes were made of hand-blown glass and prohibitively expensive. As they became more affordable, they became status symbols, with families boasting of owning one. Traditional healers adopted them to inject their decoctions with. In that era, a patient might get three hundred shots in a lifetime, and the barrels and needles were often not sterilized between patients.)

Another multiplier was the economic collapse of the former Belgian Congo after independence in 1960. In the early 1900s, the Belgians had permitted only African males with work passes to live in the capital, Leopoldville (named after Belgium's colonialist nineteenth-century king and renamed Kinshasa when the country became Zaire). But communities of *femmes libres* ("free women") existed on the city's edges. They were the equivalent of camp followers, providing cooking, laundering, companionship, and sex, usually for just a few men each. The colonial authorities saw the *femmes* as a necessary evil; it taxed them and ran medical clinics where they were treated for venereal diseases. (Those clinic records are among

Dr. Pépin's many sources and show that penicillin injection campaigns to fight syphilis triggered hepatitis outbreaks, providing further evidence of his syringe theory.)

After independence, the country fell into factional violence, tens of thousands of Belgians fled and the economy broke down. Thousands of desperate Congolese women moved to the capital. Bordellos known as "flamingoes" proliferated, and competition meant women were forced to service many men each night to make a living. With clinics unstaffed and antibiotics unavailable, STDs, which cause sores that make heterosexual transmission more likely, proliferated. Kinshasa became an ideal environment for HIV.

A charitable intervention by the United Nations probably moved the disease to its next network: Haiti. The Belgians had permitted almost no Congolese outside the priesthood to be educated, so when they left, the country had no professional class. From Haiti, the UN recruited about 4,500 administrators, civil servants, teachers, doctors, lawyers, engineers, and other professionals. They spoke French and were well educated and happy to earn better wages than they could at home. A few of them—or possibly even just one—carried the virus from Zaire to Haiti.

In Haiti, it spread slowly among heterosexuals, but eventually found its way into two high-risk networks. Many gay American and European men visited the island because it was touted as a sex tourism destination by the Spartacus International Guides catering to gay men. Additionally, the capital, Port-au-Prince, contained the Hemo-Caribbean blood collection center, which was owned by the head of Haiti's feared secret police, the Tontons Macoutes. In the 1970s, the center, which was known to have lax hygiene standards, exported 1,600 gallons of blood plasma to the United States each month.

The blood-clotting factors needed by hemophiliacs were made by pooling serum from many donors. One contaminated donation could turn an entire batch infectious. Before HIV tests were developed in 1985, contaminated clotting factor killed roughly 4,000 of the 10,000 hemophiliacs in the United States. Tainted whole blood also killed more than 5,000 Americans who received transfusions during surgery or childbirth, including the tennis star Arthur Ashe and the Hollywood activist Elizabeth Glaser.

In the United States, the virus also reached another network: people who injected drugs. (In its early days, the networks affected by AIDS were sometimes referred to as "the 4 H's," meaning Haitians, hemophiliacs, homosexuals, and heroin users.)

Once tests were developed, they reduced the risk of infection from transfusions and clotting factors to near zero. It took years or decades longer for state legislatures to approve programs distributing clean syringes to drug users, but those measures eventually reduced the virus in that network to very low levels. The virus still circulates among gay men, but at much lower levels than it previously did because of widespread antiretroviral treatment and the daily use of pre-exposure prophylaxis, or PrEP (drugs like Truvada that prevent infection). It also persists in Haiti at higher levels than it does on most Caribbean islands.

To my mind, the best way to fight discrimination is to focus on getting rid of the disease as fast as possible. The virus is the enemy; whoever its first victims happen to be are not. When the virus is beaten, the risk of stigma recedes.

Chapter Nine

THE MISSED OPPORTUNITIES

We are very much on the lookout for military attacks. Spy satellites cross our heavens, the Arctic Circle is rimmed with radar stations, submarine-detecting hydrophones line the seabed. If only our pandemic sentries were so wide awake.

As a subscriber to disease-alert services, I see new outbreaks reported from somewhere in the world almost every day. Most are not terribly threatening. They can include anything from Xanthomonas wilt in bananas to Hendra virus in horses.

Many turn out to be false alarms. A "mystery pneumonia" in a rural Argentine hospital that killed six people in 2022 turned out to be Legionnaire's disease. The guests who began dying one by one after a West African wedding ultimately turned out to have shared a lethal batch of homemade alcohol. A spate of deaths after a South Asian wedding turned out to be caused by a cooking pot made from a steel drum that had previously contained pesticide.

Many outbreaks begin with an odd pattern of unexplained deaths in a remote area. It may not even be noticed until it reaches a city, where the threat becomes magnified. Between 1976 and 2012, there were 17 Ebola outbreaks, none of which killed more than 300 people. In 2014, the virus reached the capitals of Liberia, Sierra Leone, and Guinea, exploding and killing 11,000.

Ideally, we want to catch those clusters as early as possible. Unfortunately, our current watchdog systems have inherent flaws.

In theory, the WHO should be the clearinghouse for all alerts. It has GOARN, the Global Outbreak Alert and Response Network, created in 2000. It has the International Health Regulations, which require countries to report any outbreaks of a long list of notifiable diseases.

Since 2017, it has also had the Epidemic Intelligence from Open Sources program, or EIOS, a computer network that gathers thousands of news reports from all over the world, translates them, and pushes them through algorithms to determine which are important.

But in practice, the WHO's systems have not worked very well. I can't think of a single serious outbreak I learned of first from them.

After Covid was well under way, a search showed that EIOS had received early notice of pneumonia deaths connected to a seafood market in Wuhan, and the agency had reacted within twenty-four hours. But the process was slowed by inherent flaws.

One is the bureaucracy: a WHO officer in China who hears something worrying must report it to the regional office in Manila, which may or may not report it to headquarters in Geneva. When I was in regular contact with the WHO, life in Geneva seemed to go dormant at 5 p.m. If I didn't know whom to call directly, the media office would sometimes say, "Well, the person you want has gone to dinner and can't be disturbed. Call back tomorrow." I'm generalizing unfairly because some dedicated officials did return calls quickly, and some previous WHO directors-general tolerated torpor that recent ones do not. But swift reactions have historically not been the agency's forte.

Also, the bureaucracy has many silos: separate officers for each disease, for emergencies, and for the media. Each expects to be consulted, which slows responses.

But the most important limitation is that the WHO is a UN

organization. As with a London gentlemen's club, management defers to the members. If it hears of an outbreak in a member country, it must first ask that country for information. Although countries are legally obligated to report, some don't—or they lie. There is little the WHO can do about it. It can complain via the media, hoping to shame the country into compliance. But that's risky, since the member country can retaliate by cutting its annual "dues" paid to the WHO.

For more than twenty years, Canada had a respected disease-alert system, the Global Public Health Intelligence Network, or GPHIN (GEE-fin). At one time, it issued about a dozen warnings a month and was a major contributor to the WHO system. But it went dark about six months before Covid began.

GPHIN was founded in the 1990s after an outbreak of pneumonic plague in India triggered a staff panic at Toronto's airport, where many travelers landed. It originally used computer algorithms to search the web for outbreaks, then added a dozen epidemiologists speaking several languages as analysts. It looked not just at news articles but at factors like local sales of antiviral drugs and even price movements in hog futures, which might indicate a swine flu outbreak. In 2009, it was praised for its early detection of H1N1 swine flu in Mexico, and it later helped spot the 2014 West Africa Ebola outbreak.

But then, as Toronto's *Globe and Mail* described: "Over the years, with no major threats materializing, the government grew weary of GPHIN." Its budget was pruned; its epidemiologists were shifted to other jobs. In 2018 its analysts were forbidden to send out alerts without senior managerial approval; notices that once appeared in fifteen minutes now took several days, rendering it all but worthless. Its last alert—about an unexplained outbreak in Uganda—was in May 2019, mere months before Covid broke out.

China has an internet-based pneumonia-tracking system known as the Viral Pneumonia of Unknown Etiology, which might have been useful during Covid—if doctors had used it. According to a study by Michael

Worobey, an evolutionary biologist who investigated Wuhan's first cases, VPUE was set up after the 2003 SARS epidemic and run by China's CDC. Clinicians were supposed to log on and describe cases of viral pneumonia they could not explain.

However, many were unaware it existed. In Wuhan, Dr. Worobey said, the first alert about a mystery pneumonia was on December 29 by Dr. Xia Wenguang, a vice president of the Hubei Provincial Hospital of Integrated Chinese and Western Medicine. The local health agency, which, as I described in Chapter 1, was vulnerable to pressure from the mayor's office, issued an alert the next day. Nothing was posted on VPUE until January 3. "Although mechanisms like China's VPUE system are potentially invaluable," Dr. Worobey wrote, "they will fail without widespread buy-in from health care providers and rapid data sharing from local to central authorities."

A small, independent disease-alert service, Flutrackers.com, has existed since 2006. It is sometimes the first to spot small outbreaks or to track worrying genetic changes in viruses uploaded to public data banks. But it's unwieldy. Because it is a discussion forum for many topics that interest its moderators, from disease-related polls and politics to "pandemic gardening," it can be hard to sift out what's important.

I'd like to think that, as the world's premier public health agency, our American CDC has the best surveillance system and the fastest reaction times. But during my career, I've been shocked at how long it can take them to get moving.

The Zika epidemic was a particularly trenchant example. I first heard of Zika on December 28, 2015. It was between Christmas and New Year's, which is usually a "slow news" period. I was in the office searching for something to use in my weekly three-hundred-word Global Health Update item. I found a brief article by a CNN stringer in Brazil and read it with growing horror. Brazil had declared a state of emergency because hospitals in a few northeastern cities had seen a wave of hundreds of newborns with microcephaly. A deputy health minister, the article said, had asked Brazilian women to put off having babies. I was stunned. Outside of Mao's China, I had never heard of a government asking its women to stop having children.

Up to nine months earlier, the article said, many of the mothers had been infected with Zika, an African virus never before detected in Brazil and previously considered mild. The government was looking into whether it could be the cause.

I checked the CDC's website. It had a Zika page, but with little information. It noted that the virus had recently been detected in Polynesia and South America and that some cases had been diagnosed in the United States in returning travelers. It said nothing about microcephaly—nor about Guillain-Barré syndrome, some cases of which had been detected in Polynesia two years earlier. It did speculate that imported cases could cause the virus to spread within the United States.

With my deadline rapidly approaching, I made a quick phone call to the only doctor I knew in Brazil—a plastic surgeon who also had a company that made diagnostic tests—and wrote a brief item. Then I alerted my editor that we had a big story to follow up on and asked the foreign desk if our Brazil bureau chief, Simon Romero, and I could work together. I also emailed a CDC media contact asking for an interview with a Zika expert as soon as possible.

The next afternoon, I had an interview with a Colorado-based CDC specialist in mosquito-borne diseases. She knew about Zika, but appeared unworried, almost blasé. Based on the spread of dengue, which was also transmitted by *Aedes* mosquitoes, she expected Zika to reach Puerto Rico and probably parts of Florida, Texas, and the Gulf Coast. She didn't want to talk about Brazil or the possibility that the virus caused microcephaly. "Information is pretty limited, so it's hard to comment," she said. I asked if the agency would issue a travel warning, perhaps specifically for pregnant women. She said no, it would for now stick with the current Level 1 alert, which had been in place for Latin America and the Caribbean for years because of dengue and chikungunya. It was just "Avoid mosquito bites."

Simon interrupted his Christmas vacation to report. His powerful story arrived that evening. He interviewed the deputy health minister, who reiterated his suggestion that women in the affected areas avoid pregnancy. He quoted Gleyse Kelly da Silva, a young mother in Recife whose daughter had been born with microcephaly four months earlier. "I cried for a month when I learned how God was testing me," she said. Simon's story made the front page. From then on, the *Times* was driving the story forward.

It was midwinter. Tens of thousands of vacationing Americans were headed to the Caribbean, among them hundreds of young women who were pregnant or trying to get pregnant. Puerto Rico had hundreds of thousands of women of reproductive age in the path of the virus.

Some pregnant women with vacation plans—including one of my *Times* colleagues—started calling me to ask whether they should go. I would point out that I was not a doctor and not qualified to give medical advice. But then I'd say that no, I thought they should absolutely not go to the Caribbean—even though at least one caller told me her ob/gyn had said, "It's fine! Don't worry about it." (She called back weeks later to say she had stayed home as her extended family had vacationed in Fajardo, Puerto Rico. It later turned out that Fajardo had suffered a big Zika outbreak during the time she would have been there.)

I called cruise lines to ask if they were canceling itineraries or asking pregnant passengers not to book. Their lobbying association sent me an anodyne statement saying the CDC had not changed its alert level, so they would stick to their protocol: advising guests going ashore to wear mosquito repellent and long sleeves.

Every day for two weeks, I asked the CDC what was taking so long. At one point I was so fed up that I ended up screaming at a media rep—one I actually liked—demanding to know what the holdup was. The conversation ended with me throwing my headset in disgust; my science desk colleagues, who had been forced to listen to me shouting, gave me a standing ovation.

To prod the agency, I wrote an article saying it was internally debating whether to issue a warning. It seemed clear that it was stalling until the ambassadors of every affected country could be officially informed that the U.S. government was about to drop a bomb into their winter tourism business.

Finally, on January 15, it issued an alert telling pregnant Americans to "consider postponing" travel to Zika-affected areas. It advised pregnant American women living in such areas and those considering pregnancy to "consult a doctor." That was a euphemism. The agency, perpetually fearful of congressional conservatives, was never going to publicly suggest that women use birth control or consider abortion.

One day later, the first American baby was diagnosed with Zika-related microcephaly. It had just been born to a woman in Hawaii who had lived in Brazil during her pregnancy.

To my mind, the world's most effective disease-alert service is one that is completely unofficial, unattached to any government or UN agency and staffed mostly by volunteers. The one that first raised the alarm about Covid: ProMED.

ProMED was created in 1994 by the Federation of American Scientists as the Program for Monitoring Emerging Diseases and is now under the auspices of the International Society for Infectious Disease. It began as a forty-member email list, an experiment in whether the internet—then brand-new—could be used to spot emerging diseases in far-flung places. It now relies on a worldwide network of hundreds of volunteers, many of them working or retired epidemiologists, clinicians, veterinarians, parasitologists, plant biologists, and members of other specialties. They file alerts to moderators who collate them, add explanatory information, and send them out to tens of thousands of subscribers, including many science journalists. Their alerts cover not just human disease but animal and plant ones too, because some pathogens jump species. ProMED is funded by donations and is guided not by government fiats but by the consciences and standards of its moderators.

On December 30, 2019, one of those moderators, Dr. Marjorie Pollack, got an email from a colleague who kept up with Weibo, the Chinese social media platform. It reported rumors of clusters of cases of a mysterious viral pneumonia in Wuhan and added what appeared to be a document from the Wuhan municipal health commission saying the clusters were linked to a seafood market. Dr. Pollack kept digging until she found a Chinese business news website confirming the commission's report and put out an alert just before midnight.

The WHO's alert process took longer. On December 31, its country office in China noticed a media report about the Wuhan health commission's alert and informed the WHO Western Pacific regional office in the Philippines. In Geneva, its EIOS system picked up the ProMED report before it heard from Manila. On January 1, the WHO requested more information from China; it did not receive confirmation from China until January 3.

That was not the first time ProMED had led the way. In 2003, it arguably was the first to try to alert the world to SARS. The media paid little attention to SARS until the WHO put out a global alert on March 12, but on February 10, ProMED posted its first request for information about rumors that cities in southern China were battling a mysterious pneumonia. That request, I learned later, was made by a ProMED subscriber, Dr. Stephen O. Cunnion, a retired U.S. Navy outbreak specialist. Dr. Cunnion had a friend who had a friend who belonged to a teachers' chat room in Guangdong. On it, teachers were nervously discussing reports of pneumonia deaths and hospitals filling up. The discussion even included an odd and very specific detail: vinegar was disappearing from grocery shelves and the smell of boiling vinegar was everywhere. A rumor had arisen that the fumes kept the mystery pneumonia at bay.

The outbreak had actually started many weeks earlier, and there were vague rumors of it inside China as early as November 2002. By February, Beijing was orchestrating an intense cover-up.

Along the way, there were several missed opportunities because officials assumed that any respiratory illness, especially in China, would involve influenza. Their fear was that the H5N1 bird flu first detected in humans in a 1997 Hong Kong outbreak would become more transmissible. H5N1 was clearly very dangerous: there were only 18 confirmed cases in 1997, but 6 of them had died.

On November 20, Dr. Klaus Stöhr, a WHO flu expert attending a conference in Beijing to discuss what flu strains should be used in the following year's vaccine, heard of several unusual staff deaths at a Guangdong hospital. To "be on the safe side," he told me later, he asked for tissue samples. But he ordered tests only for influenza, and nothing unusual turned up.

On November 27, Canada's GPHIN picked up a media report from China of a flu outbreak closing schools and factories in Guangdong. But its algorithm didn't realize the importance of the report and did not pass it on.

At about the same time, an American equivalent, the Global Emerging Infections Surveillance and Response System, or GEIS, picked up similar reports. But they described the cause as a B-strain influenza, and China's routine reports on its flu season said many cases were of B strains but total caseloads were within normal parameters. So GEIS discounted the report.

On February 10, 2003, after ProMED had raised the issue, the WHO's Outbreak Center in Geneva sent an official query to China, as protocol required.

The replies they got were either shocking misdiagnoses or blatant lies. On February 11, Beijing admitted that Guangdong had experienced an outbreak of respiratory disease, but said it was over, had hospitalized only 300 people, and killed just 5. It was attributed first to mycoplasma and then to chlamydia, two common bacteria that can cause pneumonia but rarely spread fast. Then there was silence; Beijing stopped answering.

Also, some obscure reports from China suggested bird flu might be on the loose. In December, wild birds had died of H5N1 inside Hong Kong's Botanic Gardens, not far from southern China. On February 5, without explaining why, the Chinese subsidiary of the company making the anti-flu drug Tamiflu took out ads saying its product worked against bird flu.

On February 12, flu specialists at the University of Hong Kong cooperating with the WHO attempted a sort of medical commando raid:

they caught a train to Guangdong, where some had friends or relatives working in local hospitals, and quietly asked them for tissue samples from dying patients. They did get a few, but also initially tested them only for influenza, not coronaviruses.

On February 19, the WHO and the CDC sent two investigators to China. The government stonewalled them, putting them up in a Beijing hotel for two weeks and giving them routine briefings, but not permitting them to travel to Guangdong. In early March, they left in disgust.

What ultimately revealed China's secret was a superspreader event. On February 21, Dr. Liu Jianlun, who had treated pneumonia patients in Guangdong, came to Hong Kong for a family wedding and stayed at the Metropole Hotel. He is thought to have suffered coughing fits in the elevator and possibly to have vomited in the hallway outside his room and then cleaned it up himself; twenty-three other Metropole guests, including seven from his floor, became infected. Over the next week, they spread the virus around Hong Kong and to Hanoi, Singapore, and Toronto. In one Hong Kong hospital, a former Metropole guest infected 112 staff and patients after he was placed on a nebulizer that spread a fine mist from his lungs into the ventilation system. In Hanoi, another former Metropole guest infected seven workers at a garment factory he owned and twenty-two in a hospital. One of that hospital's doctors, Dr. Carlos Urbani, described the clinical signs of SARS in great detail. He also caught it and died.

With major outbreaks under way in Hong Kong and Hanoi, the WHO put out its March 12 alert. Dr. Malik Peiris, chief of virology at the University of Hong Kong, finally identified the new pathogen as a coronavirus.

China did not admit the full scope of its problem until late April. By that time, Beijing's own outbreak was bigger than Guangdong's. Premier Wen Jiabao fired the national health minister and Beijing's mayor and said there would henceforth be severe penalties for covering up cases.

SARS ultimately infected about 8,000 people in 29 countries, killing about 10 percent of them. But because victims had to inhale large doses of virus to get infected and because it was not transmitted until patients were obviously symptomatic, it could be controlled by rapid case isolation and consistent use of personal protective gear.

By July, the WHO declared the epidemic over. The fiasco led to the creation of the International Health Regulations, which—at least on paper—require countries to report outbreaks.

And China is by no means the only nation to try to hide an outbreak.

The appearance in Saudi Arabia of the coronavirus that eventually was named Middle East Respiratory Syndrome, or MERS, triggered a cover-up at so many levels that there has never been a complete record of its spread during its first two years. The virus, which is even more deadly than SARS—it kills about a third of those infected—was first recognized in 2012 only because an Egyptian microbiologist working in a hospital in Jeddah, Saudi Arabia, Dr. Ali Mohamed Zaki, could not figure out what had killed a sixty-year-old pneumonia patient. Without seeking permission, he sent a sample to a lab in the Netherlands for analysis.

After he published what he had found—first on ProMED and then in greater detail in *The New England Journal of Medicine*, Dr. Zaki was fired and deported. That was followed by a series of fights over patent rights and authorship of papers between the Saudi health ministry, the Dutch lab, and other researchers. It was eventually established that MERS is a bat coronavirus that is picked up by camels and then passed on to humans.

Meanwhile, there were repeated outbreaks at hospitals and dialysis clinics in several Saudi cities. Even teaching hospitals made basic mistakes like housing a dozen patients in the same room, letting patients' families crowd hospital halls, and failing to give their staffs protective gear. Only in 2014 did the country react from the top, when the king fired the health minister and his deputy. Their replacements acknowledged that there had been more than 700 cases and nearly 300 deaths, many of which had never been reported.

During those years, people returned infected from the Middle East to more than a dozen countries, including the United States. Some infected others in turn. South Korea had a particularly big outbreak.

"This is an alarming systemic failure and speaks volumes about such a closed society," a *Washington Post* editorial said. "People and institutions react out of fear and keep painful information secret from each other."

The world needs independent disease-alert services that are *not* controlled by either a national government or a UN agency. They are too prone to either bureaucratic thumb-twiddling or actual suppression of news.

The other essential element, of course, is journalists. All too often, the world remains unaware that a killer is loose until it reaches a country with a free press. That's how the 1918 flu became the "Spanish flu." Its geographic origin is still obscure; it may have begun in China or even in Kansas. But during the closing days of World War I, as it felled thousands of soldiers, American, British, French, and German military censors suppressed the news to keep up morale back home. Only when it reached Spain, which was neutral and had no press censorship, was its full extent revealed.

Chapter Ten

THE "NOT ME" DENIALISM

When a new disease erupts, it is usually greeted not with alarm but with inertia. People have a hard time accepting that the danger is real. That initial skepticism can cost many lives.

By February 2020, videos of bodies lined up at crematories were being leaked out of Wuhan. Satellite photos showed mass graves in Iran. In northern Italy, coffins were stacked on church pews.

And yet, there was little acceptance of the obvious: it would reach the United States, and many Americans would die. Even experts took a wait-and-see attitude, noting that China's analysis of the first 45,000 confirmed cases said 81 percent were "mild." That was true, but the study defined "mild" as everything from minor cold symptoms to pneumonia not severe enough to warrant hospitalization. In other words, the remaining 19 percent who weren't "mild" were fighting for their lives. But listeners heard "mild" as if it were the sniffles.

On March 11, just before going into lockdown, I recorded another *Daily* podcast with Michael Barbaro. He again asked what I was doing to stay safe. I had become even more careful than I was when we had last talked on February 27. I was riding the subway wearing one glove to hold the pole, while I used the other to touch my phone. (He didn't ask, but I was not wearing a mask. Almost no one did then.) I sprayed surfaces I had to touch with a bottle of hydrogen peroxide—something Michael teased me about after his producer told him I had sprayed the podcast studio.

We knew people were dying, but millions of Americans still thought it was ridiculous to cancel events like the March Madness college basketball championships, the Comic-Con convention, or the South by Southwest music festival.

In every pandemic I had ever covered, I said, people would not accept that a threat was real until it had hurt them or someone they knew personally. As a nation, we were failing to believe because we had not yet had our "Rock Hudson moment." He asked me to explain the reference.

Rock Hudson was a heartthrob movie star of the 1950s and 1960s. He was most famous for his romantic comedies with Doris Day, but on-screen he had kissed nearly every starlet in Hollywood.

By 1985, however, he was clearly very ill—gaunt as a specter and shaky as he walked. In a TV special with Doris Day, he was barely coherent. Rumors spread because he so much resembled the men dying of AIDS who were then a common sight in the gay neighborhoods of San Francisco and New York: skeletons helped down the streets by friends. His publicist, however, insisted that he had liver cancer.

Late that year, Mr. Hudson went to France for treatment. For reasons that are not clear, his new French publicist revealed that he was being treated for AIDS. A firestorm of publicity erupted—much of it ridiculous. Actresses he had kissed thirty years earlier were asked by reporters whether they were afraid he had infected them.

President Ronald Reagan had also been a Hollywood leading man in the 1950s, and he and Rock Hudson were old friends. He called Mr. Hudson to check on him. Mr. Reagan had taken office in 1981, the same year AIDS was first recognized. By 1985, it was killing more than 8,000 Americans a year. During those four years, however, he had never acknowledged the threat, never even uttered the word *AIDS* in public. Homophobia was then so routine that his generation was uncomfortable with the idea of men having sex with men. Sex itself was considered unfit for polite discourse; my grandmother's dictum was that you never brought up sex, politics, or religion at the table. (I loved my grandmother but dinner conversation at her house was not exactly scintillating.)

But as soon as it touched someone he knew and identified with, President Reagan changed. That September, he mentioned AIDS in a speech. Rock Hudson died a few weeks later, and Congress authorized $220 million to find a cure for AIDS.

Mr. Hudson's illness also made many Americans drop old stereotypes, such as the notion that all gay men were effeminate. It finally dawned on them that, if HIV could kill Rock Hudson, someone they knew or even someone in their family might be at risk.

Denialism—the sense that "it can't happen to me"—has been the norm in the early stages of every disease I've covered.

During the Zika epidemic, I attended a class in a local welfare office in a suburb of San Juan, Puerto Rico, where a doctor instructed young pregnant women in how to avoid infection so they would not have brain-damaged babies. The advice was to avoid mosquito bites by wearing long sleeves and pants, staying indoors, and using insect repellent. Billboards and TV and radio spots gave the same messages, but the class existed so a medical professional could reinforce it face-to-face in the same office where pregnant women and young mothers got infant formula and food stamps.

After the class ended, I interviewed several of the women. One wearing a long skirt said her mother nagged her every morning to cover up. But most of the others had bare arms and legs, and one wore tiny shorts and a tube top, her belly sticking proudly out between them. I asked her if she wore repellent. She wrinkled her nose and said no, she hated the smell. What did she think of the advice to wear more clothes than she did? "Oh, no—it's so hot here," she said, fanning herself. "I can't." What about mosquitoes? I asked. "I don't worry—I slap them fast, like this!" she said, slapping herself all over.

Others had different excuses. One said she lived on her building's eleventh floor and mosquitoes never flew that high. Without disagreeing with her—mosquitoes can breed on a tall building with balconies like hers—I asked if she ever went downstairs. "Of course," she said. "But I'm careful."

After the class, I went back to the doctor's office. I was stunned that so few of the women seemed to take her advice seriously. Hadn't they, I asked, seen the pictures from Brazil of the microcephalic babies? "Yes, I'm sure they have," she said. "But it's very hard to get people to change their habits."

Then she dropped her voice and said, "I should be more careful. Please don't put this in the paper because I haven't told anyone yet, but I'm pregnant myself."

"What??!!" I said. "You're wearing a miniskirt!"

"Yes, I know," she said. "I really shouldn't."

My fixer—herself a former TV reporter—laughed and scolded me: "You *cannot* ask a Puerto Rican woman not to look good."

Even the doctor was in denial.

In 1990, Dr. Nthato Motlana, an anti-apartheid activist and Nelson Mandela's personal physician, described another of his patients, a young black businessman. It was clear from the opportunistic infections he suffered that his immune system was collapsing. Dr. Motlana suggested an HIV test. His patient exploded: "That's white man's propaganda!" he said. "I'm not homosexual!"

At the time, that was common thinking among black South Africans. The rest of Africa had been ravaged by AIDS for more than a decade, but South Africa had been partially cut off by the boycotts imposed in the 1980s to protest apartheid. Also, the disease had started in central Africa and was still working its way south.

As a result, at that time very few black South Africans knew anyone with the disease. Of the country's first 215 AIDS deaths, almost all were gay white men; about 10 percent of them had worked as flight attendants on South African Airways, which through much of the 1980s had flown to the United States and Britain because the Reagan and Thatcher administrations had ignored the anti-apartheid boycott.

By the 1990s, the virus was racing through the African population but, because of its long incubation period, was not yet showing its effects. During apartheid, the African National Congress and the Pan Africanist Congress had maintained guerrilla armies in exile in countries where the epidemic was raging. The borders had reopened in 1990 after negotiations between Mr. Mandela and President F. W. de Klerk. The exile armies returned—some bringing the virus.

During the 1994 elections that made Mr. Mandela president, many leaders of those exile groups ended up in Parliament. In 1996, a friend who edited South Africa's most liberal newspaper told me that he had been told off the record that two-thirds of the new parliamentarians were taking antiretroviral drugs, which was costing Parliament's generous health insurance plan a fortune. He was never able to confirm that tip, and when I asked him about it in 2022, he said he could not remember who had given it to him. I mention it as a rumor of historical interest, except to note this: a 2008 study by the UN Commission on HIV/AIDS and Governance in Africa noted that the speaker of Zambia's Parliament said 35 members of his body had died of AIDS between 1984 and 2003, and the speaker of Malawi's Parliament said it had lost 28 members to AIDS between 1999 and 2003.

Denialism is most dangerous when it infects a country's leader.

By 1985, after HIV tests were developed, it became clear that what was then known as "slim disease" in Africa was, in fact, late-stage AIDS. Initially, many African presidents insisted that their countries had no cases at all, which was ridiculous.

The notable exception was Yoweri Museveni, president of Uganda. He had sent many of his army officers for training to Cuba, where HIV testing was mandatory. Fidel Castro took him aside at a meeting of the Non-Aligned Nations to alert him that a third of his officers were infected.

Mr. Museveni, who had come to power in a coup, quickly grasped the ramifications of a third of his army dying, and what sky-high HIV rates would do to Uganda. Soon afterward, he created the ABC campaign, which stood for Abstain/Be Faithful/Use Condoms, and then the Zero Grazing campaign, meaning "don't graze your cow in your neighbor's pasture" (that is, don't sleep with your neighbor's partner). Uganda became a model for the rest of Africa.

In sharp contrast to Mr. Museveni's attitude, Thabo Mbeki, who succeeded Mr. Mandela as president of South Africa, repeatedly questioned whether HIV caused AIDS. Until 2006, his government refused to buy antiretroviral drugs, either to treat dying patients, or even in the small amounts needed to prevent pregnant HIV-positive women from passing the virus to their babies.

The consequences were tragic. In 2008, soon after Mr. Mbeki was pushed out of office, a study by Harvard researchers estimated that his policy had cost 330,000 South Africans—including 35,000 babies—their lives.

In 1999, as widespread HIV testing revealed that South Africa had a huge AIDS epidemic brewing, Mr. Mbeki made a speech in which he described antiretroviral drugs as "toxic." In conversations with friends, he revealed that he sat up into the night doing research on the web (then unusual because search engines were rudimentary) and had found sites claiming that AIDS was a myth invented by pharmaceutical companies to enrich themselves by selling drugs at astronomical prices.

In the West at the time, denialists insisted that gay men were dying not from a viral infection but from "consequences of the gay lifestyle," such as anal sex with multiple partners, bouts of syphilis and other STDs, the use of amyl nitrate "poppers," and exhausting all-night disco dancing—all of which, they said, broke down the immune system. When it was discovered that AIDS was common in Africa while anal sex, poppers, and disco were not, the denialists modified their theory to say that the immune system could also be degraded by poverty and parasitic infections.

After Mr. Mbeki's 1999 speech, reporters sought comment from the country's top AIDS experts, almost all of whom were white. They were harshly critical.

Mr. Mbeki, a cerebral but thin-skinned man living in Mr. Mandela's enormous shadow, was given to seeing conspiracies everywhere. He was a vocal proponent of the "African Renaissance," saying Africans would "be our own liberators." He was also deeply offended by the suggestion that promiscuity spread the continent's epidemic, which he said fed Western stereotypes about Africans being oversexed.

He responded to the criticism first with anger, and then by convening a thirty-three-member Presidential Advisory Panel to "explore the causes of AIDS" (even though it had been sixteen years since HIV had been determined to be the cause). To it, he appointed well-known denialists. The panel split; the doctors on it gave the conventional view that HIV caused AIDS, while the denialists argued that it was a condition needing treatment with vitamins, massage, music, yoga, spiritual care, homeopathy, Ayurvedic medicine, and other alternative therapies. Although 1,500 South Africans a day were testing positive, some denialists argued that the epidemic was a false rumor and testing should simply stop.

In July 2000, soon after the panel issued its report, the 13th International AIDS Conference was held in Durban, South Africa. As the host, President Mbeki gave the opening address. Before he did, five thousand conference participants signed the "Durban Declaration," which was published in *Nature* magazine. It stated that HIV caused AIDS and antiretroviral drugs suppressed it. In his speech, Mr. Mbeki rejected that view and claimed it was caused by poverty, other infections, and poor nutrition. Hundreds of delegates walked out. By contrast, they loudly applauded Nkosi Johnson, a tiny eleven-year-old in a suit and sneakers who had been born with HIV and whose mother had died of AIDS. In his speech, Nkosi said, "I hate having AIDS because I get sad when I think of the other children that are sick with AIDS. I wish the government can give AZT to pregnant HIV mothers." As he spoke, Mr. Mbeki and his entourage walked out. Nkosi died six months later.

Later that year, Mr. Mbeki's combative spokesman, Parks Mankahlana, died at age thirty-six in his parents' home. He was well-known to every journalist in the country, and they watched him waste away in his waning months. Newspaper editors agonized over how to handle his death. Some, reflecting the government line, simply gave no cause. The *Mail & Guardian*, a frequent critic of government policy, reported that Mr. Mankahlana's confidants had said he was dying of AIDS. African National Congress stalwarts angrily denied this; his widow said he had died of heart failure and anemia. Two years later, the ANC admitted that he had had HIV but insisted that what killed him was the antiretroviral drugs he took. They also claimed Nkosi Johnson had been killed by "drugs he was forced to consume."

Mr. Mbeki frequently said he knew no one who had died of AIDS. When anyone tried to rebut that by naming South Africans who had, Mr. Mbeki would retort that there were many causes of pneumonia or tuberculosis or whatever opportunistic infection the patient had finally succumbed to. His health minister, Dr. Manto Tshabalala-Msimang, became known as Dr. Beetroot because she denied public hospitals permission to distribute antiretrovirals and said the official treatment for AIDS was garlic, lemon, beetroot, and African potatoes. (The African potato, *Hypoxis hemerocallidea,* is not related to the *Solanum tuberosum* potato we use to make french fries. The African plant is used in traditional medicine to treat everything from testicular tumors and impotence to insanity to heart disease.)

As South Africa's epidemic grew into the world's biggest, the ruling ANC split over the issue. Ambassadors overseas complained that other governments wanted to talk only about Mr. Mbeki's inexplicable position. Mr. Mandela, then in retirement, would not directly criticize Mr. Mbeki out of party loyalty, but he made jokes about the need to admit being wrong. He also admitted that members of his own family had died of AIDS and donned an "HIV-Positive" T-shirt at public events calling for the government to approve antiretrovirals.

Eventually, Mr. Mbeki stopped discussing his views in public. But in 2002 he sent colleagues a rambling 114-page email attacking the "mainstream thesis" on HIV. Much of it was drafted by Peter Mokaba, a former head of the party's militant Youth League, who was himself to die of AIDS a few months later. It included a sarcastic monologue lashing out at racial stereotypes. "Yes, we are sex-crazy!" it read. "Yes, we are diseased! Yes, we spread the deadly HI virus through our uncontrolled heterosexual sex! In this regard, we are different from the [United States] and Western Europe! Yes, we, the men, abuse woman and the girl-child with gay abandon! Yes, among us rape is endemic because of our culture! Yes, we do believe that sleeping with young virgins will cure us of AIDS! Yes, as a result of all this, we are threatened with destruction by the HIV/AIDS pandemic! Yes, what we need, and cannot afford because we are poor, are condoms and antiretroviral drugs! Help!"

As noted, epidemics lead to accusations of racism, and there is no question that stigmatization and racism play big roles in Africa's epidemic. But epidemics are not stopped by denying the truth. There is no question that rape is a major problem in South Africa nor that the rumor that sex with a virgin cured AIDS circulated for years and led to horrifying examples of child rape.

Mr. Mbeki was ultimately forced out of office in 2008 by a revolt within his party. His temporary successor, Kgalema Motlanthe, fired Dr. Tshabalala-Msimang and replaced her with an AIDS activist. The next president, Jacob Zuma, was constantly mired in corruption scandals—but he did upend Mr. Mbeki's policies and provide antiretroviral treatment to his people.

I have seen countries get past denialism that emanates from the very top of the social pecking order. It's not always clear why it happens. There is often a slow buildup of overwhelming evidence and fierce public criticism, but it may be hard to know why reform arrives. Autocrats rarely explain their changes of heart.

As I mentioned, China's 2003 denialism about SARS led to the International Health Regulations, which require reporting outbreaks to the WHO. In January 2020, although there was an initial cover-up in Wuhan, it was far briefer than the SARS cover-up had been.

The Saudi regime also once underwent a semipublic change of heart, although it was about polio and occurred earlier than its MERS cover-up.

In late 2004, polio was hovering on the brink of eradication; there had been fewer than 800 cases worldwide. At the time, I very much hoped to write the disease's obituary, so I regularly checked the Global Polio Eradication Initiative's website for new case clusters.

I was studying a map of them when I noticed something strange. Most diseases spread in rough circles outward from the index case, or in a series of circles as index cases fly from one city to another. But the new ones were appearing in a straight line from West Africa due east along the southern edge of the Sahara. Then they took a sharp left and went north.

It was the year after several Muslim-majority states in northern Nigeria had stopped all polio vaccination because of rumors that the vaccine was a Western plot.

Suddenly I had an epiphany: these small outbreaks were probably being seeded by pilgrims headed for Mecca. Rich pilgrims can afford to fly. Poor ones take buses, and some camp along the way and seek work to earn money to continue their journeys. I checked another map and learned that there are few roads crossing the Sahara Desert, but several paralleling its southern edge and then turning north to Khartoum and Cairo. An offshoot from those led to Port Sudan, where the last case had been detected. Port Sudan is the embarkation point for ferries across the Red Sea to Jeddah, Saudi Arabia's chief port city.

While I was reporting the story, cases of polio paralysis turned up in Jeddah—the first appearance of the virus inside Saudi Arabia in many years. Then one was reported in Mecca itself.

Initially, WHO media representatives put me off, declining to discuss the issue. But after a couple of days, I was able to reach Dr. Bruce Aylward, a Canadian emergency response specialist who was then in charge of the WHO's polio eradication efforts. He confirmed my suspicions and told me that the Mecca paralysis case was of a child in a Nigerian family illegally camped in the hills outside the city.

When I wrote, I raised the specter of polio spreading to other countries. The hajj was then drawing about two million pilgrims a year.

My story did not make our front page, but the Saudis definitely noticed it. A few days later, I got an email from our Middle East bureau chief warning me that I was being attacked on the front page of *Al-Watan*, the government paper, under a headline in red ink: "New York Times Tries to Blacken the Hajj."

The story featured WHO representatives rapidly backpedaling. *Al-Watan* quoted them as saying they did not believe the pilgrimage would spread the virus and suggesting that I was prejudiced against Islam. (Dr. Aylward had already told me my story had been completely accurate, even if it embarrassed the agency.)

A few weeks later, Yemen, which borders Saudi Arabia, experienced its first polio outbreak in years. Genetic sequencing—then a new science—showed that it was the Nigerian strain. Then cases of paralysis turned up thousands of miles away in Indonesia—again, of the Nigerian strain.

The only logical explanation was that Mecca had become a focal point for spreading the Nigerian strain.

Quietly, the Saudis changed their policies. In 2005, in their annual list of hajj regulations, they ordered all pilgrims from countries with known polio outbreaks to arrive in Jeddah with a certificate showing they had been vaccinated.

Unscrupulous travel agents, however, soon began selling "hajj packages" including airfare, accommodations, and forged vaccination certificates. Beginning in 2009, the Saudis went further: every pilgrim from any country with polio cases had to swallow a dose of vaccine as soon as he or she got off the plane.

The kingdom also acknowledged that the disease had effectively become a Muslim problem. It was by then found almost exclusively in Muslim countries or in Muslim regions of mixed countries. Not long afterward, for the first time, they began donating millions of dollars to the global polio eradication drive.

Chapter Eleven

THE TOXIC FATALISM

Denialism's bleaker cousin is fatalism, which exerts a mysterious force. Denialists refuse to believe in a disease. Fatalists do believe—but just won't save themselves.

It's hard to explain why impending danger can be met by malaise, but I've felt it myself. On backpacking trips when I was young, there were times when I could see rain and lightning headed my way, but just could not make myself set up my tent or hunt for a cave. I felt too tired. As soon as the storm hit, I'd get a burst of energy and do something—but by then I'd be soaked. Confused by my own stupidity, I put it down to the drop in barometric pressure before the storm. It made me torpid.

Sometimes that seems to happen to whole populations.

In September 2021, I attended a symposium about the spread of Covid in Africa and was startled to learn that South Africa's efforts had ground to a halt with less than 30 percent of its populace vaccinated. Months of vaccine shortages had been replaced by a surplus of doses. The country had lived through three lethal waves of the virus and suffered more deaths per capita than anywhere else on the continent. It was facing the dangerous Delta variant that had emerged in India five months earlier. But demand for vaccine had simply dried up, said Dr. Stavros Nicolaou, chief executive of Aspen Pharmacare, which was distributing the Johnson & Johnson vaccine, one of two the country had then approved.

The problem, he said, was not outright resistance. In polls, only about 14 percent of South Africans said they would never accept a vaccine. Nor was it access. By then the country had plenty of doses and, although some of its rural areas are remote, its network of paved and gravel roads is quite good and the health ministry had sent teams on foot to the most distant villages. It was also broadcasting public service announcements in eleven local languages.

The problem was "vaccine apathy." People knew the shots were available and had no serious objections—but were just not motivated to get them.

"We have a surge when each new age group qualifies for the vaccine," Dr. Nicolaou said, "but then it plateaus very quickly. We've reached only half the people we'd planned."

Two months later, in November 2021, the world was facing a new variant, Omicron, with fifty mutations from the original virus. It had first emerged in South Africa and reinfected many there who had survived one bout. It was so worrying that much of the world summarily cut off flights from Johannesburg and Cape Town. President Cyril Ramaphosa was furious that his country was being punished for telling the truth.

Yet South Africa *still* could not vaccinate more than a third of its population. By then, it had such a huge surplus of vaccine that the health ministry had asked Johnson & Johnson and Pfizer to stop sending shipments. There were 17 million doses in stock and only 106,000 injections each day. The plan had been to ramp up to 300,000 a day, but the country had never gotten close.

By then, the term *vaccine apathy* was common. One poll showed that 72 percent of the population had no objections to vaccines; they just weren't eager for them.

Part of the hesitation was that their rollout had been a confusing mess. When vaccines were first approved in Europe and North America, South African political leaders—echoing those in many donor-reliant countries—expressed outrage because wealthy nations bought more doses than they needed while Covax, the UN-backed agency collecting doses for the Global South, was going begging.

In early 2021, the health ministry received a million doses of the AstraZeneca vaccine from India. Then it summarily rejected them because a small and unimportant study suggested they might not protect against the Beta variant then circulating. They were resold to the African Union for use elsewhere in Africa.

By that time, Aspen, Dr. Nicolaou's company, had signed a deal with Johnson & Johnson to import vaccine in bulk and put it in vials. Then it was discovered that J&J's Maryland plant was shipping contaminated batches. By August it was reported that the Aspen plant had been forced to destroy 30 million doses—enough for half of all South Africans.

That poisoned the waters. In May, Pfizer started shipping what was to be 30 million doses. But South Africa asked it to stop because no one was accepting them. The same thing happened in nearby Zimbabwe, Malawi, and Namibia, which get much of their news from South African outlets.

Ultimately, vaccine apathy spread throughout Africa. By late February 2022, the Africa Centres for Disease Control and Prevention asked all vaccine companies to stop sending doses, even though only about 14 percent of the continent had been vaccinated.

"Let's pause and avoid the risk of sending so much that it gets expired," Africa CDC's director, John Nkengasong, told *Politico*. "It's like buying a whole basket of food just to put it on your kitchen counter. If you cannot use any, it will rot. But if you do that in smaller pieces, then you still get to the end goal with the same amount of food on your kitchen table."

Admittedly, many African countries faced major logistical challenges. Rural areas lacked refrigerated warehouses. Blackouts were common. Some countries lacked syringes, alcohol pads, and trained vaccinators and had received a mishmash of donated vaccines, exacerbating the storage problems.

But by far the greatest limitation was that most people were just not afraid enough to care. There had been only about 250,000 recorded Covid deaths among 1.4 billion residents of sub-Saharan Africa, which was one-seventeenth the U.S. death rate. Malaria and AIDS each killed more than twice as many as Covid did. People who worried about putting food on the table each night faced bigger threats than Covid.

Fatalism is also sometimes a response from devout religionists who believe life and death are in divine hands. Many Christian Africans belong to Pentecostal congregations and march to Sunday services in tunics beneath medieval-looking banners. Among them, vaccine refusal was high. Their argument that it thwarted God's will was the same one used in Britain in the eighteenth century against smallpox vaccination.

I heard the same sentiment from devout Muslims when I covered polio campaigns. "My child's fate is in Allah's hands," one Pakistani man said as he turned a vaccine team away from his house. I remember an exchange early in the pandemic between a CNN reporter and a woman on her way into a Cincinnati church that was defying Ohio's ban on public gatherings, including religious services. Wasn't she, the reporter asked, nervous about getting infected? "I'm covered in Jesus' blood!" she answered. "They could get me sick, but I'm not—because I'm covered in Jesus' blood!"

Fatalism is "one of the greatest challenges in global health," Dr. William H. Foege, one of the leaders of the drive to eradicate smallpox, wrote in his 2011 memoir, *House on Fire.* (Before he was recruited by the smallpox campaign, Dr. Foege was a Lutheran missionary doctor in Nigeria; he later became director of the CDC.)

In India, he said, devout Hindus refused the vaccine because they feared angering the moody smallpox goddess Shitala Mata, who sent epidemics when she was enraged and comforted victims with cooling water when she was pleased. In Hindu art, Shitala Mata is portrayed astride a donkey with a pot of water and a broom to sweep epidemics in or out.

Nigeria's Yoruba tribe has an even more fearsome smallpox god,

Shapona, who has a sharp-pointed head and carries a monkey skull, said Dr. Donald R. Hopkins of the Carter Center in Atlanta, who fought smallpox and neglected tropical diseases for decades and also became director of the CDC. Through the slave trade, Shapona made his way into voodoo, Santeria, and other Caribbean religions, where he was known as Babalu. (When Desi Arnaz, Lucille Ball's Cuban bandleader husband Ricky on *I Love Lucy*, beats his conga and cries, "Babalooo-ayeh!" he is summoning the smallpox god.)

The starkest expressions of fatalism I remember arose during interviews I did in 2001 in bars in Hlabisa, a black township in the Zulu homeland north of Durban.

AIDS by then was killing thousands of South Africans every month. Antiretroviral drugs were unavailable under the Mbeki administration then in office, so every infection was effectively a death sentence. Yet most men refused to wear condoms. As part of a series looking at how AIDS affected one small township, I asked why. One bar I visited was just an empty garage with a pool table, with the owner selling beer and pint bottles of cheap Richelieu brandy.

"Because if you are a man, you are born to die," Albert Msimango, twenty-five, told me. "It is like Shaka said: 'We are Zulus. The men must go forward and get something.'"

What he meant was that a boy was not a man until he faced death. Shaka, the Napoleon of southern Africa, had created the Zulu empire in the nineteenth century by conquering and absorbing nearby tribes. His armies fought in regiments by age. (There is still a Zulu tradition that you are born into an *impi* or regiment of your peers and expected to attend ceremonies with them.) No regiment was allowed to marry or father children until its members had proven themselves in battle. The punishment for impregnating a woman could be severe, although young people were allowed to practice nonpenetrative "thigh sex."

Most of the bar's patrons agreed with Mr. Msimango. There was general cynicism about condoms; the government-issued ones were cheap and tore easily. Thanks to Mr. Mbeki, some were skeptical that AIDS even existed. Every man knew someone who had died of AIDS symptoms, but they chalked their deaths up to tuberculosis, pneumonia, or just "bad lungs" or "bad blood."

The KwaZulu-Natal province had been so violent for so long that fatalism was almost inevitable. More than 10,000 had died in the tribal and factional massacres in the run-up to the 1994 elections. The police and the apartheid government had pitted Zulu nationalists against Mr. Mandela's African National Congress, which was mostly Xhosa and other non-Zulu tribes. One bar patron was in a wheelchair because a bullet had severed his spine. Two others were police officers in an area where officers were often ambushed and killed for their guns. A slow death from AIDS seemed remote compared to the risks they took every day.

"We are not scared of death," one officer said. "I don't see the importance of AIDS."

Also, they added, some men—not them, but some—practiced a truly sinister form of fatalism. "Some men with AIDS say, 'I don't want to die alone,'" Khaya Manyanga, a hospital X-ray technician, said. "So they go out and spread it."

That echoed something Randy Shilts, a *San Francisco Chronicle* reporter covering the early days of AIDS, had reported years earlier in his book *And the Band Played On*. He claimed that Gaetan Dugas, a gay Canadian flight attendant, was "Patient Zero," who introduced the virus to America. (In 2016, genetic testing of stored blood samples disproved that theory. The virus had arrived in the United States years before Mr. Dugas did.)

Mr. Shilts portrayed Mr. Dugas as sexually insatiable—and a sadist. In the years before his death in 1984, he wrote, Mr. Dugas ignored his doctor's warning to stop infecting other men. He kept going to bathhouses and by his own estimate had about 250 partners a year.

"When the moaning stopped, the young man rolled over on his back for a cigarette," Mr. Shilts wrote of one encounter in the Club Baths in San Francisco. "Gaetan Dugas reached up for the lights, turning the rheostat slowly so his partner's eyes would have time to adjust. He then made a point of eyeing the purple lesions on his chest. 'Gay cancer,' he said, almost as if he were talking to himself. 'Maybe you'll get it too.'"

Chapter Twelve

THE FAILURES TO UNDERSTAND CULTURE

Diseases spread when culture is misunderstood. Western scientists have been working for nearly forty years to find a way to protect African women against HIV and have not yet succeeded (although they are getting closer).

African women are at extraordinarily high risk. More than 60 percent of the infections on the continent are among women. As a result, over 50 percent of people with HIV around the world are female—a fact that tends to astonish Americans used to thinking of AIDS as a disease of gay men. Girls in African high schools are infected six to ten times as often as their male classmates are. Why? Because they're not getting it from their classmates. They're being infected by older men—through rape, through incest, but mostly through "transactional sex." Vulnerable girls are constantly pressured to have sex with teachers in return for good grades, with minibus drivers in return for rides to school, with "sugar daddies" in return for clothes or money to buy food for their siblings.

Western scientists, aware of the situation, keep coming up with one innovation after another, only to see each fail in clinical trials.

Only one failed because it truly did not work—a vaccine. The latest failure was in August 2021 in the "Imbokodo" trial of a new Johnson &

Johnson vaccine. (*Imbokodo* is the Zulu word for the grooved stone used to grind grain into flour and is a reference to women's strength.)

That failure was frustrating but not a surprise: scientists have been trying for forty years to make an HIV vaccine. The chief obstacle is the speed at which the virus mutates. The measles vaccine invented in 1963 still works. Influenza viruses mutate so quickly that flu shots must be reformulated annually. But HIV mutates as much *in a single day* as flu viruses do in a year.

Other innovations for African women have been relatively simple, commonsense ways to block or neutralize the virus. The problem has never been the technology; all of them worked. Not just one—*all*. The problem is that women wouldn't or couldn't use them. They signed up for clinical trials. They took the new inventions home. They swore to the nurses doing trial interviews that they had used them. They even turned in evidence that they had.

But when researchers realized that they needed to confirm those interview statements—usually by taking blood samples or vaginal swabs—they found that most of the women had not used the interventions. They were flushing them down the toilet or throwing them in the trash. As a result, they were getting infected.

Why?

For cultural reasons. The power of culture cannot be ignored.

As soon as it became clear in the 1980s that AIDS was killing African women, cries to protect them arose. The first solution offered was the obvious one, one that had worked for fifty years for many American women who feared pregnancy or disease: condoms. That was controversial in itself—both in African culture and American culture.

The Christian conservatives in Congress who backed the creation of George W. Bush's President's Emergency Plan for AIDS Relief (PEPFAR) initially were unwilling to pay for condoms. They would spend $350 in taxpayer dollars to treat an infected woman for a year, but not $5 for enough condoms to protect her for that long. They instead insisted that

PEPFAR advocate only abstinence and marital fidelity. Liberals mocked them, saying conservatives refused to face reality.

As mentioned earlier, President Museveni of Uganda became the first African leader to endorse condoms. As a born-again Christian, he had allies among Mr. Bush's backers. His "ABC" approach was subtle: First, *a*bstain. Then, *b*e faithful. Then, if you must, "*c*ondomize." Mr. Bush, defying his conservative backers, ultimately endorsed ABC and let PEPFAR buy condoms.

Numerous problems soon arose, however. The cheapest condoms, sold in bulk for three cents each, came from China. But their foil packets often had butterflies, penguins, or other cute logos, which had zero appeal to men from other cultures. In Cuba, the solution was to have the makers repackage them for straight men with pictures of male hands clutching female breasts and for gay men with pairs of male buttocks side by side. American aid officials, however, were not about to risk the wrath of congressional conservatives that way. They paid for an ad campaign creating a new brand: "Goalkeepers." Prominent goalies on national soccer teams were paid to endorse Goalkeepers as the brand that "keeps the ball out of the net." In South Africa, British aid money paid to create a TV soap opera, *Soul City*, which featured African characters in roles as young professionals, rather than in the old apartheid-era stereotypes of maids, gardeners, and hustlers. It was the first to openly discuss AIDS. *Soul City*–brand condoms were marketed.

Then difficulties arose with the goods. Although condoms are easy to manufacture—rods of the right length and circumference are dipped repeatedly in liquid latex—they require careful quality control. Latex, the sap from rubber trees, is almost as fragile as milk. If it's the wrong consistency or temperature, the condoms will tear. Donors bought condoms where they were cheapest—China, South Korea, and Malaysia. But most African governments could not afford to send inspection teams to factories in Asia or do "burst tests" on random batches. The suppliers quickly realized that they could foist their iffiest batches off on African customers. The word spread that condoms broke and were not to be trusted.

They also didn't catch on for other reasons. The first was that, initially, they were just unfamiliar. In a 1990 article in the *Sowetan*, the newspaper of Johannesburg's vast black township, Soweto, a reporter asked women how they felt about condoms. Many were against them, even disgusted by the idea. Sex, they said, must be "flesh to flesh."

One, a teacher, said, "I want sperms not rubber. I would fire [my boyfriend] if he wanted to use the damn thing." Another said she had never met a man who suggested one, but if she did, "I will tell him not to come and waste my time. Just imagine the whole night with rubber in you." A third said "sperms have proteins and I need those proteins."

Another problem was that, even after condoms became familiar, they were seen as something used only by sex workers and the promiscuous. A woman who asked a man to wear one would not just face the usual male complaints about decreased feeling. He would accuse her of cheating or suspecting him of cheating, or even implying that he had HIV. "And he will hit you," Goodness Mbikozi, an HIV advocacy worker, told me. "Definitely, he will hit you."

A third problem was that science education was so lacking that girls knew little about their own anatomy. I was told several times that girls feared condoms because of rumors that, if they came off, they could "get lost inside," cause infections, or even "wander around" until they were coughed up, choking them.

Some aid agencies gave up on getting average women to accept condoms and focused on getting them to sex workers. That reinforced damaging stereotypes, but made sense from a public health standpoint: sex workers were an important vector. Early studies showed that HIV cases followed highways and sprang up first in towns with big truck stops. Truck stops inevitably had bars, pool halls, restaurants, and sleeping rooms for truckers, and truckers had cash, so working women frequented them. (In some countries, including Thailand and Cambodia, condom distribution backfired because the police treated possession of a condom as evidence that any woman they detained was a prostitute.)

When I interviewed African sex workers, however, they told me that, even when condoms were plentiful, it was hard to get customers to use them. When she started working at truck stops in 1988, a woman named Thandi told me only 2 out of 10 customers would agree to wear one. By the time we spoke in 2001, black South Africans were dying in droves—and yet only about 7 of 10 men would wear them, she estimated. They would pay up to twice as much for sex without one. If a man had several women to choose from, he would haggle, asking who would do it without one.

"If we have made enough money, we try to tell him that he must wear one," Thandi said, adding that she made about $65 in a good week. "But if we do not, we try to ask him."

And if he still says no? I asked.

"I will think twice, and then I will do something with him."

Nosipho, who sold sex for about $6 per customer at a taxi stand, said she got free condoms from a nearby clinic. If a man tried to use one of his own, she would insist he open the foil cover in front of her—because some men would jab or bite holes into them.

Why in the world, I asked, would they do that, since they clearly knew the risk? She shrugged. "They want to use their own body." To them, sex with an intact condom was not real sex.

In 1999, donors tried introducing the female condom. In theory, it was an ideal solution. Women didn't have to reveal it; they could just quietly insert it. It was made of polyurethane, which was tougher than latex. Dual rings held it in place.

But it had serious drawbacks. First, at 62 cents each, female condoms were twenty times as costly as male ones. On the other hand, they could be washed and reused a few times, which cut the price per use. Also, they were not nearly as invisible or undetectable as advertised; the opening hung outside the labia.

In Cape Town, I went out with Glynis Rhodes, an educator from SWEAT, the Sex Workers Education & Advocacy Taskforce, as she introduced female condoms to the young women working on Somerset Road, where the price was $25 for sex with a condom and up to $50 without. Most were teenagers who appeared high as they stood in gaggles waving at passing cars. They had never heard of female condoms and were skeptical. Or they just giggled when Ms. Rhodes opened them and pantomimed how to use them.

One thirty-nine-year-old woman named Fazilin, however, was an advocate. She came from a conservative Muslim family but worked on Somerset because she had six children and a jobless husband to support. (She told her family she worked in an all-night restaurant, she said.) Fazilin had common sense and charm. The younger women clearly looked up to her. "I've tried it with about fifteen okes," she said, using South African slang for "blokes." "It's quite great."

However, it worked best if men were drunk or high. "When they aren't, they can see it, they can feel it, they can smell it," she said. When a drunk customer insisted on not using a condom, though, she would excuse herself and slip briefly into a bathroom. "They never know," she said, "and they think they got flesh-to-flesh, so I charge them double."

Unfortunately, thanks to programs like SWEAT's, the female condom became firmly associated with sex work and never caught on.

In 2007, the WHO endorsed male circumcision as a weapon against HIV. Three clinical trials in Kenya, Uganda, and South Africa had found that circumcision reduced the risk of male infection through heterosexual sex by about 60 percent. Scientists were not sure why, but foreskins suffer small tears during intercourse and they also contain many Langerhans cells, immune-system sentinels that attach to viruses.

It took a while for circumcision to catch on in Africa—except among Muslims, of course, and in tribes like the Xhosa in South Africa and Kikuyu in Kenya where boys are circumcised as part of manhood rituals. Nonetheless, as rumors slowly grew that women preferred circumcised men and that sexual sensation was greater, men began volunteering for the operation. Between 2015 and 2022, PEPFAR paid for about 8 million circumcisions. Even that number, however, was too small to seriously dent the epidemic.

In 2010, a huge breakthrough was made in preventing HIV in gay men.

The worldwide iPrEx study found that taking a daily antiretroviral pill called Truvada cut HIV risk by 99 percent. If taken without fail, it was a nearly perfect substitute for a vaccine. Partners in PrEP, a 2012 trial, found similar results. It was the best prevention news in decades. Studies began immediately to see if it would protect African women too. Truvada's main ingredient was an antiviral, tenofovir. To see if women could use the drug locally rather than swallowing a pill that dosed their whole body, a tenofovir-containing vaginal gel was created. It came with a thin, discreet applicator. Other scientists created a silicone ring impregnated with slow-release dapivirine, a similar antiretroviral, that could be inserted and left under the cervix for a month.

Great efforts went into ensuring that the new technologies killed HIV but not sperm, since many women still wanted to be mothers.

One by one, each of these clever innovations failed.

Clinical trials conducted at multiple African study sites enrolled as many as 5,000 volunteers. In initial interviews, many hesitated because the products were unfamiliar, but then became enthusiastic. In some trials, women kept 95 percent of their clinic appointments—far more than the 2,500 men in the iPrEx study had. In interviews, they swore they were following all protocols.

The final results, however, were a bitter failure. The women who supposedly had used the methods were infected with HIV at roughly the same rate as women given placebos. But it was not because the methods failed. It was because most of the women hadn't used them.

The researchers were shocked when they realized how far participants had gone to deceive them. About 90 percent told nurses they were taking their pills or using the gels. They turned in empty applicators and pill bottles. Counts suggested that 86 percent were complying.

But when stored blood samples taken during the trial were analyzed, it became clear that most had not told the truth. Only about 30 percent of participants had *any* detectable tenofovir in their blood.

Dr. Ariane van der Straten led follow-up interviews with hundreds of women. Many admitted throwing out their pills or squirting the gel down the toilet. One gave hers to a friend who was a sex worker. Another hid hers to take later if they turned out to work, but her sister-in-law threw them out.

"No one expected they would go to such contortions to appear being adherent when they were not," Dr. van der Straten said.

When asked why, most women said they were afraid their husbands or boyfriends would find the preventive pills or gel and accuse them of having HIV. Some feared gossipy neighbors would say they were infected—or needed protection because they slept around.

Also, the waiting rooms had been abuzz with rumors. Some were that the drugs would "rot the uterus" or cause liver cancer or infertility. Some claimed the doctors were injecting them with HIV or taking blood samples to use in witchcraft. Young single women, petrified by such tales, were the least likely to be adherent, Dr. van der Straten said.

When asked why they had stayed in the trial, women gave several reasons: They were paid $10 to $15 per visit, nominally for travel expenses. That was a lot of cash when most earned only a few dollars a day. They got regular checkups, monthly gynecological exams, and free contraception. Some brought their children along and the doctors, wanting to keep their subjects happy, treated them, too. Also, the study clinics were clean, the staff were polite, the doctors were kind, and the pharmacy never ran out of drugs. All of that was a far cry from conditions in the public hospitals the women normally had to use. In addition, the younger women were afraid the trial nurses would yell at them if they knew they were cheating. They had no idea what the blood tests could reveal.

Similar patterns were found in 2016, in the trials of cervical rings. Older women who got rings containing dapivirine had one-third fewer infections than those using placebo rings. But once again, the youngest and most vulnerable women—those aged eighteen to twenty-one—got almost no protection. They were afraid of being caught with the rings, so they unwrapped them, hid them, and brought them back unused.

The failures changed the way such trials were run. Payments were recalibrated to reimburse expenses rather than induce women to join. Blood tests became more frequent. Women got encouraging pep talks.

To increase support from male partners, the trials sponsored movie nights and soccer matches with free food. Men got pamphlets explaining the technology and how it could protect them and their children too.

For the few women who used the interventions correctly, they worked fairly well. For example, tenofovir gel, used daily, reduced HIV risk by 66 percent. It also prevented genital herpes, which is caused by an unrelated virus that tenofovir can kill.

But stigma—the inevitable cultural flaw—overwhelmed the medical triumph. The WHO endorsed the dapivirine ring for women at high risk and for "key population groups." "Key population groups" is WHO-speak for women who sell sex or use drugs. In press releases, it avoids even defining the term for fear of associating it with sex work.

After earlier trials failed, investigators tried oral PrEP. For women who actually took it daily, it worked quite well, reducing risk nearly to zero. But as of late 2021, only about 300,000 South Africans were using it—a drop in the bucket compared to how many were at risk.

"In the communities, people don't understand that antiretroviral drugs are also used for HIV prevention," explained Sibongile Tshabalala, national chair of the country's Treatment Action Campaign. "If you are a woman living with a man or have multiple partners, it can be difficult to take daily PrEP because of stigma."

By late 2021, scientists and activists were in sharp disagreement about PrEP in Africa. The former considered it a failure because so many women couldn't or wouldn't take it. But activists like those at the Treatment Action Campaign were still enthusiastic. Even if women used it imperfectly, they argued, it was still protective during crucial life moments. For example, young women cycled on and off PrEP depending on whether or not they trusted their current sexual partners.

The cultural battles that PrEP had triggered in the United States were repeated in Africa. When PrEP was first introduced here, there was an almost puritanical backlash by a few vocal gay leaders who still preferred condoms or "sero-sorting" (having sex only with partners of the same HIV status). They dismissed Truvada as a "party drug" and stigmatized early adopters as "Truvada whores." Some doctors even refused to prescribe it for their patients because it protected only against HIV, not against syphilis or gonorrhea; they kept advising condoms.

Then there was a backlash against the backlash. After the CDC endorsed PrEP in 2014, Adam Zeboski, a twenty-six-year-old counselor for the San Francisco AIDS Foundation, designed a "Truvada whore" T-shirt. "People are either very supportive or very offended," he told me. "By reclaiming the 'Truvada whore' term, we're taking the power away from those who use it against us."

Something similar had happened long ago, in 1960. A drug named Enovid, which the FDA had previously approved for infertility, was re-registered for a very different use: birth control. It was soon known simply as "The Pill," and eventually triggered the sexual revolution. Before that happened, however, there were ugly fights. Doctors and pharmacists resisted giving it to unmarried women, saying it would encourage premarital sex. Churchmen railed against it. Many young women would not use it because it was tantamount to admitting they were easy. Slowly, the tide turned. Pioneering feminists like Margaret Sanger and her wealthy backer Katharine D. McCormick stood up to the vilification. Madison Avenue created ads featuring Andromeda, the princess of Greek mythology, nude and breaking free of her chains.

Some of the moralists' dire predictions did come true: premarital sex increased; so did gonorrhea. Rare but dangerous side effects, including blood clots, emerged. But there was no stopping it—the revolution arrived anyway.

As of this writing, the big hope for women in Africa is "long-acting injectables." Studies showed that injections of cabotegravir every two months are almost 90 percent more effective than oral PrEP because compliance is far better.

The fact that women prefer the shot did not surprise researchers with long experience in Africa. Depo-Provera, a form of birth control delivered as a shot once every three months, is unpopular among American and European women because of its side effects: irregular periods, headaches, depression, acne, weight gain, extra facial and body hair or hair loss, and osteoporosis. But in Africa, Depo is very popular. Its big advantage is privacy. Women whose husbands or lovers may be furious that they don't want more children can visit a clinic and get it with no one the wiser. If current studies on some newer antiretroviral drugs like lenacapavir and islatravir work out, there may one day be a six-month shot or an implant good for a full year.

In early 2022, my successor on the *Times* global health beat, Stephanie Nolen, reported wonderful news: AIDS wards in Africa were finally emptying out. Infection rates among women were dropping rapidly.

It was not, however, because women were, at last, personally protected. It was because so many infected men were finally on antiretroviral drugs. Even if the men were merely saving their own skins, suppressing their virus to undetectable levels protected their partners, too. They could not pass it on.

That principle, known as "Treatment as Prevention," had been proven effective as far back as 2006 in studies in Canada. But poor countries could not adopt it because buying the drugs and getting them to everyone who was infected cost so much—more than they could afford and more than donors were willing to pay. Even now, many African countries cannot afford to find, test, and treat everyone infected. By mid-2022, only 29 million of an estimated 38 million people in the world with HIV—about two-thirds of whom are in sub-Saharan Africa—were on treatment. About 1.5 million are still newly infected each year.

That's enormous progress since I started covering the disease in the 1990s, when only a few hundred wealthy or politically connected Africans had a prayer of survival. But there's still a long way to go—and women in Africa won't be safe until they can protect themselves at will.

Chapter Thirteen

THE CANCER OF RUMORS

In the fall of 2015, the nightmare broke out almost simultaneously in numerous maternity hospitals in northeastern Brazil. Obstetricians who normally saw one or two children with microcephaly in their intensive care units each year were suddenly seeing a dozen or more. Desperate mothers were asking what was wrong with their babies.

Looking at the newborns was disorienting. From the eyebrows down, their faces looked normal and placid. But above, what was usually a bulbous forehead protecting the growing brain was missing. They resembled the troll dolls of the 1960s: above and behind their eyebrows was a depression filled with hair. Scans showed very little behind the babies' sloping foreheads. Some had a rind of gray matter with large fluid-filled gaps. Some had midbrains, but their frontal lobes had never grown. The most severely affected had just the nubs of brain stems.

Many who survived birth died soon after, killed by seizures that cut off their breathing or by slow starvation from being unable to swallow. Some had enough intact brain matter to be able to follow a light or react to sound—but doctors knew they would never walk or talk, never recognize their mothers, never smile for pleasure, never retain a memory.

Soon it was soon clear that, whatever had struck the babies of Recife, Fortaleza, Salvador, and other northeast Brazil cities was spreading outward to next-door countries and to islands in the Caribbean.

From the first, Brazilian doctors suspected that the most likely culprit was the obvious one: about nine months earlier, northeastern Brazil had suffered a major outbreak of a virus never before seen in the Western Hemisphere: a mosquito-borne African virus named for the Zika Forest in Uganda, where it had been discovered in 1947.

However, although Zika virus had long been known, it had hardly been studied. No one had ever previously suggested it could hurt fetuses. Other viruses definitely do; the brain damage suffered by the Brazilian babies resembled that done by rubella (German measles) before vaccines were developed, but was even more severe.

Zika virus had left Africa and turned up in Asia at least as early as the 1960s, but between 1947 and 2007, only 14 cases were diagnosed. Molecular testing for it did not exist, and the mild rash and bloodshot eyes that were its most common symptoms went unrecorded because almost all other mosquito-borne diseases were more serious. If it caused microcephaly in Asia, it went unnoticed. Fetal brain damage has many causes, including rubella, cytomegalovirus, toxoplasmosis, maternal alcoholism, drugs, and industrial toxins. Those ills were more likely to strike the poor, and poor women in Asia often gave birth at home. Babies with serious deformities might simply have been hidden away and never officially counted.

At some point, the Asian strain began island-hopping across the Pacific. A 2007 outbreak on Yap Island in Micronesia was investigated by a CDC team: it washed rapidly through the population, infecting about 70 percent of all islanders in a few months, and then disappeared. It caused rashes, fevers, headaches, and the bloodshot red eyes of conjunctivitis but no long-lasting effects, the CDC said. In 2013, it hit French Polynesia, where scientists from France's Pasteur Institute found that a few adults had developed Guillain-Barré syndrome, a usually temporary form of paralysis. They noticed no effects on fetuses or babies.

The next big outbreak was in northeast Brazil in early 2015. (It was initially assumed that it had reached Brazil either during the June–July 2014 soccer World Cup or during an international canoe race in Rio a month later in which several teams from South Pacific nations had participated. Later, however, researchers decided the virus was probably introduced by a single player, staff member, or traveling fan of a soccer team from the island of Tahiti, part of French Polynesia, which had played a match in Recife in June 2013 during the FIFA Confederations Cup, a prelude to the World Cup. The virus probably circulated silently until early 2015 and then surged during a hot wet spell hospitable to mosquitoes.)

As soon as news about the microcephalic babies emerged from Brazil, wild rumors began springing up, rumors that it was *not* Zika virus that had caused the microcephaly—it was something else.

There were so many that my *Times* science colleagues and I finally compiled a long list of them, with the evidence showing why each was wrong. (Other diseases had spawned rumors, but never so many that we had to catalog them.)

What surprised me was that I wasn't hearing just from the usual tin-foil-hat-wearers. Bizarre claims were sent to me by intelligent people I knew. One was a respected Yale expert in mosquito-borne diseases. One was a retired *Times* reporter, a Harvard graduate. Another came from a group of doctors working in rural Brazil.

The tone of some letters was condescending. They weren't so much raising questions as scolding me for "falling for the conventional wisdom." Others sneered that, as a *New York Times* reporter, I should publicize the "real cause."

In retrospect, it felt like a watershed moment. It was the first time I remember that so many readers seemed to assume that carefully thought-out statements from scientists were just lies. The Zika outbreak seemed to normalize the proliferation of conspiracy theories about disease.

Among the rumored "real causes" of the microcephaly were:

- The weed killer Roundup sprayed on crops.
- Pyriproxyfen, a larvicide sprayed into drinking water tanks in the Brazilian favelas to kill mosquito larvae.
- Genetically modified mosquitoes that had recently been released in Brazil in an experimental attempt to control dengue virus.
- A new whooping cough vaccine.
- A bad or expired batch of rubella vaccine.

Another rumor, one that had surprising staying power, was that there was actually no epidemic of microcephaly at all, that Brazil was simply inept at keeping accurate statistics.

Brazil typically reported about 150 cases of microcephaly a year; it was suddenly reporting about 2,700. The rumor's proponents claimed that it was just the first time Brazil had noticed the problem and done a careful count. A variant of that rumor was that the government had changed by one centimeter its definition of how small a head constituted "microcephaly" so that thousands of babies with normal but small heads were now being wrongly labeled microcephalic.

From a distance, it's easy to see the various agendas at work: anti-vaccine activists blamed vaccines, anti-GMO groups blamed genetically modified mosquitoes, environmentalists blamed pesticides, people who disdained Brazil assumed incompetence. The rumors all sounded "science-y," so they fooled people with little science education.

There was never any truth to any of them.

Roundup had been sprayed on crops all over the globe for decades.

There was some evidence that long-term exposure might cause cancer in agriculture workers, but not fetal damage. In any case, many of the affected Brazilian mothers were city dwellers with no contact with Roundup.

Pyriproxyfen had been long used in Brazil to kill mosquito larvae in neighborhood water tanks and in household rainwater barrels. But it targets an enzyme found only in insects, not in vertebrates. It is used in many countries, and the WHO rates it as safe for drinking water when used at correct doses. In the United States, it is sold as a flea treatment for pets and as a flea-killing carpet spray. Babies have crawled in it for years.

The transgenic mosquitoes had been released more than 1,000 miles away from the affected northeastern cities. Mosquitoes travel less than half a mile in their lifetimes. Similarly modified mosquitoes had been released in Australia and Indonesia with no ill effects. Also, all the released mosquitoes were males, which can't bite people because they lack the needle-sharp proboscises that females need for blood meals. Males spend their brief lives sipping flower nectar.

The whooping cough vaccine used in Brazil had been in use around the world for years, and was used all over Brazil, not just in the northeast. No bad or expired batch of rubella vaccine was found, and the mothers had not had rubella, which is easy to diagnose.

On the question of the miscount: the Brazilian government had indeed changed its definition of microcephaly by one centimeter during the outbreak. But it had *tightened* it, not loosened it, so that only babies with heads less than 32 centimeters around, rather than 33, were considered microcephalic. Nonetheless, the numbers of microcephalic babies were still through the roof.

More to the point, multiple reporters had interviewed numerous Brazilian hospital pediatricians—well-educated, highly trained doctors in charge of neonatal intensive care units in several cities. They all said the same thing: "In my whole career, I've never seen so many babies with microcephaly." News photographers found waiting rooms crammed with young mothers in shock, cradling babes with tiny heads and blank faces.

Yet many Americans either refused to believe it was happening or insisted there was some nonviral cause.

Ultimately, months of work did prove the virus was to blame. Epidemiological studies showed that many mothers had had Zika symptoms early in pregnancy and that increases in microcephaly and Guillain-Barré followed Zika outbreaks. Autopsies on miscarried and aborted fetuses found the virus in their brains. Studies in which pregnant mice or monkeys were deliberately infected with Zika showed the virus crossing their placentas and attacking the radial glia cells, which form the scaffolding of the developing brain.

And, of course, nine months after the Zika outbreak ended, the flood of damaged babies suddenly stopped. The weed killers, larvicides, transgenic mosquitoes, vaccines, and other "real causes" were still in use, but microcephaly ebbed anyway.

(The threat then faded. After 2017, very low-level circulation of the virus persisted in Africa, Asia, and the Americas, but there were no more explosive outbreaks. Travel warnings to pregnant women were slowly canceled. Researchers assume that the virus had infected most inhabitants of the tropical latitudes it reached in 2015–16, leaving them with long-lasting immunity. If most female babies born in those regions now get it and recover from it in infancy or childhood, before they reach their childbearing years, there will—with luck—never again be an epidemic of Zika microcephaly. An unlucky pregnant tourist might get it, but there is so little circulation that the chances of that are now extremely low.)

Does any of this sound familiar?

Every pandemic is beset with rumors. Over the course of my career, however, the rumor mills just seemed to get more frantic, more insistent with each new outbreak. The amount of time spent debunking them grew. The disdain for science, the accusations that medical scientists were not humanitarians but elitists conspiring to enrich themselves, just seemed to grow.

In her book *Stuck: How Vaccine Rumors Start—and Why They Don't Go Away*, Heidi J. Larson, director of the Vaccine Confidence Project at the London School of Hygiene & Tropical Medicine, traces the roots of many anti-vaccine rumors and why they appear again and again.

The storm of rumors surrounding Covid was by far the most intense I ever covered—for an obvious reason: many of them were spread by the president of the United States and by cable news hosts with millions of viewers.

They began almost as soon as the virus in Wuhan was discovered. Interestingly, this time there was never any real doubt that the virus caused the illness. But every other aspect of the disease was called into question.

Early on, I got emails insisting that Covid was no worse than seasonal flu, and the low death rate on the *Diamond Princess* proved that. There were rumors that it didn't infect black people, because Africa had few cases, so melanin must be protective. Rumors that it was a Chinese bioweapon or the result of Chinese scientists selling dead lab animals in wildlife markets. Rumors that it contained snake genes or HIV genes. Rumors that China was faking its numbers, that it actually had 3 million cases in January, not 80,000.

When it reached our shores and Americans started dying, rumors spread that it could be cured by the malaria drug hydroxychloroquine or the deworming drug ivermectin or the antibiotic azithromycin or the plant pigment quercitin or vitamin D or zinc or some combination of the above. Veterinary stores sold out of ivermectin-containing horse paste. Poison control centers were overwhelmed with calls from people taking it. Doctors were threatened with violence by the families of hospitalized patients for refusing to prescribe it.

The rumors that greeted vaccines were even more absurd. That they had never been tested. That they reduced fertility or swelled testicles. That they were secretly infused into Covid test nasal swabs, so merely taking a test would inoculate you. That they magnetized you.

Rumors like those scared nearly a third of the American population away from vaccines, with fatal consequences. By as early as May 2021, 99 percent of all Covid deaths were among the unvaccinated, according to a data analysis by the Associated Press.

(That extreme disparity between deaths among vaccinated versus unvaccinated people eventually narrowed. By early 2023, the unvaccinated were only four times as likely to die of Covid as the vaccinated. By then, however, most deaths were of patients who were elderly and had life-threatening comorbidities like cancer or heart disease. Also, by then most of the unvaccinated had endured one or more previous bouts of Covid, which left them roughly as immunologically protected as the vaccinated. Also, evidence emerged that vaccine protection waned with time.)

It was all horrifying—but, sadly, par for the course.

In rumors about epidemics, some elements always seem to turn up. One reliable chestnut is the "evil billionaire" trope. For Covid, it was Bill Gates and George Soros. Gates was accused of hiding microchips in vaccines so his company, Microsoft, could track everyone in America. Soros was accused of triggering the pandemic to benefit pharmaceutical companies his hedge fund owns shares in.

In an earlier era, the "evil billionaire" was John D. Rockefeller, founder of Standard Oil and the world's richest man.

In the early twentieth century, Dr. Charles Wardell Stiles, a parasitologist at the U.S. Department of Agriculture, discovered that millions of Americans in the Deep South were infested with hookworms, which attached to their intestines to suck their blood, leaving them dull-witted and anemic. He named the worm *Necator americanus*, the "American killer." Magazines called his discovery the "germ of laziness" and attributed to it everything from the economic backwardness of the South to the Confederacy's defeat. (The worm enters through the feet, and up to a third of the Confederate Army went shoeless at times. A persistent legend about the Battle of Gettysburg is that it was triggered when a southern foraging party raided the Pennsylvania town because of rumors that it had a warehouse full of boots.)

Dr. Stiles appealed for help to Rockefeller, who created a Sanitary Commission with a $1 million budget. With its backing, Dr. Stiles urged southerners to adopt major behavior changes: Take regular doses of thymol, a worm-killing thyme extract. Build outhouses instead of defecating outdoors. And wear shoes all day, every day. Unfortunately, he hailed from a family of haughty New England Methodist ministers, and many southerners were offended by the tone of his advice. The rumor grew that he was helping Rockefeller only because the oil magnate had secretly bought up shoe companies.

Also routine are rumors that any given outbreak began with a lab leak. A 2022 article speculated that the West Africa Ebola outbreak that killed more than 11,000 people began in a Tulane University lab studying hemorrhagic fevers in Kenema, Sierra Leone, rather than from bats in a village in Guinea ninety miles away. In 2009, the WHO debunked a briefly widespread rumor that the swine flu then circulating had been manipulated in a lab; the rumor was started by a retired Australian virologist who believed—incorrectly, the agency said—that the virus had a mutation triggered by being grown in eggs. In 2011, a paper from the University of Leeds speculated that the lethal 1916 New York City polio epidemic was started by a leak from a Rockefeller Institute lab that was trying to make a more virulent polio strain in order to better infect the monkeys used in vaccine research.

Another evergreen trope is that the vaccine is a genocidal conspiracy by a rival ethnic or religious group. Such a rumor almost destroyed decades of efforts to eradicate polio.

In 1988, the businessmen's service club Rotary International declared that its "gift from the 20th century to the 21st" would be the eradication of polio by the year 2000. The World Health Assembly, an annual convocation of the world's health ministers in Geneva, endorsed the grand gesture.

It seemed doable, and probably for less than $500 million. The oral Sabin vaccine drops could be given by anyone with a few minutes training. It took several doses to fully immunize a child, but that could be accomplished with repeated rounds of immunization. The vaccine, which was not patented, cost pennies to make and there was no such thing as an overdose.

Rotary members around the world raised hundreds of millions of dollars, recruited and trained millions of volunteer vaccinators, and lobbied health ministers to make polio eradication a priority.

In 1999, the campaign was short of its goal but got a late boost when the Bill & Melinda Gates Foundation donated $50 million and Ted Turner's United Nations Foundation kicked in $28 million more. By 2000, it had achieved stunning success. Two billion children had been reached, and cases of polio paralysis had plummeted by more than 99 percent. In early 2001, there were fewer than 500 in the whole world. Victory was in sight.

Then, almost imperceptibly, the effort began crumbling. Logistical problems mounted, as did expenses. Fatigue with repeated immunization rounds set in. Mothers complained that the authorities seemed to care only about polio while their children were dying of measles, cholera, and other ills. In some places, mothers assumed the heavily promoted vaccine would protect their children against everything, including malaria and vomiting. When it did not, they felt betrayed. Some governments lost interest.

In September 2001, after Islamic terrorists crashed jetliners into the World Trade Center and the Pentagon, the drive's problems multiplied a hundredfold.

The United States invaded Afghanistan and then Iraq. A mere decade after the Cold War between capitalism and communism had ended, a new enmity was forged: the West and Islam were pitted against each other as bitterly as they had been centuries before in the Crusades.

By then, most regions where polio still circulated were Muslim. The vaccines suddenly became suspect. By 2003, as described by Dr. Larson in *Stuck* and by other journalists and scholars, rumors originating in northern Nigeria led to a catastrophic setback.

Nigeria is divided; the north, converted to Islam in the fourteenth century by Arabic-speaking raiders, is dominated by Hausa-speaking Muslims.

The south, colonized by Britain, is dominated by Christian Yoruba and Ibo. In 2002, an ugly presidential election was won by a Yoruba-speaking born-again Christian, Olusegun Obasanjo. He soon declared sharia law unconstitutional.

Nigeria's polio campaign became a pawn in the struggle; lucrative jobs in it went to southerners with political connections, infuriating northerners. Dr. Datti Ahmed, a northern physician who was president of the Supreme Council for Sharia in Nigeria, threatened civil war. The terrorist group Boko Haram, whose name means "Western influence is forbidden," was founded in the north that year.

In 2003, Dr. Ahmed claimed in newspaper and radio interviews that "modern-day Hitlers have deliberately adulterated the oral polio vaccines with anti-fertility drugs . . . and viruses which are known to cause HIV and AIDS."

The vaccines, he said, were "corrupted and tainted by evildoers from America."

He also recalled that in 1996, the drug company Pfizer had conducted a clinical trial in the northern city of Kano of a new antibiotic named Trovan. Pfizer was testing it against the lethal bacterial meningitis that struck Africa's "meningitis belt" every year during the hot, dry months. At least one child in the trial had died—not unexpectedly, since many died in each year's outbreak. But some local medical experts claimed Pfizer had lacked ethical-board approval for its trial and had not obtained clear consent from the children's families. That had morphed into a rumor that Pfizer was using Nigerian children as guinea pigs.

Dr. Ahmed's rumors spread widely and vaccine refusal became common. Eventually, the governors of three northern states with majority-Muslim populations halted all polio vaccinations while they convened a panel of experts to investigate the rumors. That process ended up taking almost a year.

(Some rural West Africans also have a pre-Christian, pre-Muslim belief about paralytic diseases like polio: that they are caused by a female spirit,

Shan-inna, who consumes victims' limbs. Because traditional healers are paid to either expel Shan-inna or mollify her with gifts, some of them were also hostile to the vaccine, which threatened their livelihoods.)

As is often the case, the rumors had kernels of truth, which then became wildly distorted in the retelling.

The source of the AIDS-related rumor was easy to spot. It sprang from the controversial 1999 book *The River* by the science journalist Edward Hooper. Mr. Hooper's central thesis was that the source of human AIDS was an experimental polio vaccine created by Hilary Koprowski, director of the Wistar Institute in Philadelphia. That vaccine, later improved upon by Albert Sabin, was tested on more than a million children in the Belgian Congo between 1957 and 1960.

At the time, it was assumed that AIDS had originated somewhere in the Congo during the same time period. The earliest known viral sample had come from an autopsy tissue slice stored in Kinshasa, the former Leopoldville, since 1960.

Mr. Hooper's thesis depended on his belief that the Philadelphia vaccine virus had been expanded by brewing doses in another Congolese city, Stanleyville, in vats containing a broth of chimpanzee cells. Those cells, he argued, could have been infected with the chimp immunodeficiency virus that is the precursor to HIV. After his book was published, however, numerous studies debunked his thesis. Tests on stored vaccine stocks showed that they had not been grown in chimpanzee cells and did not contain HIV or its simian equivalent. Molecular clock dating showed that HIV began infecting humans in the 1920s, decades before Dr. Koprowski invented his vaccine. Genetic testing showed that the viral strain in chimpanzees in the Stanleyville region was not the one that had become the human strain.

Neither Mr. Hooper nor anyone else had suggested that the vaccine in use in 2003—a modified version of the Sabin oral vaccine—contained HIV or any other dangerous virus. But Dr. Ahmed and alarmist journalists conflated the two ideas.

The antifertility rumor had multiple roots. In Africa, rumors that vaccines cause sterility went back at least to the 1950s, when vaccination campaigns by colonial authorities were suspected of being plots to lower African birth rates. (The same rumor had attached itself to colonial school milk handouts, vitamins, and malaria medicines.) Such rumors outlasted colonialism. In Cameroon in 1990, for example, the government offered tetanus vaccine to girls and young women, but not to males. Medically, that made sense: many newborns die of neonatal tetanus, and antibodies from the mother are protective. But because Cameroon had previously offered vaccines to both sexes, rumors arose that it was a government plot to sterilize women.

Next-door Nigeria was ripe for such rumors. In the 1980s, President Ibrahim Babangida had tried and failed to slow down the country's explosive birth rate by limiting each woman to four children, and the rumor arose that the government was surreptitiously adding birth control drugs to children's vaccines. In 2003, that rumor naturally attached itself to the government-backed polio vaccine.

A polio worker told me about being shouted at as she oversaw the delivery of vaccine from the UN Children's Fund. "Look!" a man in the crowd had yelled, pointing at a box. "It even says 'Sterile.' Do you think we're stupid?"

Making matters worse, scientists at a Nigerian university claimed to have found estrogen—the main ingredient in birth control pills—in the vaccine.

I asked a vaccine expert if that was possible.

"Well, it's grown in a broth of fetal calf serum," he answered. "And calf blood contains some hormones. So, yes, in theory, if you used a sensitive enough test, you might find some estrogen. But it would be at far smaller amounts than you find in breast milk, for example. And we know that breast milk doesn't make babies sterile."

Other scientists theorized that the water used in the testing might have been contaminated with trace amounts of estrogen, since the hormone is in urine, and sewer lines and drinking water lines sometimes leak into each other in crowded slums. But, again, it would have been in amounts far too low to affect fertility.

The expert panel went overseas to inspect vaccine factories. Ultimately, they recommended restarting vaccination but sourcing all of Nigeria's vaccine from a plant in Indonesia because it was also a Muslim country.

But by the time the governors rescinded their stop-vaccination orders, the virus had been spreading in Nigeria for nearly a year and, as I described in Chapter 10, eventually reached Mecca. By 2005, eighteen formerly polio-free countries had suffered new outbreaks, and genetic sequencing confirmed that all were of the Nigerian strain.

The rumors about the vaccine spread to Pakistan and Afghanistan, two other conservative Muslim countries that had never ended polio transmission. There, another ugly twist was added.

In poor countries, maps with household addresses often simply do not exist. Millions of villagers live in mud-walled compounds. Millions of urban slum-dwellers have only tents or shacks. Millions more are migrant laborers perpetually on the move. Without addresses to record, vaccination teams used crude methods to keep track of which families they had visited. They marked children's fingernails with silver nitrate or permanent ink that took a few days to wash off. On the outside wall of every compound or house they visited, they scrawled in chalk how many children they believed were inside and how many they had vaccinated. They also had a symbol for "household that refuses."

It was done to tell follow-up teams which houses to visit. But on the Pakistan-Afghanistan border, where American drones were killing Taliban leaders, the rumor spread that the teams were marking the houses for drone strikes.

Then, in 2011, the CIA made everything far worse. In its hunt for Osama bin Laden, it zeroed in on a compound in Abbottabad, near Pakistan's national military academy, where he was rumored to be living with his wives, children, and grandchildren.

To confirm that the family was inside, the agency hired a local physician, Dr. Shakil Afridi, to run a fake vaccination campaign. He recruited nurses to visit nearby houses claiming to be from the government and offering shots against hepatitis B. The plan was to eventually enter the suspect compound, inject vaccine into the children, and aspirate back a few drops of blood to test for bin Laden DNA. The CIA already had some closely linked DNA because bin Laden was one of fifty-two children of his Saudi father's multiple wives. Some of his siblings were cooperating with Saudi authorities and one sister had been hospitalized in Boston.

The effort failed because bin Laden's wives shooed away the vaccinators. (The scene is portrayed in the movie *Zero Dark Thirty*.) The CIA eventually found other ways to confirm bin Laden was inside, and on May 2, 2011, Navy SEALs landed in the compound and killed him.

The hepatitis B vaccination campaign was unveiled two months later during Pakistan's investigation of the raid. It became a huge setback for polio eradication. After the campaign had spent years trying to convince Muslims that vaccines were *not* a Western plot, the CIA had used a vaccine as part of an assassination plot.

Doctors Without Borders, other aid groups, and the deans of public health schools wrote open letters of protest saying the tactic endangered the lives of humanitarian workers. The CIA's response was indifference. When I wrote about it, a CIA spokesman called me to take issue only with my calling it a "fake" vaccination campaign. It had, he said, used real hepatitis B vaccine, so it was a "real" campaign.

The backlash grew slowly. Some villagers chased away vaccination teams. Then Taliban leaders in two mountainous border provinces banned all vaccination in their areas until drone strikes stopped. The WHO tried to negotiate, arguing that it had no control over American drone pilots—to no avail.

In late 2012, the killings began. In December, two months after Taliban gunmen shot Malala Yousafzai, a schoolgirl advocating for girls' education, two-man assassination teams on motorcycles stalked and shot dead nine polio vaccinators in three Pakistani cities over three days. Most of those killed were women, and several were related because families typically worked in their own neighborhoods, where they were known and trusted. They were easy to spot going house-to-house with their white boxes on shoulder straps.

The killings were a shock, even in Pakistan. Previously the Taliban had stripped, humiliated, and even stoned individual women who defied their rules. But carefully coordinated assassinations of women who were only protecting their neighbors was something new. The country's vast polio campaign, which had been so effective that it had driven paralysis cases down to only 52 the year before, was suspended and plunged into crisis. As many as 225,000 vaccinators were now terrified to venture onto the street.

President Asif Ali Zardari and his daughter Asifa, who had declared it their personal mission to drive out polio, pledged to provide protection. But when I went out with vaccination teams in Karachi and Peshawar in 2013, it was clear that the whole operation was still vulnerable. Local officials made sure the teams I observed were escorted by jeeps full of officers with automatic weapons. They closed off traffic to whole neighborhoods while the vaccinators made their rounds.

But that was just for show. When we returned to the vaccine distribution center at day's end, I could see how other teams fared. One group of women arrived with dusty sandals after a long day on foot. They were accompanied by a lone potbellied sergeant dyeing his gray hair with bright red henna. His only weapon was a billy club. A UNICEF doctor confirmed that most of the teams had only that level of protection. "What can a stick do against a gun?" he asked cynically.

Since then, the campaign has been periodically shut down by bursts of killings. As of early 2023, more than 100 vaccinators and their police escorts had been killed in Pakistan. In Afghanistan the picture is murkier; the Afghan Taliban claims to favor vaccination, but local leaders have their own ideas. More than 2,200 assassinations took place in the years before the Taliban took power in Kabul, but how many were polio workers is unclear.

Yet the campaign staggers on, because families are so desperately poor that a few dollars can tempt them to take chances. In Pakistan, pay for vaccinators in the most dangerous areas has been steadily raised, and Rotary International pays consolation money to families whose loved ones are killed.

Rumors turned Rotary's "Gift to the 21st Century" into an expensive nightmare. The latest five-year plan issued by the polio eradication initiative envisions eliminating polio by 2026, at a cost of over $1 billion a year.

The WHO recognizes that rumors often kneecap its efforts. It has sometimes formed "rumor teams" to try to quickly debunk the most extreme. In the early 1980s, these teams followed up on reports of smallpox popping up after it had been eradicated. (Often, the problem was simply misdiagnosis by local doctors seeing patients with chickenpox or similar diseases.) In the early 2000s, rumor teams chased reports of avian flu outbreaks in Asia. In 2019, the Ebola outbreak in the Democratic Republic of the Congo proved a huge challenge. The eastern border regions abutting Rwanda, Uganda, Burundi, and Sudan are full of displaced people speaking many languages and often deeply suspicious of the Congolese army and police. Tribes raised their own militias, and fratricidal violence was common. The WHO paid local people to listen to local radio stations and monitor social media to report circulating rumors. Local dignitaries considered "trusted messengers"—usually religious or tribal leaders—were asked to go on the air and debunk them.

Modern developments, including twenty-four-hour news, the internet, and social media, have made rumors a more powerful force. News was once filtered by editors at wire services, newspapers, radio, and TV stations who at least tried to weed out obvious lies or have reporters check them out. (In my youth, there were only three national television networks: ABC, CBS, and NBC. The Federal Communications Commission kept close tabs on their news programs, which lasted only an hour each evening.)

Soviet and Russian disinformation campaigns have existed for decades, but they previously had more difficulty planting rumors. For example, the rumor that the AIDS virus was a bioweapon invented in the U.S. Army lab at Fort Detrick, Maryland, to kill black people was concocted by the KGB, the Soviet intelligence service, according to defectors from that era. But the KGB had to spread it via a very roundabout route: In 1983, it planted an anonymous article in a Communist Party newspaper in India. It was weeks until the rumor got enough traction so that the well-known anchorman Dan Rather mentioned it on CBS. And, of course, he did so skeptically and quoted American intelligence experts dismissing it as ridiculous.

Russia's intelligence services are still at the same game. In September 2022, *The New York Times* reported that they were spreading rumors that the United States secretly manufactured bioweapons in Ukraine, trained birds to fly pathogens into Russia, and ran laboratories in Nigeria making monkeypox more transmissible.

But there has been a breakdown in the morals of public discourse. Many public figures no longer find it dishonorable to lie to get what they want. Instead of slinking away when caught, they double down, repeating the lie and attacking anyone—especially journalists—who questions them.

Americans seem to me to be more gullible than we once were, more ready to believe absurdities like the ideas that vaccines would be released with no testing or would magnetize recipients. We also appear more cynical: voters no longer drub out of office politicians caught lying. Presidents have lied, of course. Dwight Eisenhower's State Department lied about U-2 spy flights. John F. Kennedy had his brother Robert say he did not have Addison's disease and, in office, he lied about military intervention in Cuba. Lyndon Johnson lied about the Tonkin Gulf incident in Vietnam. Richard Nixon lied about bombing Cambodia and in saying no one in his White House was involved in Watergate. Ronald Reagan lied about trading arms for hostages. Bill Clinton lied about his affair with Monica Lewinsky. But those lies were so rare that they became front-page news when they were exposed. Some were excused as necessary for national security. Some led to angry denunciations by voters, and in Nixon's case, to his resignation. The idea that we would one day elect a president from whose lips fact-checkers would ultimately tally more than 30,000 lies was unthinkable.

That cynicism toward truth, coupled with very low levels of science education in many Americans, creates fertile ground for rumors. When those rumors are believed, and cause listeners to eschew lifesaving measures, lives are lost.

Chapter Fourteen

THE DESPICABLE PROFITEERS

When I was at the *Times*, as soon as any disease became headline news, I would get messages from people claiming to have the cure. It was usually a scientist, or a media rep hired by one. The scientists would pour on the medical jargon in a sort of "We science guys understand this stuff, right?" tone. The media reps would instead start with flattery, professing to be longtime fans of my work.

There was a pattern. Often the first message was vague and urgent—"Please call me, I have a breakthrough I must discuss with you! This is an exclusive to you only!" The note might suggest I'd win a Pulitzer if I broke the story.

Usually, I would reply by asking what the miracle cure was and what evidence they had that it worked. They typically replied with results from animal tests or from a small trial in which a few patients did better than expected. If it was published, it was usually in a journal I'd never heard of. In other words, nothing even close to the gold standard: a large trial in which the participants are randomly sorted into one group getting the treatment or a "control group" getting a placebo and in which both the participants and the doctors are "blinded" as to who is on treatment or placebo, and which is overseen by an independent ethics committee and then later reviewed by independent peers.

If I replied, "Thanks, but your small study is not enough to go on, and I can't abuse the enormous pulpit of *The New York Times* by touting something with thin evidence behind it," the author usually would express regret that I was unconvinced, promise to send more evidence—and then suggest, not terribly subtly, that they might contact my competition.

Sure enough, I would often soon see a story—usually in a local TV station or an outlet without a science staff. The headline might be noncommittal and in the form of a question: "Is Compound X the Cure?" Sometimes the inventor would forward these to me, as if to say, "See? They understood."

If the disease itself was big news, word of the alleged miracle cure might spread until I or one of my colleagues was effectively forced to cover it—either debunking it or saying some doctors were interested, some were skeptical, but, in any case, most wanted to wait for clinical trial results.

Alternatively, if I kept ignoring the blandishments—or if I did look into the purported cure hard enough to conclude that it probably could *not* work, and wrote that—I would often get one last furious note: "You're just like the rest! You're a tool of Big Pharma! People will die because of you!"

I don't mean it would always end that way, but it often was like a brief love affair gone bad: introduction, flattery, seduction, disappointment, fury.

Typically, the "miracle cure" was something already on the market, but whose supposed powers only the author recognized. Often it was a vitamin or mineral or food supplement, or perhaps a known disinfectant like a bleach or a silver compound or ozone or ultraviolet light. Or a prescription medicine normally used for another condition. Sometimes it was a mystery drug whose contents the inventor refused to reveal.

When facing crises, we humans crave quick solutions. When we're scared, we accept ideas that in normal times would seem silly.

Then, having grasped at a straw—and perhaps having been mocked for doing so—we double down. We bat away anyone who doubts us.

Every epidemic generates a new set of nostrums.

But that's just a symptom of a much more pernicious trend: every epidemic is exploited by profiteers.

Some hope to get rich and/or win a Nobel Prize. Some hope to become famous and collect donations to their 501(c)3 nonprofit advocacy organization. Some want to discredit valid treatments because they threaten their lucrative business selling fake cures.

A vitamin always seems to be in the mix. When I was young, Linus Pauling—who had won not one but two Nobel Prizes, in chemistry and in peace—became famous for touting megadoses of vitamin C as the cure for everything from the common cold to cancer. Today, for reasons beyond me, vitamin D seems to have taken its place in endless YouTube posts as the designated cure-all.

Vitamins are essential to health, but there is no proof that they prevent infectious diseases. (Vitamin C prevents scurvy and vitamin D prevents rickets, but those are not transmissible; they are simply deficiencies of those vitamins.)

Because vitamins, minerals, botanicals, amino acids, probiotics, and some other compounds are considered "dietary supplements," they are exempt from the strict approval and oversight standards that the FDA imposes on prescription and over-the-counter drugs. It is illegal for the supplements industry to make medical claims for its products, but it constantly subverts the spirit of such regulations by calling its stuff "immune-boosting" or using words like *mega-male*, *testo-enhancer*, or whatever.

In the rare cases when the FDA does step in, the abuses can be shocking. For example, in July 2022, the agency announced "voluntary" recalls of two brands of honey. Dose Vital honey claimed to be 95 percent honey with added "caviar powder" and "tongkat ali," which is alleged to be a Southeast Asian aphrodisiac. Royal Honey VIP claimed to be "the ultimate power source." Both secretly contained generic Viagra or Cialis.

During the 2014 Ebola outbreak, I got notes asking me to write articles about various patent medicines. Most turned out to be mild bleaches or silver compounds. Yes, strong bleaches kill pathogens, and you can safely gargle with a weak bleach like hydrogen peroxide. Yes, silver has antibacterial properties, and silver nitrate is a topical disinfectant. But it's not safe to drink or inject or inhale large amounts. None had been tested in Ebola patients. It was unnerving to see supplement makers push such toxic products, as if African lives didn't matter.

Indifference toward African lives came out even more sharply during AIDS. When the disease was first exploding across South Africa in 1997, researchers from the University of Pretoria claimed to have invented a cure, which they named Virodene P058. The subsequent "Virodene scandal" lasted five years and deeply undermined the credibility of the Mbeki administration.

The chief inventor, Olga Visser, was neither an HIV specialist nor a virologist. She was a cryonics specialist working with two Pretoria heart surgeons, Dirk du Plessis and Kallie Landauer. Together they claimed to have frozen rats' hearts and then thawed and restarted them—a claim greeted with skepticism by other cryobiology experts. Her husband, Siegfried Visser, was a businessman. Through the country's health minister, Dr. Nkosazana Clarice Dlamini Zuma, they got an introduction to Thabo Mbeki, the country's deputy president, who had not yet become the AIDS denialist I described earlier. Mr. Mbeki invited them to address the cabinet, where they presented several AIDS patients who said Virodene had reversed their symptoms. The cabinet gave the Vissers a standing ovation; they asked the government for $1 million for further research. A simultaneous press rollout had also been arranged; local newspapers and TV stations given exclusives by the researchers did breathless adulatory pieces about Virodene. (I was stationed in Johannesburg then and remember being stunned when sudden news of a "mystery cure" for AIDS that I had never heard of appeared on the front page of several newspapers.)

The Medicines Control Council, the country's equivalent of our FDA, was outraged to discover that the researchers had done human experiments without its permission. Its leaders also publicly denounced the decision to let doctors appeal directly to cabinet ministers who had no medical backgrounds. Mr. Mbeki lashed back, saying Virodene was potentially an "African solution to AIDS" and he would not rest "until the efficacy or otherwise of Virodene is established scientifically." Because of the enthusiastic press coverage, desperate South Africans began demanding the drug. The Virodene team portrayed itself as the nemesis of the Western pharmaceutical companies then charging astronomical prices for the new HIV drugs.

Within weeks, it leaked out that Virodene was actually dimethylformamide, an industrial solvent similar to dry-cleaning solution and used in plastics manufacturing. It was known to cause liver failure and cancer. It was also not chemically related to any known antiretroviral, and the Vissers could not explain how it supposedly inhibited the AIDS virus. The surgeons were disciplined by their university for not seeking ethical approval for human testing, and the medicines council banned all human testing until toxicology research was done. That set off a long public battle between the council's leaders and Mr. Mbeki and Dr. Zuma. When it reached the courts, evidence emerged that the Vissers and their partners had proposed giving 6 percent of their company to the ruling African National Congress. Mr. Mbeki denied that any such promise had been made. In early 1998, Dr. Zuma fired the senior members of the Medicines Control Council and had them locked out of their offices. An arbitration tribunal prevented her from dissolving the council, but it ceased to function, and a backlog of hundreds of unapproved drugs built up.

After failing to get permission to do human trials in Botswana, the Vissers shifted to Tanzania, where the Ministry of Defense agreed to test it on 64 HIV-infected soldiers in a military hospital. Who paid for the trials was never revealed, although investigative reporting in *Rapport* and the *Mail & Guardian* suggested that $3.5 million was funneled through businessmen with close ties to Mr. Mbeki.

To bolster their publicity efforts, the researchers sought to have Luc Montagnier, who had won a Nobel Prize in Medicine as a co-discoverer of the AIDS virus, test Virodene. He sent a letter saying that, based on what he had been told by the Vissers, it appeared to clear viral loads surprisingly fast; but he did no research. (Like Dr. Pauling, the late Dr. Montagnier in his declining years made increasingly bizarre pronouncements, such as claiming that DNA emitted electromagnetic radiation, that autism can be treated with antibiotics, and that Covid vaccines would slowly kill vaccinees. The tendency of some Nobel winners to embrace bizarre ideas, usually late in life, has a name: "Nobelitis.")

Meanwhile, in the middle of the scandal, the Vissers went through a bitter divorce, with accusations of infidelity and violence. Court documents suggested that they had formed opposing companies with different backers, each claiming to own the rights to Virodene. In 2002, it all collapsed. The trial in Tanzania—which did have a control group—concluded that Virodene did nothing to slow the progress of AIDS. A few months later, although Mr. Mbeki did not repudiate his denialism, his government dropped its opposition to antiretroviral drugs and began distributing nevirapine to HIV-infected mothers to keep their children from getting infected.

A close parallel had taken place in Kenya a few years before. Starting in 1990, Dr. Davy Koech, director of the Kenya Medical Research Institute, and his colleague Dr. Arthur O. Obel claimed that low-dose interferon helped their AIDS patients gain weight and sometimes cleared the virus. (In high doses, interferon, which the body naturally produces to trigger the immune system, has been used to treat hepatitis B and cancers. But it can have serious side effects.) They named it Kemron, and Kenyan president Daniel arap Moi soon took up the cause, claiming 50 patients had been cured. Western AIDS experts were skeptical, especially since the institute had not done a placebo-controlled study. The researchers struck back angrily, suggesting that lingering colonialist condescension toward Africa underlay the doubts. The *Amsterdam News*, a Harlem newspaper, denounced the "racist white press" for "cabalistically [ignoring] this amazing discovery." Desperate Kenyans spent their life savings trying to get the tablets, which had to be imported from Japan. Americans with AIDS flew to East Africa to outbid them. Counterfeits proliferated. In 1993, the researchers added an herbal supplement they called Pearl Omega and marketed the combination as a two-drug regimen.

Eventually, the WHO sponsored formal studies of interferon in Africa comparing it to the early antiretroviral AZT and to placebo; the National Institutes of Health did similar trials in the United States. None found any effect. Kemron and Pearl Omega were discredited.

But there was a crucial difference: Kemron had appeared before antiretroviral triple therapy existed, at a time when HIV sufferers had no hope. It did find adherents in the West and was for a while distributed at American HIV clinics run by the Nation of Islam, but it vanished when triple therapy proved successful. Virodene, by contrast, appeared well *after* triple therapy was shown to work. The South African government wasted five years pursuing it and that delay, compounded by Mr. Mbeki's stubborn denialism, as I noted earlier, probably cost more than 300,000 South Africans their lives.

Our domestic struggle with hydroxychloroquine and ivermectin during Covid is well-known.

In Wuhan, desperate doctors tried everything their pharmacies had that might work: dexamethasone and other steroids; antivirals like interferon, favipiravir, remdesivir, lopinavir, and ritonavir; the anti-flu drug oseltamivir and a Russian anti-flu drug arbidol; antibiotics like azithromycin; and traditional Chinese medicines. And the antimalarial chloroquine and its analog hydroxychloroquine.

The Chinese never completed clinical trials on any drug. The principal reason was that their draconian lockdowns worked so well that they ran out of patients. Also, as was explained to me by Dr. W. Ian Lipkin of Columbia University's Center for Infection and Immunity, the Chinese government funded research in ways that fostered dog-eat-dog competition rather than collaboration. At the time, the lead author of any paper published by *The New England Journal of Medicine*, the *Lancet*, or *Science* would get a $100,000 government bonus. Therefore, hospitals often would enroll their own patients in trials but not pool their data with rivals. The result was studies too small to draw conclusions from.

As the virus moved west, doctors in Europe tried the same remedies. An iconoclastic French doctor, Didier Raoult, became instantly famous after publishing a small study claiming to have cured 100 percent of his patients with a combination of hydroxychloroquine and azithromycin. Fox News hosts touted his study, suggesting that a miracle drug would quickly end the lockdowns they despised; President Trump echoed them. Finally, the British National Health Service organized the Recovery trial, linking 176 hospitals with 12,000 enrolled patients, and the WHO organized the Solidarity trial, linking 500 hospitals in 30 countries. In the United States, the NIH organized trials, but they proceeded slowly, for two reasons. First, we have a fragmented medical system, so hospitals argued over which protocols to follow. Second, President Trump publicly defended the drug and also pressured the FDA to authorize it for emergency use. That made it difficult to enroll patients in trials because they faced a 50 percent chance of getting a placebo, which desperately ill people will not risk. Many demanded hydroxychloroquine and, if they were rebuffed, would go doctor-shopping until they found one who would prescribe it.

Ultimately, the British and WHO trials reached similar results: Steroids like dexamethasone that eased lung inflammation did cut death rates. Nothing else did. (This was, of course, well before vaccines, monoclonal antibodies, or Paxlovid.)

Not everyone is motivated only by money, of course. Another form of reward is what I think of as the "Semmelweis Effect": the iconoclast who bucks conventional wisdom and proclaims himself an unrecognized genius surrounded by idiots. Everyone who has studied medicine has heard the story of Dr. Ignaz Semmelweis: a senior obstetrician at the prestigious Vienna General Hospital. The hospital had two birth wards, one run by midwives and one by doctors and medical students. Women in the doctors' ward were three times as likely to die of "childbed fever" as those in the midwifery ward. The doctors often came to their ward straight from dissecting corpses in the autopsy room. Germs were still unknown, but Dr. Semmelweis deduced that his students were carrying some sort of "morbid poison" from the corpses to their patients, and in 1847 he began requiring them to wash their hands with chlorinated water. Deaths in the medical ward plummeted. However, other doctors were infuriated by his implication that their unsanitary habits had killed hundreds of their patients, and some mocked him. Dr. Semmelweis, who was erratic and prickly, flung insulting letters back until he lost his post and a subsequent one in Budapest. His mental health failed, and he died in an asylum at age forty-seven after being beaten by its guards.

Semmelweis, of course, was right. Self-proclaimed Semmelweises, not so much.

The false hopes raised by the fervent backers of hydroxychloroquine later gave way to false hopes raised by the backers of ivermectin. Even as the pandemic faded away, some doctors were happy to prescribe such drugs for a fee. A relative of mine who survived two bouts of Covid later came to regret having been vaccinated and found a website offering to help her "detox from the jab."

The protocol was as follows:

- **Repent and say prayer (Click to download prayer).**
- **Take our CoviCleanse, which is a four-day detox.**
- **Use CoviLyte daily for a week.**
- **Register for a telehealth visit to get ivermectin.**

The site, DrStellaMD, sent patients to Dr. Stella Immanuel, one of "America's Frontline Doctors." In mid-2020, those doctors gained fame for holding a news conference in white coats outside the Supreme Court denouncing lockdowns and masks. They raised doubts about vaccines and defended hydroxychloroquine. They later switched to defending ivermectin. Dr. Immanuel was a part-time Christian pastor who had given sermons saying women's problems like endometriosis were caused by having sex with demons while asleep. She also said witches were treating patients with "alien DNA" and planned to destroy the world using abortion, gay marriage, and children's toys.

In March 2023, an analysis of prescription data by the medical news outlet MedPage Today found that, in 2021, Dr. Immanuel had written 69,000 prescriptions for hydroxychloroquine and 32,000 for ivermectin. The average HCQ prescriber, such as a rheumatologist prescribing it for autoimmune disease, wrote 561, the MedPage authors said. The average prescriber of ivermectin wrote 15 prescriptions for it a year.

The founder of America's Frontline Doctors, Dr. Simone Gold, was later imprisoned for taking part in the January 6 Capitol riot. She pled guilty to entering the Capitol and making a speech in Statuary Hall opposing vaccine mandates and lockdowns. After her release, she was sued by her charity's own board, accused of misusing millions of dollars in donations to buy a Florida home and expensive cars for herself and her boyfriend, a former underwear model.

America's Frontline Doctors was distinct from the Front Line COVID-19 Critical Care Alliance, another ivermectin-prescribing group. For months during the pandemic I received weekly emails from their media rep. At first they exhorted me to cover ivermectin's miraculous powers, then suggested I investigate the government's ivermectin cover-up. The last ones denounced me as part of the problem.

Profiteering doesn't require selling false cures. Some industries merely downplay disease threats that could cut into their profits.

In 1918, as flu began killing Americans, health experts advised closing baseball stadiums, theaters, burlesque halls, restaurants, saloons, schools, and other public gatherings. A few cities, notably St. Louis, did so rapidly, and suffered lower levels of mortality. Others succumbed to pressure from business owners to stay open—which came along with pressure from the Wilson administration to sell war bonds.

Philadelphia's city fathers debated whether to cancel a Liberty Loan parade set for September 28, 1918. They had been warned—a small "Win the War for Freedom" parade by soldiers and shipyard workers in Boston on September 3 had spread disease into that city's civilian population. Also, 600 sailors in Philadelphia's shipyard were already hospitalized, a few dying each day. But Wilmer Krusen, the city's public health director, fearful of causing panic and under pressure to keep up bond sales, let the parade proceed. It was two miles long and more than 200,000 Philadelphians crowded Broad Street to watch. Within seventy-two hours, every bed in the city's thirty-one hospitals was filled. Soon more than 2,500 residents were dying each week. Bodies were left in the streets for police wagons to collect; a military morgue unit was brought in to handle the dead; Holy Cross Cemetery hired a steam shovel to dig mass graves. When the epidemic ended two years later, Philadelphia had been the hardest hit of all American cities.

Decades later, during the AIDS epidemic, it quickly became clear that gay bathhouses, bars, cinemas, and bookstores with private cubicles or darkened rooms for group sex were foci for transmission of the virus.

Randy Shilts, the *Chronicle* reporter who would go on to fame with *And the Band Played On*, described the culture of the baths in an article in the *New York Native*: "By the mid 1970s, promiscuity was less a lifestyle than an article of faith. . . . Before long an entire subculture and business network emerged catering to drugged out alcoholic gay men with penchants for kinky promiscuous sexual acts."

The long battle between San Francisco's City Hall and the sex industry is well described by the Columbia University bioethicist Ronald Bayer in 1989 in *Private Acts, Social Consequences*. Dr. Bayer called Mr. Shilts, who died of AIDS in 1994, "a strong antagonist of the bathhouses, the sexual culture they fostered, and the timidity of gay political leaders."

The fight opened schisms between politicians, health officials, and civil libertarians. It also split the gay community. Some, like Mr. Shilts, wanted the baths closed. Others argued that sexual freedom was at the core of gay identity and "letting the government into our bedrooms" would set gay rights back a century. The most libertarian argued that if some men wanted to knowingly risk death, as sky divers and mountain climbers did, it was nobody else's business. They denounced Mr. Shilts as a sex-hostile traitor collaborating with homophobes; he was spat upon in the street. The counterargument, of course, was that some victims never realized they were at risk, including women married to men they didn't know were bisexual, and the children they bore.

Others argued that closing the baths would shift sex to private house parties or back to the parks and piers where men met before—and where they had sometimes been attacked by muggers or homophobes.

The fight also had puritanical aspects. Only some gay men visited the baths and even fewer practiced "kinky promiscuous sexual acts." But lurid news stories describing glory holes, anal fisting, sex involving urination and defecation, sadomasochism, and bondage horrified many Americans in the era of Ronald Reagan and his Moral Majority supporters.

The owners of the bars and baths were wealthy and influential. Their ads supported the *Bay Area Reporter*, the local gay newspaper. They mounted a public relations drive to portray their establishments as symbols of gay liberation and to deny that the still-mysterious illness was related to sex.

"I used to live in the Portrero District, and one of the bathhouses was on my route home—its parking lot was always full," said Dr. Dean F. Echenberg, who was then the city health department's director of communicable disease control and had served as a flight surgeon during the Vietnam War. "The owners were taking out ads saying 'Don't believe the city health officials. Come on down and fuck your brains out.' They knew what they were doing—making money and not caring that people were dying as a result. That's what pissed me off so much."

By 1984, the virus that caused AIDS had not yet been found, but many gay men realized that they were at risk and that sex played a role in the spread. Diagnoses of rectal gonorrhea, an indicator of the frequency of anal sex, had risen rapidly in the 1970s. They plummeted after AIDS was described in 1981—presumably because many scared men tempered their behavior. But then they leveled off and stayed constant.

"The gay community wasn't stupid," Dr. Echenberg said. "Most men were practicing safe sex. After 1981, the people still going to the bathhouses were being taken in by the owners' propaganda."

It was becoming clearer that there was a correlation between visiting the baths, having multiple partners, and HIV infection. Many of the men dying in Ward 86 at San Francisco General Hospital—the nation's first AIDS ward—admitted to multiple encounters in the baths. In a 1984 survey at a city-run STD clinic, men who said they found more than 65 percent of their partners at the baths had a mean of 866 lifetime sexual partners, which was more than four times as many as men who did not visit the baths. The men surveyed had been chosen because they had all given blood samples between 1978 and 1980 as part of a trial of a new hepatitis B vaccine—in other words, even before AIDS was known to exist. Later tests on those blood samples found HIV antibodies in 53 percent of them, which suggested that, by the time AIDS was even discovered, as much as half the city's gay men were already infected. "It was as if I saw a freight train coming right at us and I could do nothing about it," Dr. Echenberg said.

By 1984, San Francisco mayor Dianne Feinstein was adamant that the baths be closed. Her health director, Dr. Mervyn F. Silverman, was initially hesitant, but his deputy, Dr. Echenberg, favored closure. He worked with the city attorney's office on an order that could withstand constitutional challenges, sent investigators into the clubs to take notes on exactly what sex acts occurred inside, and had epidemiologists survey gay men about their risk behavior.

That October, Dr. Silverman ordered fourteen baths, clubs, theaters, and bookstores closed as public nuisances. The owners fought back. One month later, a court ruled against outright closure, but ordered the owners to prevent risky sex on their premises and remove the doors to cubicles.

The owners, whose reputations were suffering from the publicity, especially as more of their former customers died each month, offered to negotiate. "They wanted sex with condoms, but I said I wasn't going to have my guys pulling people apart to see if they had condoms on," Dr. Echenberg recalled.

Ultimately, the owners agreed to new rules and to hiring bouncers to enforce them. Mutual masturbation was permitted. Oral and anal sex and any contact with urine or feces was forbidden. Cubicle doors were allowed to stay but had to be small enough for the bouncers to see that only one man was inside. The clubs also had to distribute pamphlets about safe sex.

"So, we didn't close them, but we agreed they could stay open if they were just jack-off clubs," Dr. Echenberg said. "I remember the night I drove home when we'd closed the bathhouses. I drove by that lot and it was empty. I just felt good—very, very, very good. Hot damn—we did it! We had beat them."

To my mind, the most dangerous profiteers by far are the prominent anti-vaxxers.

Opposition to vaccines goes back centuries. In Britain, for example, acts of Parliament passed in 1853 and 1867 making smallpox vaccination mandatory led to the establishment of the Anti–Compulsory Vaccination League in 1869. In 1885, the league sponsored a demonstration in Leicester that drew tens of thousands of protestors, some holding signs with exhortations like "Keep Your Children's Blood Still Pure."

The movement has waxed and waned ever since. Its popularity depends upon how much terror a disease engenders. In the 1950s, the fear of polio was so great that vaccine demand survived even the "Cutter Incident," in which batches of Jonas Salk's vaccine from Cutter Laboratories in California contained live virus that caused 40,000 cases of polio. About 200 children suffered paralysis and 10 died.

The modern anti-vaccine movement emerged in the 1990s after autism rates suddenly soared in wealthy countries. That surge is still unexplained, but many experts believe it is a combination of more screening, broader diagnoses of "autism spectrum" traits, more births to older parents, and the survival of more very premature infants.

In 1998, a British transplant surgeon, Dr. Andrew Wakefield, suggested a link between autism and the measles-mumps-rubella vaccine. He theorized that the vaccine somehow triggered "leaky gut" bowel disease, allowing unspecified compounds to get into the blood and reach the brain.

His study of a dozen children, published in the *Lancet*, caused an uproar. Terrified parents stopped vaccinating their children. Pediatricians tried to convince them otherwise, but it took ten years to produce convincing studies disproving his nonsensical theories. Ultimately, sixteen studies from Britain, Denmark, Finland, the United States, and Japan between 1999 and 2019 showed that neither the vaccine itself, nor "vaccine overload," nor thimerosal, an antifungal preservative, nor any other aspect of vaccination triggered autism.

In 2010, Dr. Wakefield's medical license was revoked by the British General Medical Council, which found him guilty of serious misconduct, including needless lumbar punctures on disabled children, and of concealing the fact that he had been paid by lawyers who were suing vaccine companies. Other investigations found that he had plans to market his own measles vaccine and a test for the condition he claimed to have identified, "autistic enterocolitis." Mr. Wakefield moved to the United States, remains a champion of the anti-vaccine movement, and portrays himself as a victim of the medical establishment.

The modern anti-vaccine lobby has exploded since then. It portrays itself as a movement of concerned parents but is really an industry underwritten by unscrupulous entrepreneurs. Some profit by selling "immune enhancing" vitamins as alternatives. Others claim to treat "vaccine damaged children" with chiropractic, homeopathy, chelation, hyperbaric chambers, or hydrogen peroxide nebulizers. Science reporters are routinely escorted out of their conferences, but they always record how the exhibition halls are filled with sales booths for quack cures.

Anti-vaccine "charities" like Robert F. Kennedy Jr.'s Children's Health Defense sell books and solicit tax-deductible donations.

The consequences of the anti-vax industry's lies are far-reaching.

Obviously, they cost many lives during the Covid pandemic. I've already described how measles returned to New York in 2019 because some ultra-Orthodox Jewish families were convinced to stop vaccinating. More than 100 children were hospitalized. In 2016–17, something similar happened to Somali children in Minnesota. When autism appeared to be on the rise there, anti-vaccine activists began campaigning. They so scared many Somali families that measles vaccination rates dropped from 92 percent in 2004 to 42 percent in 2014. Two years later, there was a measles outbreak, mostly among Somali children, more than a dozen of whom were hospitalized.

In 2022, vaccination rejection led to the return of polio transmission to the United States, something not seen since 1979. It paralyzed a young ultra-Orthodox man in a New York suburb who had not been out of the country recently. A CDC investigation found that the virus strain was identical to strains circulating in ultra-Orthodox neighborhoods in Israel and North London, and that some Hasidic neighborhoods had vaccination rates below 40 percent.

I cannot see how Hasidic community leaders allow that to happen. I've met children crippled by polio in both Nigeria and Pakistan, and it was heartbreaking. In Kano, Nigeria, two-year-old Omar Ahmed dragged himself into the cement courtyard of his house as I interviewed his parents. His spindly legs, covered with calluses, trailed limply behind him. His father, Aminu, and his mother, Hadiza, were both also childhood polio victims. Hadiza walked by entwining her bad leg around a crutch. Both of Aminu's legs were withered, so he used a rag to tie them in the lotus position and got around on six-inch wooden hand crutches, with which he could hoist himself off the ground and swing his pelvis forward. Nonetheless, he was a leader in his community. He was president of the Kano State Polio Victims Association and ran its welding shop, which made hand-cranked wheelchairs from bicycle parts. He played soccer on a skateboard, punching the ball with his fists, and had coached his city's "polio football" team to three national championships. He even owned a motorcycle.

He and Hadiza had six children. Omar was the only one affected; he was born during the year when three northern states—to Aminu's great frustration—had suspended polio vaccination.

In Karachi, Pakistan, two-year-old Musharaf limped along a hospital corridor on a bowed leg as I interviewed his father, Usman. (Usman would not give his last name because he came from the Swat Valley, which was then a Taliban stronghold, and he feared being killed for meeting an American reporter.) Usman had vaccinated his first three children but then turned vaccinators away from his house after the CIA's vaccination plot against Osama bin Laden and because American drones had killed people he knew. Usman too had a leg bowed by polio. His limp was even more severe than his son's, and walking made him grimace in pain. Angry as he was at Americans, he said he had come to regret not letting Musharaf be vaccinated: "I know now I made a mistake."

How any parent could risk this happening to their child is beyond me—and it shocks me that any religious leader would witness it without condemning it.

In 2021, Kennedy, Dr. Joseph Mercola, and other leading anti-vaxxers were labeled the "Disinformation Dozen" by the Center for Countering Digital Hate, which accused them of generating more than half the vaccine misinformation on social media. It called on media companies to cancel their accounts or post warnings.

To me, that seems far too feeble. Facebook, Twitter, Instagram, and TikTok are not the guardians of public health. They're run by mercurial executives with their own opinions, and TikTok is under the influence of a foreign government. They have deep conflicts of interest in that their platforms increase viewership by promoting controversy. Also, they sell ads, including to anti-vaccine campaigns.

I think medical associations and the government should be far more aggressive about this issue. Freedom of speech does not include the right to market lies that kill American children. Federal and state prosecutors should investigate the industry. The Internal Revenue Service should scrutinize its tax-exempt status. Those making false claims for their supplements should have their assets seized like other drug dealers. Doctors who tout false cures or denigrate approved vaccines should have their licenses revoked. If their patients die, they should face manslaughter charges.

There is precedent for this. In the 1930s, in the name of free speech, we tolerated the German American Bund and the Silver Legion, even as they spread the lies that Hitler was America's friend, that Nazism would save the world from communism, that FDR was in thrall to Jews, and that George Washington was our "First Fascist."

But when we entered the war and Americans actually began dying in the fight against Hitler, the nation's patience ended. Congress held hearings, prosecutors investigated, the leaders' financial frauds were exposed. The Legion's founder was imprisoned for sedition. The Bund's German-born founder was imprisoned for embezzling and tax evasion and later deported to Germany.

We lost more than a million Americans to Covid. The anti-vaccine industry caused and profited from many of those deaths. In my opinion, they should face severe consequences.

Chapter Fifteen

THE RARE POLITICIANS WHO OUTWIT SCIENTISTS

To fight an epidemic, it's sometimes better to be good at psychology than to slavishly follow the science. Scientists may advise one policy path, only to have politicians ignore them—and the politicians turn out to be right. That may be because politicians have had years of experience at something most scientists know little about: crowd psychology. By talking to constituents, by speaking in front of audiences, by reading polls, by watching votes, they develop a feel for how people behave. If you can't anticipate and control groupthink, you can't beat a pandemic. But there is an art to it.

In early 2020, numerous experts said average Americans should *not* wear masks. This mistake later cost them dearly in credibility. At the time, the known science was on their side, and they offered many scientific-sounding reasons for their advice: surgical masks, they said, were not protective enough because they left gaps where air could slip in. N95s, which filtered out 95 percent of all particles, were better but supposedly didn't work unless they were "fitted" by a professional and could not be worn with beards. Some argued that masks gave wearers a false sense of security, so they might venture too close to sick people or neglect handwashing. They warned that masks collected viral particles on the outside and wearers might get infected while removing them. And they emphasized that no one should buy masks because hospitals needed them—which was a valid point. Doctors and nurses in many hospitals were having to reuse protective gear for days on end.

Of course, most of the prevailing wisdom from those days turned out to be false. Scientists initially assumed that most transmission was from large droplets and the surfaces that people coughed those droplets onto, such as hands, doorknobs, subway poles, or groceries. As a result, they were skeptical of masks and backed frequent handwashing instead.

From a scientific point of view, that made some sense. When the pandemic began, published studies on masks were rare and fairly iffy. The two I knew of were from Canada's McMaster University. The first, done on a mere 43 nurses in Toronto hospitals during the 2002–03 SARS epidemic, concluded that nurses who wore masks when entering patients' rooms were better protected than nurses who wore none. The second, done on 448 nurses during the 2008–09 flu season, concluded that inexpensive surgical masks were neither better nor worse than N95s at preventing flu.

And, naturally, with the best-known studies having been done on hospital personnel, there was an unspoken assumption that masks were only for them.

Asian countries, on the other hand, had a completely different tradition. Masks during flu season had been normal for years. They were also common in Asian cities as protection against air pollution and in farm fields as protection against dust. Surgical masks were routinely available.

So, when the pandemic began, Asian countries imposed universal mask use with little pushback. (When it was needed, enforcement could be harsh. I remember watching a Chinese TV network video of an elderly lady being chased down a street by a police drone, its loudspeaker berating her for going maskless.)

In the United States, early in the pandemic, masks were vanishingly rare, even on New York's crowded subways. The only people I ever saw wearing them were Asian; in previous years, a few Asian Americans wore them in flu season. I suspect that, from the first reports out of China until lockdowns began in March 2020, there was an unspoken racist dynamic at work—that masks were seen as "an Asian thing." It was not until February 4—a month after the first reports from China—that I saw anyone who wasn't Asian wearing a mask on the train. (I remember the date because it was so unusual that I surreptitiously snapped the wearer's picture with my phone.) It seems hard to believe now, but mask-wearing did not become common in New York until late March, as people began venturing out of lockdown. On March 13, on an episode of *The Daily* podcast called "Learning to Live With the Coronavirus" and recorded the day I went into lockdown, I described what I was personally doing to stay safe: I washed my hands frequently and avoided people who were coughing; I was having second thoughts about riding the subway or taking an airplane. Michael Barbaro and I did not even discuss wearing a mask.

Nearly two decades before, I had been in Taiwan when mask use first became normalized there. It happened *not* because of scientific data but because a politician bucked scientists' advice.

It was during the 2003 SARS epidemic. Most Taiwanese did not wear masks then, but hospital doctors did. (Standard N95s then had a horizontal seam and resembled duckbills, with an unintentionally comic result: every news conference I attended with the country's top doctors looked like a row of very serious mallards leaning into microphones.)

The behavior of local TV reporters showed how little they understood the risk. They did not wear masks during the press conferences, which were held in poorly ventilated hospital meeting rooms with doctors who had just come from tending SARS patients—a situation in which it would have been smart to wear a mask. But just before their on-air stand-ups—which they did outdoors in the breeze—they would pop one on. It was classic "hygiene theater."

At that time, the prevailing scientific opinion in Taiwan was that only medical personnel and people who were currently infected with SARS should wear masks. Even the director of Taiwan's CDC said it was pointless for anyone else to wear them.

Technically, that makes *some* sense. To substantially lower the risk within any crowd, any restaurant, or any subway car, the best use of a single mask is to put it on the infected person. Because masks absorb droplets, a well-fitted one is much better at keeping aerosolized particles *in* than it is at keeping them out. But there is no way to know which person in a crowd is infected. And even if someone knows he is sick and is blatantly coughing, he will never put on a mask unless everyone else is wearing one, too. When only the sick person must wear one, the mask becomes a leper's bell announcing that the wearer is contagious. Who would tolerate that? In Taipei, no one.

The epidemic, however, was spreading rapidly. Taipei's mayor saw the dilemma and ended it with one stroke. Understanding his constituents better than the head of Taiwan's CDC did, he declared that no one could enter the subways without a mask. Police officers were posted at turnstiles to enforce the new rule. Within days, virtually everyone was wearing one. Infections slowed down. The mayor, Ma Ying-jeou, later went on to be elected president of Taiwan.

Of course, as with all such decisions, it had unintended consequences. The first was a mask shortage—just as we would face seventeen years later. Hospitals ran out. Desperate doctors and nurses appealed for more.

At first, a few were sent by friends and relatives overseas. (At the time, the United States was a source of masks to Asia, not the other way around.) Then, as big shipments arrived, they piled up in warehouses. That was partly because customs agents were overwhelmed, but mostly because the importers were holding them back, hoping the government would cancel import duties, which would increase their profits. That drove price gouging; masks in Taipei, when they could be found, were briefly $20 each.

Another forceful political move had to be made. The government declared it illegal to charge more than $3 per mask and threatened stiff fines for price gouging. And it gave the speculators an ultimatum: clear their masks through customs within forty-eight hours or see them seized. The shortage quickly ended.

After 2003, because SARS had spread so far—China, Hong Kong, Taiwan, Singapore, Vietnam—the wearing of masks became normalized in much of Asia. (Canada, too, had 251 SARS cases, mostly in Toronto, but masks did not become normal there.) Additionally, from 2004 to 2008, Asia had regular avian flu scares. Although the H5N1 virus that caused it never went pandemic, it killed about 60 percent of the 300 people known to have been infected during those years, so it caused people to be more scared of flu season than they were in the West.

In the United States in 2020, none of those lessons were known. Dr. George Gao, head of China's CDC, told his American counterpart, Dr. Robert Redfield, that he thought the biggest mistake Americans were making was not wearing masks. His advice was ignored.

On March 28, the WHO insisted that the virus was "not airborne," which was both incorrect and confusing. It was transmitted by touch but also by sneezes and coughs that traveled at least a yard through the air, the WHO said. To most laymen that means "airborne." The agency's mistake was failing to distinguish between "droplet transmission," which is infection by big, wet drops that fly out of the mouth but fall to the ground a few feet away, and "aerosol transmission," which is by tiny droplets that can hang in the air and even slip through vents into adjoining rooms. Measles is so transmissible that just a few virions—viral particles—in a minuscule droplet can infect. Most common colds need many times more virions, meaning bigger droplets, to infect.

Also, the virus's mutability was underestimated. Initially, Chinese scientists said it was less infectious than SARS, which was probably never true—they did not yet know that there were many asymptomatic cases. Moreover, every few months, the virus became *more* transmissible: the D614G or "European" strain that was dominant by June 2020 was more transmissible than the original Wuhan strain. In late 2020, it was outcompeted by the Alpha strain, first found in Kent, England; and then by the

Beta strain, from South Africa's Nelson Mandela Bay area; and then by the Delta strain, first seen in Amravati, in central India. Delta dominated most of the world until late 2021, when Omicron emerged near Pretoria, South Africa. (Southern Africa may have generated multiple variant strains because so many people there suffered from untreated or poorly treated HIV. An immune system mounting a prolonged but weak attack puts the virus under pressure to mutate rapidly to evade a succession of different antibodies.) The Omicron subvariants that emerged later were many times more transmissible than the Wuhan strain and perhaps as infectious as measles. By then, however, transmissibility was almost impossible to measure because so much of the population had partial immunity from vaccination or previous infection.

In early 2020, it took time for mask studies with convincing data to be done. Physicists in Japan used flashing lasers to show how clouds of microdroplets emanated from people who were not coughing, but merely talking or laughing. The clouds drifted at head height through unventilated rooms. Fabric studies showed that masks with asymmetric weaves and mild static charges could absorb most such microdroplets. The Czech Republic adopted early universal masking like that in Asia and saw cases drop rapidly. (Its masks were hand-made because so few were available.) Eventually, epidemiological studies from many places, including Germany, and even Arizona and Kansas, concluded that the spread was slower in cities where residents masked up.

That new body of evidence strongly suggested that masks *did* work—as common sense and years of experience in Asia suggested they would. Most experts, including those who had initially rejected mask-wearing, came around and strongly endorsed them. Also, hospital shortages disappeared as new supplies began to flow.

But by then, many Americans were utterly fed up with lockdowns, isolation, job losses, income disruptions, and the whole miserable pandemic experience. The constantly shifting mask advice confused and irritated them.

Politics supercharged the issue. President Trump initially disdained masks as unmanly. Cable news hosts who supported him mocked scientists for changing their minds. Even when the president gave in—after repeated superspreader events within the White House itself—he reveled in publicly doffing his mask, as he did on the White House Portico after being released from the hospital after a serious bout with Covid. Governors who admired him avoided mask mandates or lifted them quickly. Governors who despised him—like New York's Andrew Cuomo—imposed them.

The rest of that history is well-known. The red state versus blue state battle over mask mandates continued for years and became a national flashpoint. There were demonstrations outside state capitols and public mask burnings. Cashiers and security guards were actually shot dead over the issue, and many were involved in fistfights. Interestingly, New York City, where masks became truly routine indoors after it was hit hard in early 2020, suffered quite a bit less infection than the rest of the country during the deadly winter wave of 2020–21 and the Delta wave of fall 2021. Not until Omicron arrived in January 2022, by which time mask use in the city had noticeably declined, did New Yorkers again suffer hospitalizations and deaths proportional to the rest of the country.

Even at this writing, three years later, politicized battles over mask studies continue. (Many epidemiological studies suffer from confounding factors: Are people who wear masks also more likely to isolate themselves from other people? More likely to be vaccinated? Also, mask studies have the same flaw as condom studies: It is very hard to know if your study subjects who report wearing them were actually doing so. People constantly render masks useless by pulling them away to speak, eat, or smoke.)

As in Taiwan in 2003, fashion also clouded the picture. The first masks there were simple white and blue surgical and N95 forms. Then brand names sprouted everywhere. For my daughters, I brought back a collection of Hello Kittys, Paul Frank Monkeys, Nike Swoops, Chanel Cs, Burberry plaids, and so on (all presumably counterfeit). Eighteen years later, the same thing happened in the United States: President Trump and his entourage wore intimidating dark colors with the presidential seal affixed. Fashion houses like Prada sold $700 masks, and more were counterfeited. Masks with exhalation valves were briefly popular because they were comfortable and suggested the owner was an athlete—and then were banned because the valves spewed infectious particles. Some men would only wear neck gaiters, which looked macho but were all but useless at particle absorption. Throughout 2021, I enjoyed watching thousands of patterned, colored, and be-sloganed cloth masks drift by, each reflecting the wearer's personality. (I usually wore one from the Getty Museum that was based on Impressionist color theory.)

By late 2022, cloth masks had lost some credibility because they had symmetric weaves and no static charge. By early 2023, the small fraction of New Yorkers still wearing masks were once again in dull, monochromatic N95s or disposable surgical ones. The pandemic "ended" for me in February 2022. By then, I'd been vaccinated four times and had had a mild bout of Covid in December 2021. It seemed likely that, if I got it again, it would just be another common cold, so that's when I stopped wearing masks, even on subways, planes, and in the gym. Everyone's pandemic ends at his or her own pace. (I did get Covid again, in October 2022, but it was even milder.)

The mask battle was an exhausting spin cycle of science, politics, and fashion. However, it has normalized mask-wearing for many people in this country as SARS did in Asia twenty years earlier. Most Americans will presumably never return to the utter indifference to masks that we felt in early 2020.

In 2021, another struggle took place between scientists and politicians, this time over "booster" shots. The politicians ignored the scientists—and were ultimately proved right.

By mid-2021, preliminary data from Israel suggested that the protection from two shots of the Pfizer mRNA vaccine wore off after about six months. Later data from Britain reached the same conclusion.

Israel and then Britain began giving out third doses of vaccine: first to immunocompromised people and health care workers, then to people over age 80, then to people over age 65, and so on until they were offered to everyone.

An outcry arose. At the time, the world's poorest countries were desperate for vaccine. Rich countries had bought up almost all the mRNA vaccines. When India, which had mysteriously suffered few deaths in the pandemic's first year, was suddenly hit hard by the Delta variant in April 2021, it held back millions of doses it had made for export. China's vaccines had fallen out of favor because they were initially released with little efficacy data and then countries like Chile and Brazil that bought them reported them to be only 60 to 70 percent effective.

Africa cried foul, and the WHO agreed. Dr. Michael J. Ryan, the WHO's director of health emergencies, said giving booster shots to vaccinated citizens of wealthy countries amounted to "handing out extra lifejackets to people who already have lifejackets while leaving others to drown."

In the United States, advocates for global health shared Dr. Ryan's view. Others argued that there was no need for boosters because two mRNA doses appeared to give more than 90 percent protection against hospitalization and death. Some went so far as to claim that protection against death was Operation Warp Speed's original goal. That was untrue. The FDA's publicly stated standard had been vaccines that were at least 50 percent effective against *infection.* These scientists and advocates pushed for delaying third doses and shipping the extras to Africa, Asia, Latin America, and the western Pacific.

But the Biden administration perceived a popular reality that scientists could not. Although nearly 30 percent of Americans were resisting vaccines, the other 70 percent were caught in a vortex of anger and fear. At that time—early fall of 2021—the Delta variant was at its peak. Hospitals in some states were as crowded as they had been during the deadly surge of the previous 2020–21 winter. Deaths, which had dropped to 200 a day in July, had again soared past 1,000 a day and were on their way to 2,000.

More than 90 percent of those dying were unvaccinated. That, however, was cold comfort to the vaccinated because their own children and teenagers were still mostly unprotected. Although schools were soon to reopen, the vaccine had just been approved for teens and was not yet approved for children. Also, it had been six months since the oldest cohorts had had two shots, and the Israeli and British data suggested that their protection was fading away. The most worried were health care workers, who had been vaccinated first; they faced the virus every day and their protection was waning.

By then, the vaccinated majority was furious at the unvaccinated minority. In their eyes, the vaccine resisters were prolonging the pandemic, keeping the economy crippled, putting innocent children in danger, and forcing the whole country to keep wearing masks.

That rage was visible on venues like SorryAntiVaxxer.com and the "Herman Cain Awards" subreddit. (The latter was named for President Trump's most prominent black supporter, who attended a Trump rally without a mask, got infected, and died.) Readers gleefully posted screenshots from the social media feeds of people who publicly sneered at masks or vaccines and then died.

The rage grew even greater when governors who had outlawed vaccine mandates in their states opened clinics where their infected constituents could get lifesaving monoclonal antibodies at no cost. The expensive antibodies were in short supply nationally, and states with anti-vax governors like Florida and Texas were using far more than their share of the national stockpile. (Even though the antibodies were based on newer technology than vaccines and had been less thoroughly tested, the anti-vax lobby never went after them and Trump supporters readily accepted them.) To stop the hoarding, the Biden administration took over distribution.

Many Americans very much wanted booster shots immediately, regardless of what advocates for poor countries wanted.

It was clear to anyone who followed politics that, if the Biden administration shipped millions of vaccine doses to Africa while forcing panicked Americans to wait, there would be a backlash even from his most loyal constituents. At the time, it seemed certain that the Democrats would lose the 2022 midterm elections and likely that Donald Trump would be president again in 2024.

President Biden said he would do both—make sure all Americans wanting boosters would get them, but also send 110 million doses to Africa. He left vague exactly how he would do that, but Americans seemed reassured.

Simultaneously, the unexpected happened: demand for vaccine across Africa dried up as vaccine apathy set in. Tales emerged of people in rural areas arriving for shots but being sent home because nurses would not open a vial for fewer than five people, and not even that many showed up. The Africa CDC asked companies to stop sending doses.

Then, on November 26—the day after Thanksgiving and at the start of the holiday travel season—the Omicron variant emerged. Despite the cutoff of flights from Johannesburg and Cape Town, it soon spread from South Africa to Britain, Norway, and Denmark and then to the United States, where it soon pushed out the Delta variant. Its fifty mutations changed the shape of its spike protein so much that two doses of the original vaccine were virtually useless against it.

Very quickly, what had been America's "pandemic of the unvaccinated" turned into a "pandemic of the unboosted." Scientists began saying they should have known all along that protection would require three doses since many other vaccines did, and predicted that "fully vaccinated" would soon mean three shots.

The clamor for third shots rose even louder, especially from medical workers and those in Omicron-hit cities like New York. From a public health point of view, the booster rollout faltered; by the time Omicron arrived in full force, only about 15 percent of Americans had gotten boosters. Psychologically, however, it was a success—Americans got what they wanted because politicians had read the tea leaves correctly while scientists clung to older assumptions and prejudices while hesitating to accept the new data from Israel and Britain.

It's a common pattern: scientists dither as they wait for rock-solid proof, while politicians are forced to act on instinct—and sometimes are proven right. It's hard to know beforehand who will ultimately prove correct, of course. But sometimes acting fast is best.

Chapter Sixteen

THE MEDIA'S FORCED ERRORS

There's a pernicious synergy between the media and public health agencies, especially in the early days of a pandemic. In the initial foggy period, journalists often hesitate to sound alarms about a threat until the agencies have made it official. (In general, media outlets are run by former White House reporters, not by former science reporters.) But the agencies often fail to act until the media—particularly *The New York Times*—makes a front-page fuss. Headlines prod politicians, who prod bureaucrats to act, which makes headlines. It's a self-reinforcing cycle.

The number of errors the news media makes in covering diseases is legion, although I hate generalizations about "the media." I'm the media; Tucker Carlson is the media; China state TV is the media. We all see things differently and are controlled by different forces.

All media pretend to be objective, and all media are biased. Usually, it's easy to see that at work—how Fox News and the *Times* handle the same set of facts, for example. But sometimes the pressures on individual reporters are not so obvious. What one thinks the story is may not match what one's editors think it is, what the White House or the competition thinks it is, and what the story *really* is—which is often discernible only later anyway.

One example I can think of comes from the late summer of 2009, during the H1N1 "swine flu" pandemic.

By August, the United States had been through ups and downs. The initial reports in April had been scary—Mexico City hospitals overwhelmed; many young adults dead; a state of emergency declared with the government asking citizens to stop shaking hands or kissing; the military handing out masks. The virus reached New York almost immediately: Mary Pappas, the nurse at St. Francis Preparatory School in Queens, found a line of sick students outside her office, some of whom had been to Cancún, Mexico, on spring break. On April 24, the *Times*' Mexico City bureau chief, Marc Lacey, and I collaborated on a front-page story. Perhaps prompted by that, Secretary of Homeland Security Janet Napolitano declared a public health emergency two days later. Most subsequent flu cases in the United States were mild, however, and, on May 1, a study suggested that flimsy testing protocols in Mexico had overestimated the virus's virulence. The rest of the media and most New Yorkers remained blasé until May 16, when an assistant school principal, Mitchell Weiner, became the first New Yorker to die of the virus. His death became the Rock Hudson moment: a dozen public schools in Queens closed, more flu stories were assigned, and their tone became more alarmist. Colleagues stopped by my desk to express their outrage at their pediatricians' refusals to prescribe Tamiflu prophylactically for their children. I would point out that the CDC publicly opposed that because it would create shortages for hospitalized patients. "Yeah, but now we're talking about *my* kids," one of my colleagues retorted.

An outbreak closed Horace Mann, an exclusive private school, generating more headlines. Then the situation calmed; the end of school and warm summer weather slowed down cases. Our coverage became less intense. I offered to go to Australia, South Africa, or Argentina to track the virus through the Southern Hemisphere winter, which could predict what would happen in the fall. But the 2009 "Great Recession" had the *Times* struggling financially. Travel budgets for many departments had been cut to near zero. I was told to make do with phone calls and stringers.

There were summer camp outbreaks, which briefly put the story back on page 1. We were covering the pandemic largely as it affected our wealthy New York readers. Work on a vaccine was under way and since flu vaccine production lines were well established, it was expected by fall.

Then August provided a perfect example of how mismatched imperatives can knock coverage cockeyed.

In midsummer, the President's Council of Advisors on Science and Technology had drafted a report. Its conclusion was alarming: it predicted that, when the virus returned in the fall, it could kill up to 90,000 Americans—three times as many as seasonal flu normally killed. Most, it warned, would be children and young adults.

But it was released in an odd, under-the-radar fashion. Dozens of science reporters, myself included, had been invited to CDC headquarters in Atlanta for a two-day seminar on influenza, something the agency had never done before. After a day of technical presentations, we were addressed by Kathleen Sebelius, the secretary of health and human services, and Dr. Thomas R. Frieden, then the new CDC director. As Secretary Sebelius spoke, a brief summary of the council's report was handed out—but it was slipped into a large pile of other press material. Neither of them referred to it. Their tone was not at all ominous; at one point, she joked about handkerchiefs coming back into fashion. They did express real frustration at polls saying most Americans did not plan to get flu shots. In the Q&A session, when they were asked how many deaths they expected in the fall, all they said was, "Some Americans will die." That vague response was the standard CDC line.

Since I was busy taking notes, I didn't read all the press material until after the meeting ended, by which time the secretary and her entourage had left. I found the summary mentioning 90,000 deaths buried on page 3 and was shocked. I went to a CDC media person to ask about it. He sidestepped. "That's not our document," he said. "It's from the President's Advisory Council. We don't have anything to do with it."

"Why did you hand it out then?"

"Just as a courtesy."

"Well, the CDC advises the president," I said. "This estimate seems wacky to me. Does the CDC believe it? This is August 24. Why is the report dated August 7?"

"I don't know. You'll have to ask the White House."

In that week, the president was on vacation in Martha's Vineyard. I was a medical reporter with no White House sources, sitting in Atlanta without even my list of contacts. This is going to sound pathetic, but I didn't own an iPhone then; my contacts list was a pile of paper that ran to over one hundred pages and, since I was expecting a boring seminar, not a big story, I'd neglected to pack a copy.

I didn't believe the 90,000 number. From everything we'd seen all summer, the virus didn't look that lethal. But I knew no one authoritative to ask who might conceivably have read the council's report. I didn't even have the report, just a press release mentioning it. I was also afraid that, if I told my editors, they'd get overexcited, as they always did about everything out of the White House. They'd tell me to write it up, I wouldn't be able to find anyone to say it was off base, and I'd be guilty of spreading panic.

In retrospect, I should have stayed up all night trying to get a copy and find epidemiologists to read it to, but it was late and I felt stuck. In those days, if you filed anything after about eight o'clock, they either tore up the front page if it was huge news or buried a six-inch version. I decided to pocket the thing, hope no other journalist at the seminar had noticed it, and work on it the next day, demanding that CDC epidemiologists tell me what they thought.

Of course, I should have known what would happen. The full report had already been leaked to *The Washington Post* and *USA Today*. (The council's media rep was a former *Post* reporter.) Their front pages the next day both had headlines predicting 90,000 dead.

My editor called me early, demanding, "Why didn't you have this?" The executive editor, she said, was furious that we'd been scooped and wanted to know why. When our night editors had seen the *Post* story, they had shoehorned a brief Associated Press rewrite of it into late editions.

I did have it, I said, but I didn't believe it. It couldn't possibly be right—but I couldn't prove that yet.

"Well, you've got to file something as soon as possible."

I spent the day in the halls of the CDC on my flip phone, trying to track down scientists, trying to get landline numbers for their vacation homes. I finally reached one of the chief authors, Dr. Marc Lipsitch, a prominent Harvard epidemiologist. He no longer stood by the report, he said. The White House had sat on it for so long that new data from South America had shown that the mortality rate was far lower than it first appeared. The 90,000 figure was unrealistic. The CDC finally let their top experts speak. They also agreed that 90,000 dead was highly unlikely.

Now I was angry. What was the plan? I asked: to slip an alarmist report to gullible reporters so they'd spread enough panic to make reluctant Americans get flu shots?

The CDC denied that, of course—but they couldn't explain why the report had been delayed, why it hadn't been fixed, and why it had been buried in their press material. It was a White House report, they repeated.

Suddenly my cell phone rang, and it was a White House press aide. She was unbelievably rude—nearly screaming at me, saying she knew what I was writing, and it was a lie. Clearly someone had passed on my questions.

"You don't know what I'm writing," I said. "*I* don't know what I'm writing yet. I'm still reporting."

"I know what angle you're pursuing," she shot back. "And it's a lie!"

"This is called reporting. I ask questions. I decide what to write when I think I know the answers."

"I'm going to call your boss!"

I really detest that kind of intimidation—which I heard from colleagues was quite common from the Obama White House under Chief of Staff Rahm Emanuel. "So call my boss," I said. "This'll be interesting."

I wrote and filed my story and headed for the airport. On the way, I got two phone calls, each from a higher level of White House attaché. Each pressed me—albeit more politely—to reveal what my story would say.

But, since I wasn't a White House reporter and didn't have to make nice with them, I told them I was furious at their bullying colleague, and they could read my story in the morning, like everyone else.

The headline on my story was "Agency Urges Caution on Estimates of Swine Flu." No one stood by the 90,000 figure. Since I had no evidence, I left out the possibility that they were trying to boost vaccine uptake. And, since it was a day late, the *Times* buried it on page 12.

One day later, the *Columbia Journalism Review* lambasted most of the media for posting "90,000 Will Die" stories. Their item ended: "A tip o' the hat goes to *New York Times* science reporter Donald G. McNeil Jr. who, on Wednesday, clarified the record and subtly chastised the media for its sensational coverage."

I showed it to my editor.

"Yeah, fine," she said. "You still should have filed the day before."

By the following spring, when the pandemic was over, only about 11,000 Americans had died.

Far more serious errors occur when sources deliberately deceive reporters. In late July 2023, this book was almost in print when I learned, from emails and Slack chats leaked by the Congressional Subcommittee on the Coronavirus Pandemic and posted on *Public*, a Substack magazine, that I was the victim of deception in the pandemic's earliest days. In February 2020, four eminent scientists whom I respected had discussed with each other various ways to throw me off the track when I asked whether it was possible that the virus had been manipulated in a lab or might have leaked from one. Their efforts affected how I viewed the controversy over Covid's origins and how the *Times* covered it. My publisher allowed me to quickly rewrite this chapter. (By the time it appears, more facts may have emerged.)

Even now, I do not pretend to be certain whether the virus jumped to humans from an animal in the Huanan Seafood Market or a culture in a Wuhan lab. Strong arguments have been made for both sides. I have always leaned toward zoonotic spillover, for a simple reason: As was true in almost every outbreak I've covered, it was first spotted by hospital doctors with every incentive to raise alarms and none to cover it up. They were sure the market was the epicenter. If it had leaked in a lab, there should have been a detectable surge among lab workers and their families, as happened in previous lab leaks. Beijing presumably knows the answer, but I fear this is doomed to be one of those long-unsettled questions like "Was Cuba behind JFK's assassination?" or "Was Alger Hiss a Soviet spy?" that will be answered only when an authoritarian state opens its archives—something I don't expect in my lifetime.

Almost as soon as the virus appeared, conspiracy-oriented websites claimed it was a bioweapon. The first such article I found was on January 26 in *The Washington Times*, a newspaper founded by the Unification Church. The only evidence it cited was that the outbreak occurred in the same city as the Wuhan Institute of Virology. It quoted an Israeli bioterrorism expert saying the lab did bioweapons research and a leak was "possible." I phoned him, and he said he was not misquoted, but it was only *possible*—he did not claim it had happened. (Such suspicions seemed logical. As the comedian Jon Stewart later put it: If there was "an outbreak of chocolatey goodness" near Hershey, Pennsylvania, would you first suspect that a steam shovel had mated with a cocoa bean? Or would you suspect the chocolate factory?) Meanwhile, other rumors were whirling. Unreviewed papers posted on preprint servers claimed the virus had originated in snakes or had HIV genes. Chinese labs were accused of selling their dead animals as food. We science reporters were frantically rushing to confirm or debunk each one.

What I did not know at the time was that some of the world's leading evolutionary virologists, including Kristian G. Andersen of Scripps

Research, Edward C. Holmes of the University of Sydney, Robert F. Garry Jr. of Tulane University, and Andrew Rambaut of the University of Edinburgh, suspected the virus had been manipulated in a lab. It had features that seemed rare in SARS-like coronaviruses, making it "loaded for human transmission," as Dr. Holmes observed in the February 2020 Slack chats. Most worrying was that it had a cleavage site that attached to furin, a protein in human cells that viruses use to "cleave" or split open to inject their genetic instructions.

On February 1, a conference call to discuss their fears was convened by Dr. Jeremy Farrar, director of Britain's Wellcome Trust, which is the British equivalent of the Bill & Melinda Gates Foundation. Drs. Anthony S. Fauci and Francis Collins of the National Institutes of Health sat in; Dr. Fauci asked the virologists to write a paper reflecting their thoughts. (That conference call and the emails were revealed starting in late 2022 when investigative reporters used the Freedom of Information Act to get progressively less redacted versions of the records of Drs. Fauci and Collins. The long silence about that important discussion has hurt the credibility of everyone involved.)

On February 3, 2020, in the middle of this maelstrom of speculation, the Wuhan Institute posted a surprising paper: among its frozen samples it had identified a bat coronavirus named RaTG13 that was 96 percent identical to SARS-CoV-2. The paper's point was to suggest that the pandemic virus had come from bats, but conspiracy theorists pounced on it as evidence that the lab had cooked up the virus.

Virologists publicly pooh-poohed that conclusion, saying it would take at least forty years of natural evolution to create a four percent difference in a virus 30,000 base pairs long. However, the emails and Slack chats released in July 2023 showed that Dr. Andersen and his colleagues initially had exactly the same fears: that Chinese scientists could have mutated something resembling RaTG13 into SARS-CoV-2 by adding a furin cleavage site and growing it in cultures of human cells or mice with "humanized" immune systems to evolve a spike protein that attached to human receptors. "The lab escape version of this is so friggin' likely to have happened because they were already doing this type of work and the molecular data is fully consistent with that scenario," Dr. Andersen wrote. They even joked that Predict, a government-funded program to detect dangerous viruses, might have started the pandemic. But they hesitated to reveal their suspicions. Dr. Rambaut suggested "limited dissemination."

I left the paper on March 1, 2021, and have not had access to my *Times* emails since. My memories of who said what in early 2020 have faded. But the leaked Slack chats show that on February 6, I emailed Drs. Andersen and Rambaut—each of whom I had interviewed for previous stories. I was "trying to check out a rumor that an editor got from a government source—that the U.S. government is trying to seriously investigate the possibility that the nCoV came out of the Wuhan Virus laboratory rather than out of a wet market." Although the rumors included "silly conspiracy theories," I wrote, was there any way to tell if a virus had been manipulated by human hands, such as sequences from other viruses inserted or unexpected deletions?

The virologists shared my emails on Slack. (Jon Cohen of *Science* magazine was also "sniffing around," one wrote.) After debating how to reply, they agreed on answers that were technically accurate but omitted all mention of their own fears. "McNeil very credible but like any reporter can be mislead [*sic*]," Dr. Garry wrote. "Don . . . pretty much nailed it," Dr. Andersen added. "Let's not tell him."

The rumors, they replied, were "demonstratively false—we would have been able to easily pick that up if that were the case, however it is not." They left out any mention of their suspicions about the furin site, the possibility that the virus's evolution had been sped up, or that they knew the Wuhan lab had done such work.

On February 16, along with W. Ian Lipkin of Columbia University, who was not on the Slack channel, they posted their paper, "The Proximal Origin of SARS-CoV-2" on the forum virological.org. Their analysis, they said, "clearly shows that SARS-CoV-2 is not a laboratory construct or a purposefully manipulated virus."

It was a tough read for any non-geneticist, including me. I began drafting an effort to turn it into plain English and interviewing other scientists to explain why most favored zoonotic spillover.

If I remember correctly, I interviewed or emailed Richard H. Ebright of Rutgers University, Stanley Perlman of the University of Iowa, Trevor Bedford of the Fred Hutch Cancer Center, Pardis Sabeti of the Broad Institute, and Peter Daszak of the EcoHealth Alliance. (I didn't yet know how involved EcoHealth was with the Wuhan Institute.)

On February 19, when I again wrote to Dr. Andersen saying I'd been asked to write a narrative of how the rumor started, he not only put me off, saying he had "nothing to add," but also boasted to the others that his reply "includes humor to deflect the fact that I'm dismissing him." He even added what he called a "very deliberate" smiley face.

Why do that? Why not admit that they initially feared a lab leak? The 140-page-long Slack conversation suggests three motives: 1) At first they truly were unsure whether the virus had been manipulated. 2) They were reluctant to give ammunition to critics like Dr. Ebright, who, Dr. Garry wrote, thought scientists who did research into making dangerous viruses even more transmissible "should be locked up." 3) They feared what Dr. Rambaut called "the shit show that would happen if anyone serious accused the Chinese of even accidental release." In the absence of proof either way, they decided to be "content with ascribing it to natural processes." Dr. Andersen said he "hated when politics is injected into science—but it's impossible not to."

In the ensuing months, as more SARS-CoV-2-like features were found in wild viruses, they became surer they were right. Nonetheless, I feel they clearly misled me early on. In August 2023, as I rewrote this chapter, I sent a draft of it to all four scientists, seeking a response. Dr. Andersen replied and repeatedly denied having misled me. He described their answers as "accurate and specific." It would have been "reckless" to tell me that they were "speculating on still-changing early hypotheses," he wrote. I did not find his answer persuasive, since the Slack chats suggest that, as of

February 6, their suspicions about viral engineering were still very much alive. But readers can read the emails and chats for themselves.

I'm disappointed, both in them and in myself, that I was so easily taken in. On the other hand, it's one thing to be lied to by a politician and fail to check it out. But on viral evolution, to whom do you go for a second opinion? At their level, there are precious few experts. If Albert Einstein assured you that nuclear fission is harmless, whom would you trust to quote saying, "Einstein's dead wrong?"

I worked on the origins story intermittently from February to April. It was then no one's top priority because the pandemic was raging in New York and I was reporting the long "predict the future" articles I had been assigned. Its tentative headline was "New Coronavirus Is 'Clearly Not a Lab Leak,' Scientists Say." It outlined many reasons: Previous outbreaks like SARS were zoonotic spillovers. Coronaviruses with furin cleavage sites and pangolin viruses with a similar spike had been found, meaning both anomalies existed in nature and might be in some mystery animal. After the market was hosed down, SARS-CoV-2 was found in swabs taken from the wild-animal section, including from floors, drains, and sewers—places where coughing humans would not have deposited virus, but the sloshed-around blood of a butchered animal would. The "Proximal Origins" paper argued that the new virus's spike was so unlike those of SARS or MERS that any lab hunting for a candidate to test for an affinity for human cells would not have chosen it to experiment on. Also, the virus was studded with glycans, sugar-like molecules that act as shields against antibodies; shields would more likely appear if the virus evolved inside an animal with an antibody-producing immune system, not in a lab.

My story never ran, for two reasons: Inside the *Times*, we had a fierce debate. Washington-based national security reporters had sources insisting it *was* a lab leak. But their sources were anonymous, offered zero evidence other than "take our word for it," and, to me, seemed clearly part of the Trump administration's campaign to blame China instead of admitting its own failures. (With one exception: a science colleague had a non-administration source—also anonymous—who knew the Wuhan lab and felt its safety procedures were shoddy.)

My sources, by contrast, were respected scientists, spoke on the record, and laid out their arguments in exhaustive detail. They seemed more credible. The other reason it never ran was that it was four thousand words long and full of jargon like "polybasic cleavage site" and "RNA-dependent RNA polymerase gene." My overtaxed editors just didn't want to struggle with it.

At some point—probably in early April—my Washington colleagues drafted an article quoting their anonymous sources. They were shown my draft; they reduced my detailed arguments to two short "Some scientists disagree . . ." paragraphs. When I was allowed to see their draft, hours before it was to be published, I exploded. I wrote a note accusing them of downplaying my reporting because it had "too many big words." I was told off for my tone, but their article was held. I can only surmise that their sources then went to Fox News, which soon ran something similar.

Had I known that the "Proximal Origins" authors initially suspected a lab leak, would my approach have been different? Of course. Did my ignorance—and my insistent advocacy—tip the balance of *Times* coverage away from the lab-leak theory? I don't know because I don't attend Page One meetings, but it probably contributed to what happened next: the *Times* essentially dropped the topic for a year. It seemed decided, and we had other priorities: the battles over lockdowns and masks, the prospect of 100,000 deaths, Mr. Trump's own bout with Covid, the vaccines—and, eventually, of course, the presidential election and the January 6 Capitol takeover.

Over the course of the next year, however, important facts emerged. No close SARS-CoV-2 ancestor was found in wild or domestic animals. Other scientists noted what the "Proximal Origins" authors played down: the virus seemed remarkably well adapted to humans, suggesting lab engineering. *The Wall Street Journal*, citing anonymous sources, reported that three Wuhan researchers fell seriously ill in November 2019. It later turned out, however, that the State Department suspected they might just have had "common seasonal illnesses." In June 2023, another outlet, again citing anonymous sources, published what it claimed were the researchers' names. They denied having been sick in 2019, denied working with live viruses, and said antibody tests done in March 2020 showed they had not had Covid.

Bizarrely, China repeatedly behaved as if it had something to hide. It hampered a WHO investigation and insisted its report play down the possibility of a lab leak. It removed genetic sequences from public databases. It also raised silly red herrings, including the ideas that the virus reached China in frozen seafood or was unleashed in Wuhan by the American military during the "Military World Games."

Most important in my eyes was this: Internet sleuths translating obscure papers from Chinese virology journals had shown that RaTG13 was identical to a virus previously known as Bat Coronavirus 4991. Virus 4991 had been found in a cave where miners digging bat guano in 2012 had died of what appeared to be viral pneumonia. The Wuhan lab, investigating the deaths, had sequenced Virus 4991 and dubbed it "SARS-like." Those revelations undercut a crucial premise of the "Proximal Origins" paper. They showed that the lab suspected 4991 could kill humans, even though it did not superficially resemble SARS or MERS. So it actually *had been* a good candidate for genetic manipulation. In February 2020, when it first described RaTG13, the lab had omitted that important information. (The new name, it said, was just for convenience, and stood for "*Rhinolophus affinis* bat, Tong Guan Cave, 2013.")

It was also revealed that the lab's coronavirus chief, Shi Zhengli—regarded with awe as "Bat Woman" for her prowess at sampling bats in dangerous caves—had years of practice in making "chimera" viruses by splicing new spikes onto viral backbones to produce variants that could infect human cells. She had learned in an American lab to do that without leaving traces. All this circumstantial evidence suggested that her lab—or another, perhaps even a military one she could not control—*might* have made chimeras using virus 4991 as a backbone and then grown them in human cells or humanized mice.

In an interview with *Scientific American* published June 1, 2020, Dr. Shi said that, on December 30, 2019, when she was ordered to leave a conference in Shanghai and return to Wuhan to help analyze the new virus, her first fear was that it had come from her lab. She went through years of records to reassure herself that it had not. "That really took a load off my mind," she said. "I had not slept a wink for days." In a June 2021 interview in *The New York Times*, she reiterated that her lab had done no work that could have led to SARS-CoV-2. In a 2022 article, she said the whole virus 4991 sample had been used up in 2018.

Much depends on whether one believes Dr. Shi. Her American and British collaborators praised her as an imaginative and forthright scientist trained in the West. Wang Linfa, a virologist at the Duke-NUS Medical School in Singapore, told the BBC he visited Dr. Shi's lab in January 2020 as it was investigating the new pneumonia; its researchers had acted normally, making plans for dinners and karaoke nights, which made him feel there was "zero chance" they feared it had leaked inside. Dr. Shi has repeatedly expressed her fury at the accusations and blames anti-China bigotry. But she is also presumably under intense pressure to not undermine her government's narrative of blamelessness.

On May 17, 2021, two months after leaving the *Times*, I published an article on Medium titled "How I Learned to Stop Worrying and Love the Lab-Leak Theory." It was a play on the subtitle of the movie *Dr. Strangelove*, but a poor choice because it implied that I believed the theory. I was really arguing that it was time to stop dismissing it as crackpot nonsense and to press China to open its records. It appeared shortly after a similar article by Nicholas Wade, another retired *Times* science writer, and just as eighteen prominent scientists published a letter in *Science* titled "Investigate the Origins of Covid-19." Ten days later, the Biden administration ordered the country's intelligence agencies to do so. They reached widely divergent conclusions, which they mostly rated as "low confidence." If they found new evidence, they have not, as of this writing, shared it publicly.

In September 2021, viruses even closer to SARS-CoV-2 than RaTG13 were found in Laos. Since then, scientific detective work, much of it led by Michael Worobey of the University of Arizona, has powerfully bolstered the case for a market jump. He debunked reports that early cases had no market connections; the first was probably a seafood vendor infected on December 10; the previous "patient zero" had been hospitalized December 8, but for dental surgery; his respiratory symptoms did not begin until the 16th. Dr. Worobey and his collaborators showed that most of the positive market samples were near a single stall and from equipment used to strip fur and feathers from butchered animals. Photographs taken in 2014 had shown raccoon dogs and other exotics for sale at that stall. They further argued that a second variant circulated briefly in the market, implying two animal-human jumps. If true, that would be a dagger in the heart of the lab-leak theory, but not every virologist agrees that both variants—which barely differ—emerged inside the market instead of arriving later in infected humans. In March 2023, it was reported that some market swabs contained raccoon dog DNA. Those foxlike animals, bred on wildlife farms in China, are known to harbor SARS-like viruses.

As of this writing, in August 2023, the debate is a stalemate. Neither side has dispositive proof. If Beijing does, it is not saying so. In this country, adherents of both sides keep hurling mud. Science journalists are caught in the middle—even editors not committed to either side for partisan reasons keep demanding to know which explanation is most likely so they can assign analyses of which political candidates benefit. Under such pressures, a science reporter finds it nearly impossible to remain objective. If he commits either way and new evidence proves him wrong, he looks foolish. Worse, he will be accused of carrying water for that side. If both sides are willing to lie or mislead journalists, embarrassing errors become inevitable. And the truth never comes out.

Chapter Seventeen

THE CRISES OF TRUST AND FETISHIZATION OF SCIENCE

If the first casualty of war is truth, then the first casualty of pandemics is trust. Trust in political leaders, trust in doctors, trust in the pharmaceutical industry, trust in science. "Trust," as Dr. Frieden, the former CDC director, has observed, "cannot be surged." It must exist beforehand.

In a way, trust is anathema to democracy. We form democratic governments so we can remove from power leaders in whom we've lost faith. However, you cannot fight a pandemic without it.

Two things kill trust: Blatant ineptitude. And a history of untrustworthy behavior.

Initially, ineptitude is almost unavoidable. Health officials are often confused but desperate to be perceived as doing something, so they do *something*.

For example, when Zika threatened Brazil's major cities, the president sent in the army. Pictures of soldiers fogging residential neighborhoods filled TV news. Locals, seeing clouds of insecticide coming, rushed to shut their windows.

Did it help? Probably not. To the extent that any army is trained to fight mosquitoes, it's usually trained for jungle warfare. But the *Aedes aegypti* mosquitoes that spread Zika are an urban species. They lay eggs in flowerpots and pet bowls and follow the carbon dioxide plumes of human breath right into homes. The street fogging, entomologists said, probably just drove more mosquitoes indoors. It was hygiene theater.

During the Spanish flu epidemic, police were ordered to enforce laws against spitting. Sidewalk phlegm did not actually transmit flu, but viruses were unknown until the 1930s because they were too small to be seen with a microscope. In 1918, the prevailing wisdom was that influenza was caused by a rod-shaped bacterium known as Pfeiffer's bacillus, which had been found in the lungs of some victims of a deadly 1899 respiratory disease outbreak. (The bacterium is now named *Haemophilus influenzae*, a misnomer since it doesn't cause influenza, and it was probably a coincidence that it was in the 1899 lung samples.) Nonetheless, since it could be detected in sputum, spitting became a crime.

Covid saw its share of hygiene theater. Before it was known that most transmission was by aerosols, we spent months sanitizing surfaces and wiping groceries with bleach. I was partly responsible for that because I repeated the early conventional wisdom that "fomite" transmission from surfaces was important. On the March 12, 2020, episode of *The Daily* podcast, I described using hand sanitizer and hydrogen peroxide spray and riding subways wearing one garden glove "like an aging, completely unfunky white Michael Jackson imitator." My precautions had no particular downside, but we later learned that a mask would have been better.

In Chinese cities, teams kept spraying disinfectant clouds for three years. Doing so was hygiene theater, but China experts said local officials kept it up to prove their loyalty to President Xi Jinping's zero Covid goal.

Hygiene theatrics are common during early pandemic responses and are innocent mistakes. But they gave some American populists the excuse to shout, "See? Scientists lied!" That shook confidence in all science.

There is also a flip side to rejecting science. Some people fetishize it, mastering arcane details and becoming zealots. They are as enraged by nonenforcement as rejectionists are by enforcement, which makes for very unhappy populaces.

In the first lockdown of spring 2020, some governors mired in denialism rejected all protective measures. Others, notably California's Gavin Newsom, went further than was necessary. Closing beaches, parks, golf courses, and other outdoor venues for weeks made no scientific sense. Early data from China suggested that outdoor transmission hardly existed. In a study of 7,324 early cases, contact-tracers found only a single instance of transmission outdoors, during a long conversation between two neighbors. Later studies in Ireland and in England confirmed that the risk might be as low as 1 in 1,000 infections.

The risky aspects of opening parks and beaches—such as the potential for crowding in bathrooms or restaurants—could have been managed. The benefits of outdoor recreation far outweighed those risks.

Masks, to my mind, were completely misunderstood—and still are.

Most Americans still assume the primary reason to wear one is to protect oneself. That's incorrect. Masks are much better at keeping aerosolized particles *in* than at keeping them *out*. The best reason to wear one is to make sure the one or two potential superspreaders in the room are wearing one. Since you can't detect the superspreader (it might even be you), everyone must wear one so the superspreader inevitably has one on. Of course, they must be worn so all wearers actually inhale and exhale through the fabric; masks that are too thin or too loose or worn under the chin do nothing.

During the pandemic, as "mask science" burgeoned into a field of study, the debate grew ever more arcane. Hundreds of articles appeared: N95s versus KN95s versus KF94s versus surgical masks, cloth masks, vented masks, gaiters; single-masking versus double-masking; and so on. Average Americans became knowledgeable about the electrostatic charges and nonparallel weaves in fibers. They fretted about fakes. (In 2020 and 2021, the CDC estimated that 60 percent of the N95s it inspected were counterfeit.) TV anchors conducted endless interviews on the subject.

In the streets, a cadre of self-appointed mask police arose, using their "I'm following the science" mantra to bully others.

During the spring 2020 lockdown, whenever I went out for walks, I scrupulously stayed far from others. On the wide sidewalks of my girlfriend's Manhattan neighborhood, I would swing out in an arc if anyone approached, even stepping into the gutter if I had to. On the narrower streets near my Brooklyn brownstone, I walked in the bike lane, keeping parked cars between me and others.

It didn't matter. A masked guy alone in his car leaned out and shouted, "Get a mask, jerk!" As I passed two men chatting in a doorway, even though I was more than ten feet away, one turned and shouted a warning to the whole block: "No mask! No mask! Selfish guy!"

One of my Brooklyn neighbors stopped me on the street and—from a distance—told me my appearances on *The Daily* and interviews with Rachel Maddow, Christiane Amanpour, and Fareed Zakaria had rendered me a known quantity on our block (rather than just the guy with the bright red door, twisty vines, and exsanguinary Halloween décor). But some neighbors, she said, were unhappy. "People have noticed that you don't wear a mask."

"I don't need to," I said. "I'm outdoors. I stay six feet away from everyone."

"They think you should set an example."

"I *am* setting an example," I said. "I'm following the science. And the law." (On March 20, 2020, Governor Andrew Cuomo had issued an executive order listing precautions that New Yorkers should take, one of which was staying six feet from others.)

"Yes, well . . ." she said, clearly unconvinced and unhappy.

The mask obsession became a visual badge of people's fears and then of their politics. Even three years into the pandemic, I could not go out for a walk in New York or in my hometown, San Francisco, without seeing people wearing N95s while alone outdoors, far from any possible source of infection. In Idaho or Montana or anywhere else I went fishing, however, I could go for days without seeing one, indoors or out.

The stubbornness of such beliefs could overwhelm common sense. In the fall of 2021, I stood for about an hour at the corner of Second Avenue and 96th Street waiting for a friend to pick me up for an out-of-town trip. To pass the time, I counted how many riders racing south in the avenue's bicycle lane were wearing masks versus how many wore helmets. More than half were masked; less than a third had helmets on. This is madness, I thought—a complete failure to perceive relative risks. The chances of catching Covid while flying along on a bicycle at 20 miles an hour were almost zero. But riding in Manhattan meant constant close calls with car doors, careless pedestrians, and other bicyclists, and the lane itself was a gauntlet of curbs, cars, light poles, and other hard objects to strike your head against. I always wore a helmet.

Covid testing became an even more fertile ground for fetishization.

In the first year, most testing was in hospitals or doctor's offices. By late 2021, though, that changed. PCR swabbing could be done in a walk-in clinic or even a sidewalk tent, with results within twenty-four hours. Rapid antigen tests came in home kits.

Very few Americans understood the science, but many began talking as if they were experts. That contributed to the spread of the Omicron variant.

For correct diagnosis of seriously ill cases, PCR testing is essential, of course.

But using tests for prevention was different. Most experts agreed that rapid tests were better for that. When they were positive—but *only* when they were positive—rapid tests were almost 99 percent accurate. It took lots of virus in the nasopharynx—where the swab touched—to get a positive. So a roomful of people who had all just tested negative on rapid tests was likely to be safe, albeit *for just a few hours.* But that was enough time to hold a meeting, a wedding, or a family dinner. Even infected people who did not test positive—yet—probably did not yet have enough virus in their nose and throat to be spewing it. Germany used frequent rapid testing to make schools and other indoor spaces safer.

However, because the media ignored rapid tests for many months and kept referring to PCR tests as "the gold standard," many Americans believed they absolutely had to get PCR-tested. To get one, they would wait for hours in frigid weather with other Covid sufferers or inside clinics crowded with them—a sure way to get infected.

Also, people wrongly assumed that negative tests were accurate. I heard regularly from friends who had recently been exposed and had what to me sounded very much like Covid symptoms. But they would get one negative test, assume it had been infallible, and resume their lives, probably infecting others.

Medical students are taught that "a negative test yields *no* information," said Dr. William Schaffner, an expert in preventive medicine at the Vanderbilt University School of Medicine.

A positive test confirms a diagnosis. A negative may mean that the person tested is healthy, or that the swabbing was bungled, or that the virus hadn't yet reached the swabbed area, or that a lab technician messed up. A clinician seeing a patient with obvious symptoms but a negative test may simply order a second test.

People also misunderstood that PCR tests could multiply tiny fragments of broken virus and come up positive for weeks. Some stayed isolated for no reason.

The second reason for a failure to establish trust, as I mentioned, is a long history of distrust.

Sadly, the history of public health is filled with examples. The most infamous is the Tuskegee scandal. In 1932, the U.S. Public Health Service and the Tuskegee Institute in Alabama began a study of how syphilis affected the human body. It enrolled 600 black men, two-thirds of whom had syphilis. Most were poorly educated sharecroppers; informed consent was not collected. They were told they were being treated for "bad blood," a local term that could describe many ills.

In return for enrolling, the men got free medical exams, some meals, burial insurance, and a few other benefits. But in the 1940s, when penicillin was shown to cure syphilis, it was not offered to them. Instead, study leaders made the appalling ethical choice to follow the men until death, so they could do autopsies to see exactly how syphilis killed. They even asked local doctors to not treat men in the study. Only in 1972, when a horrified doctor leaked word to an Associated Press reporter, was the study's existence revealed. It ended abruptly, and a congressional investigation ensued. A fund for the survivors and their widows was created, and President Clinton offered a public apology in 1997.

But the damage was done. Many black Americans lost faith in the medical system. When Covid vaccines were rolled out in 2021, resistance was initially very high among black men. When doctors asked why, they often got a one-word response: "Tuskegee."

It is hardly the only egregious example in U.S. history.

In 1916, a terrifying polio outbreak began in what was then a fringe neighborhood of Brooklyn where the city's paved streets ended and Long Island's farms and estates began. Now known as the Gowanus section, it was then a largely Italian shantytown known as "Pigtown"—because it was near the city's garbage dump, where pigs, dogs, and goats rooted.

The city's first moves were to isolate and publicly shame the victims.

Orange placards with the legend POLIOMYELITIS were nailed to front doors. The small print said the inhabitants had been fined $25 for failing to report an infectious disease. No one could leave the house without a health officer's permission.

Then it got worse. City nurses accompanied by police officers forcibly removed babies and children from their families. They were taken to public hospitals for treatment—but the treatments then in vogue were worthless or even sadistic. Children were immobilized in casts until their muscles atrophied. Their legs were "oxygenated" with jolts of electricity. Some were bathed in almond meal; others were wrapped in plasters infused with mustard, chamomile, or arnica. They might be fed caffeine, kola nut juice, quinine, gold salts, or water laced with radium. Some were injected with adrenaline, the disinfectant hexamethylamine, tetanus toxin, and even strychnine.

Needless to say, none of these treatments worked and 2,000 New York City children died. With parents forbidden to visit the hospitals, many died alone. Some survivors were discharged weaker or more paralyzed than when they entered.

In the end, the forcible removals stopped only after the Black Hand—forerunner of the Italian Mafia—publicly threatened to kill a city nurse known for seizing babies.

Given such histories, it's hard to put one's finger on how a government creates trust.

If Covid vaccine acceptance rates are a guide, for example, one ends up with a dichotomy. Some democracies did quite well at convincing their citizens to take vaccines: Australia, New Zealand, the Scandinavian countries, Canada, Portugal, Chile, and Argentina. But so did some autocracies, including Cuba, Vietnam, and the United Arab Emirates. Some democracies, by contrast, did poorly—the United States, for example, did worse than most of Western Europe and Japan. We were down on a par with Saudi Arabia and Iran. But the autocracies of the former Soviet Union—Russia and most of Eastern Europe—did even worse than we did.

The defining factor in vaccine acceptance seemed to be whether citizens trusted their governments *on health issues*. Cuba may jail political dissidents, but it gives its citizens health care. The United States has free speech but leaves millions uninsured. And trust in our pharmaceutical industry is especially low because it charges Americans the world's highest drug prices while its lobbyists stop Congress from fighting back.

While it can take generations to build trust, it can be dissipated almost overnight, as Brazil and Russia showed.

Not long ago, both Brazil and the former Soviet Union had vaccine-acceptance rates over 90 percent.

In the 1960s, the Soviet government championed vaccines and advocated global smallpox eradication. But the economic crisis that followed the Soviet Union's collapse was so deep that vaccination fell apart. The state-owned measles vaccine factory closed; that disease and even diphtheria returned briefly. Trust in government declined even further during the oligarch age. In 2020, Russian scientists created a Covid vaccine, but

Vladimir Putin, eager to beat the West, named it "Sputnik" after the first satellite in space and released it before Phase III testing was finished. Many Russians avoided it.

Brazil for decades had its own vaccine industry, no anti-vaccine movement, and averaged 98 percent acceptance rates. That was shaken by President Jair Bolsonaro, who claimed that Covid vaccines could transmit AIDS and turn people into alligators. After his health minister and some doctors echoed him, vaccination rates for all diseases fell off. Polio immunization, for example, fell to 68 percent.

Building trust where it is nonexistent is one of the hardest things public health officials can do. One rare success story was the long fight against Ebola in Africa.

Since the disease was discovered in 1976, there have been more than 25 outbreaks in 8 countries. One obstacle to success has been constant: families would not bring sick relatives to treatment centers until it was too late to save them. In a few instances, they have not only hidden relatives but have also attacked and even killed medical teams trying to find them.

Why? Because for decades most people who went into the treatment units died. Until 2019, the death rate sometimes exceeded 50 percent, only marginally better than the survival rate for people who stayed home. In the 2013–16 West African outbreak, more than 28,000 people were infected, and 11,300 of them died, despite the huge international response that outbreak triggered.

Without a cure, there was just supportive care: fever-reducing drugs and rehydration to replace fluids lost to diarrhea. (Despite the stereotype of Ebola victims bleeding out, most die when the loss of fluids and electrolytes causes organ failure and cardiac arrest.)

Naturally, terrifying rumors spread. The most common was that patients were being murdered and dissected for their organs to be used for witchcraft. The longer frightened families delayed bringing in their sick, the higher the death rates inside the treatment centers grew, which just reinforced those rumors.

Also, because Ebola is so transmissible, families had to remain outside the temporary hospitals, staring at a collection of white tents staffed by what looked like space creatures: doctors and nurses in white overalls, hoods, masks, goggles, rubber gloves, rubber aprons, and rubber boots—just what you might wear if you were chopping up bodies.

To allay those fears, the medical teams tried to demystify the process. They taped pictures of themselves to their chests so patients could see what they really looked like. They hung clear polyurethane sides on the tents so families could see that their relatives were being cared for, not slaughtered. They created visiting areas by setting up rows of orange fencing a few feet apart so patients who were still ambulatory or recovering could go outside and talk to their families.

ALIMA, the Alliance for International Medical Action, invented the "Ebola cube," a sort of instant isolation unit. The patient was zipped into a soft plastic cube with a bed and supplies inside. Ports with long gloves were built into the walls so nurses could deliver some basic care without having to gown up. Families could safely sit near their loved ones and watch over them.

Burial practices also changed. Ebola corpses teem with virus, so in some outbreaks, they were quickly cremated or dropped into mass graves. That just fed the witchcraft rumors, so the policy was changed. Religious leaders were recruited to give mourners permission to forego the custom of washing the corpse and to pray from a safe distance rather than with hands on the body, as was the norm. When possible, gowned-up burial details would return bodies to their villages for proper funerals. The detail would handle the body bag and spray the surrounding ground with dilute bleach. At the last minute, the bag would be unzipped so that relatives could confirm that no organs had been stolen.

In 2019, two successful treatments for Ebola were finally developed: both were cocktails of monoclonal antibodies. (One was from Regeneron, which a year later developed a cocktail for Covid.) When patients were brought to treatment centers quickly, 90 percent survived.

At the announcement of that success, Dr. Jean-Jacques Muyembe, director of Congo's National Institute for Biomedical Research, predicted that it would change the future of the disease. Dr. Muyembe, one of the original discoverers of the virus, had pioneered the use of antibody-rich convalescent plasma as treatment, and from one batch of that plasma had isolated one of the monoclonal antibodies that worked.

"I'm a little sentimental—I'm very happy and I can't believe it," he said. "Up to now, people saw their relatives go to the treatment units and come out dead. Now that 90 percent can go in and come out cured, they will start believing it, and developing trust. The first ones to transmit this information will be the patients themselves."

At the same time, two Ebola vaccines that had taken decades to develop and test were finally deployed.

Four more Ebola outbreaks have occurred since then: one in Gabon and three in the Democratic Republic of the Congo. Each was brought under control within three or four months, and the number of confirmed cases was small: the biggest was 130 cases, the smallest just 11. (A fifth outbreak occurred in Uganda in late 2022; it infected 164 people, of whom 77 died. But it was of a rarer strain, "Ebola Sudan," for which there was then no vaccine or treatment.)

Slowly but surely, trust can be built. Ebola—one of the "diseases at the end of the road" that usually affects a broken nation's most marginalized and mistrustful people—may be headed for eradication one day.

One way to build trust is to encourage those who face the biggest threat to "take ownership" of possible solutions. The result may turn out to be quite different from the solutions originally offered by scientists.

For example, in Los Angeles starting in 1998, the porn film industry invented testing protocols to keep its actors and actresses safe from HIV. Condoms—the solution proposed by scientists—were considered not feasible because porn customers would not rent or buy films in which men wear them. They also caused chafing for actresses shooting long scenes with multiple men.

The protocols were tightened until performers were tested every fourteen days for HIV, syphilis, chlamydia, and gonorrhea. They got their results by email or cell phone text and showed them to their costars each day before shooting began. Producers had access to a password-protected site with no medical information other than a green check for "passed all tests." Between 2004 and 2012, the industry claimed, 350,000 sex scenes had been shot without a single case of HIV transmission on a set.

"Ownership" has also been effective with drug users, sex workers, and men engaged in high-risk sex.

In 2003, Vancouver, British Columbia, became the first city in North America to create a safe-injection site. It was run with the enthusiastic cooperation of provincial health officials, despite strong opposition from conservative national politicians. The medical staff came from the University of British Columbia's medical school, and a local association for addicts played an important advisory role.

The injection area resembled a theater dressing room: clients sat at a row of booths facing big mirrors. The mirrors allowed the staff nurses—who wore everyday clothes, not scrubs—to spot anyone passing out. They offered clean syringes, TB and HIV tests, as well as gynecological exams to female users who sold sex to support their habits. Upstairs, detox and methadone programs were available. In the next decade, there were more than 1,000 overdoses inside the center, but no deaths, because the nurses reacted quickly with oxygen and Narcan.

In Johannesburg, the Wits University medical school opened a free clinic for sex workers. For the sake of privacy, it had no permanent address, because the women said they could not be seen entering a known STD clinic because it would reveal what they did for a living. The doctors rented rooms in the same red-light-district hotels the women used. They held afternoon appointments because their clients worked nights and slept in. They offered child care and had a pediatrician on hand to see children. And they offered not just HIV-related services, but a full range of care.

In San Francisco, the city drove down new HIV cases by 90 percent.

Because much of the spread was driven by men with multiple partners in venues that facilitated anonymous sex, the staff of the San Francisco AIDS Foundation's Magnet Clinic wore "No Blame, No Shame" T-shirts and decorated the offices with penis-toy mobiles and posters saying things like: "How You Fuck Is Your Business. Your Health Is Ours."

"We have no stigma," said Pierre-Cédric Crouch, the clinic's nursing director. "You can come in saying you just slept with 20 guys and you don't know what a condom is, and we don't criticize you. We help you out."

In each case, trust was built by listening to the victims and trying novel ideas that worked for them—not solutions imposed by experts who were still fighting the last pandemic.

Part Four

SOME WAYS TO HEAD OFF FUTURE PANDEMICS

Chapter Eighteen

WE NEED A PENTAGON FOR DISEASE

We just survived the most lethal pandemic in a century. Now ask yourself: Who was in charge?

Ultimately, of course, it was Presidents Trump and Biden. But below them—who, exactly?

Was it Dr. Fauci, director of the National Institute of Allergy and Infectious Diseases? His boss, Dr. Francis S. Collins, director of the National Institutes of Health? Dr. Robert Redfield or Dr. Rochelle Walensky, directors of the CDC? Dr. Jerome Adams or Dr. Vivek Murthy, the surgeons general of the United States? Dr. Stephen Hahn or Dr. Janet Woodcock, the FDA commissioners?

Was it the cabinet member who was officially the boss of all of those above, Alex M. Azar II, the secretary of health and human services? His Biden administration successor? (Can you name his Biden administration successor?) Dr. Robert Kadlec, Mr. Azar's assistant secretary for preparedness and response? His Biden administration successor? (Can you name her?)

Vice President Mike Pence, who replaced Mr. Azar as head of the White House Coronavirus Task Force?

Dr. Deborah Birx or Dr. Scott Atlas or Jeffrey D. Zients or Andy Slavitt or Dr. Ashish Jha, all of whom, at different times, appeared at podiums representing the White House COVID-19 Response Team?

Dr. Brett Giroir, the "testing czar"? Moncef Slaoui or General Gustave F. Perna, the joint leaders of Operation Warp Speed?

The "Wolverines"—the secretive group of national security experts who began meeting as the pandemic began but whose existence was revealed only later?

Jared Kushner?

Throughout the worst pandemic of modern times, spanning two administrations, we had no clear sense of who was in command. We clearly lost the war in that we had the highest per capita death rate among developed nations. But, other than the presidents, we don't know whom to blame. Other than Operation Warp Speed, which did deliver highly effective vaccines in record time, we don't know who succeeded and who failed in his or her mission. For most of them, we were somewhat unsure what their missions were.

Imagine fighting a war like that. Any student of history can name great generals and successful operations, from Washington crossing the Delaware to Eisenhower overseeing D-Day. They can name officers who died or were cashiered for their mistakes, from Pearl Harbor to Little Bighorn.

Most of the health officials above became familiar faces and spoke to the press—some more than others. But every one was essentially an advisor rather than a commander. With the exception of Operation Warp Speed, their missions seemed poorly defined and overlapping. There were no clear standards for success or failure. No one was accountable.

Two years later, when monkeypox erupted, we saw the same initial confusion and leadership vacuum.

Although the first alarms were raised in mid-May, it was not until August, when we had 6,000 confirmed cases, that the White House officially put someone in charge of the response. On August 2, President Biden named as coordinator Robert Fenton, a regional administrator for the Federal Emergency Management Agency.

Previously, the White House said, the response had been "coordinated by" the National Security Council. But coordinated is not "led." As I described earlier, confusion was rampant over what advice to give, how many vaccine doses existed, and other issues. Advisory roles were played by Dr. Raj Panjabi, the council's director of global health security and biodefense; by Dr. Jha, the White House's coronavirus response coordinator; by CDC officials, including Dr. Walensky and subordinates of hers like Dr. Jennifer McQuiston; by Xavier Becerra, the secretary of health and human services, and his deputy for response, Dawn O'Connell (there are the names); and, of course, by Dr. Fauci.

At Mr. Fenton's first news conference, he seemed to largely play the role of an emcee introducing others. His relevant experience appeared to be in setting up Covid vaccination clinics. His deputy, Dr. Demetre Daskalakis, the CDC's director of HIV prevention and New York City's former head of disease control, was better known in infectious disease circles. He was openly gay, posted bare-chested photos of himself on social media, and had been profiled setting up tables outside nightclubs to get men vaccinated against sex-related bacterial infections and onto PrEP, the protection pill. After the initial briefing, Dr. Daskalakis became the more public face of the effort.

When military crises strike, this kind of confusion usually does not prevail. The armed forces have a clear chain of command from the secretary of defense down to the rifleman in a foxhole. Commanders get specific assignments. If they succeed, they often win promotion; if they fail, they're out.

The Pentagon trains for crises. They hold war games. If their side loses, they come up with a new battle plan and do it again. They move promising officers around the world to ready them to fight in different theaters. They train them not just in basics like how to assault obstacles, but even in how to give clear presentations to their troops. The Pentagon is considered highly effective at its job. It has the respect of Congress and gets vast amounts of money, even in peacetime.

For our public health bureaucracy, the absolute opposite is true. Federal and state health budgets are political footballs and frequently cut. Congress bows to the gun lobby, the tobacco lobby, the alcohol lobby, the automobile lobby, the oil lobby, the anti-vaccine diet-supplement lobby, even to the sugar and snacks lobbies. Congress has blocked or discouraged the CDC from studying deaths from guns, smoking, drinking, car crashes, air pollution, and obesity.

Across the nation, preparations for epidemics are so threadbare that they barely exist. Battle plans are drafted and then sit on shelves. Many hospitals can just barely handle a bad flu season. Work on vaccines is chronically underfunded because most of it is in the hands of private industry and vaccines are less profitable than drugs. When coronavirus vaccines had to be invented in a rush, a whole new bureaucracy with a goofy name—Operation Warp Speed—had to be whipped up. It relied heavily on technologies like mRNA and nanoparticles that were promising but had little field testing. We were extremely lucky they worked as well as they did. In monkeypox, our reliance on luck was even more obvious: a vaccine that had been stockpiled against a terrorist smallpox attack just happened to also work against a sexually transmitted disease.

Few public health leaders have obvious command skills. Most are trained as clinicians and academics, ready to treat patients and to answer technical questions, not to lead.

History is partly to blame for this. War is an affair between nations, so the laws covering it are federal, while public health in this country has historically been a local concern. The Constitution is silent on health. It was written in a century in which whether one lived or died from an illness was seen largely as a matter of luck or divine will, rather than something subject to human intervention. It was also written in an era when diseases moved at the speed of a horse-drawn wagon. As a result, the relevant health laws are almost all state ones: quarantine orders, school vaccine mandates, mosquito control, contact-tracing rules, and so on are the province of state and sometimes county officials. In the jet age, when outbreaks leap from airport to airport, that makes no sense. Most state health agencies, moreover, have been starved of funds for decades. Many, for example, can barely field enough contact-tracers to deal with routine crises like outbreaks of syphilis or food poisoning, much less a fast-moving epidemic.

Also, almost all the frontline troops are civilians. Most medical personnel work wholly or in part for hospital systems or in practices owned by corporations. Their bosses are driven by profits, not lives saved. Our litigious society also forces them to live in fear of malpractice suits.

In other words, what we have is the opposite of what we need in a crisis. It resembles what Abraham Lincoln faced as war broke out in 1861. The standing army was so small—a mere 17,000 men, mostly stationed in the Far West—that he was forced to ask for volunteers, initially for just three months. Regiments were raised by cities or rich citizens. Their wealthy or politically connected sponsors—even those with no military experience—insisted on command positions. Some trained for only two weeks. The result was chaos and defeat in the First Battle of Bull Run/Manassas. Congress was forced to organize a true national army, appoint a new commander, and authorize him to replace the inept officer corps. By the end of 1861 the North had 700,000 men under arms.

We need to be able to do better than that. We need to pass laws that will create a Pentagon-like response to epidemics. The stakes are high. We lost three times as many Americans to Covid as we did to combat in World War II.

We need a clear sense of who is in charge, who reports to whom, and who is tasked with what mission.

We need to replace the Department of Health and Human Services with an agency whose sole mission is to defeat disease—not to also oversee Medicare, private insurers, and the welfare state. Such bureaucracies are liable to be captured by the industries they regulate.

Disparate bureaucracies like the CDC, the FDA, and the NIH must be reorganized in ways that will enhance cooperation and speed up responses—perhaps modeled on the Pentagon's Joint Chiefs of Staff.

The CDC director should not change with every new administration. As we learned during the Trump administration, that encourages abuses like allowing White House operatives to rewrite articles in the agency's scholarly *Morbidity and Mortality Weekly Report*. It leads to craven silence from the director when the president claims a pandemic will just "fade away." As with the FBI, the director should come from within the ranks and serve a fixed term.

The CDC's culture must change. It is a blend of a detective agency, a university, and a management consultancy. Imagine the FBI cut to a third of its size, with no guns, handcuffs, or powers of arrest, plus an inclination to publishing scholarly papers instead of enforcing laws. Its elite Epidemic Intelligence Service excels at investigating outbreaks but then is largely limited to making suggestions as to how states might control them. Its laboratories are world-class but proved careless when speed was of the essence. For years, foreign scientists complained that CDC labs requested samples and then published papers taking the credit. During the Covid pandemic, countries like Britain and Israel did basic tasks like tracking viral mutations faster than we did.

Even more dangerous is the agency's "if it wasn't done here, it didn't happen" attitude. For years it ignored important work done by French scientists on Ebola and Zika. Its stubborn insistence on making its own Covid test and not letting private labs compete to do so cost us dearly.

The agency, or whatever replaces it, must be funded to lead rapid responses. It must work in cooperation with the private sector but have the power to manage the relationship so public health takes priority over corporate profits.

It should have its own West Point: a school that produces experts trained to fight epidemics.

It should have the power to commandeer resources and move them to where they will do the most good. As we saw in 2020, no outbreak strikes every city at once. Forcing governors to fight each other over limited supplies of masks and equipment is counterproductive. Our fragmented state and private hospital networks reacted in exactly the wrong way, by hoarding supplies and equipment. That can be stopped.

It needs the power to temporarily commandeer facilities to isolate and care for the infected so they don't infect others, and to assign tasks to different hospitals and move specialists between them. During epidemics, people still need to give birth, to have surgery, to be treated for strokes, cancer, and so on, and must be protected. In any city, one or two hospitals could handle births and maternity care, for example, while others treat pandemic victims.

It needs the power to restrict travel from epicenters to still-unaffected areas.

Medical practitioners who harm patients or put them at risk from dangerous quackery, who prescribe drugs that clearly do not work, or who help patients avoid measures that clearly do work should lose their licenses and even face arrest if necessary. Professional associations need to be empowered to suspend and revoke licenses, and the Justice Department needs laws that will punish the most egregious offenders.

This may sound archaic, but we may also need uniforms and ranks. Currently, we have a hodgepodge of leaders in the uniforms of the military, the Public Health Service Commissioned Corps, and in mufti. The surgeon general is always in uniform, top CDC officials sometimes are, the heads of the NIH and the FDA almost never are. Uniforms command respect, including from Congress. They also confer responsibility: success means visible rewards, failure ends with the equivalent of epaulets stripped off. In crises, leaders must feel an urgency to not fail.

We also need ways to compel service from medical professionals. The medical branches of the military, the Public Health Service's Commissioned Corps, the CDC, and other federal agencies lack the staff to confront major crises, and private employers resist losing employees. During the Korean War, the Doctors Draft Act required all MDs below the age of fifty-one to register for military service, and by 1952, 90 percent of the doctors with American forces in Korea were draftees. Most were inconvenienced, but some later said it was the most satisfying period in their professional lives. Since 1986, the Selective Service System has had the power to draft doctors and nurses under the Health Care Personnel Delivery System, but Congress has never authorized it to do so.

In return, we should subsidize medical education. We already face a shortage of up to 124,000 physicians in the next decade. Medical reservists could also do tours of duty in the military, Indian Health Service, or other federal agencies.

At the global level, there should be something similar. In a 2023 op-ed in *The New York Times*, Bill Gates called on all nations to support the WHO's plans to create a Global Health Emergency Corps, which would be on call to suppress outbreaks. The WHO has very few of its own medical staff and has responded to most outbreaks—like those of Ebola in Africa—by asking countries to contribute doctors and nurses. The WHO's role was largely to provide "diplomatic cover" for such missions. It might not be easy, for example, for a dozen American doctors in military-style Public Health Service uniforms to enter a foreign country and start treating its citizens. But if they arrived as part of a WHO mission, objections were rare.

Simply having an equivalent of the Pentagon and tougher public health laws is not enough. We need a better-prepared society.

Sadly, our constitution does not recognize health as a basic human right. Newer constitutions, like that of South Africa, do. The fear of being impoverished by medical bills scares Americans away from doctors. We need universal medical insurance, as is the norm in every other wealthy nation.

Along with insurance should come responsibilities. Americans should be required to get regular checkups to catch diseases in early stages. Expectant parents should be required to seek care for themselves and their children.

To combat rumor-mongering, science education needs to improve. High school curricula ought to provide basic anatomy, human biology, and medical history—including a sense of how often children died in the pre-vaccine era. They should also learn emergency skills like first aid and CPR, and how to avoid infectious disease, STDs, injuries, and chronic diseases.

Given our polarized society, I despair of such changes ever taking place. But radical changes are needed—and could work wonders.

Chapter Nineteen

WE NEED TO FIGHT GLOBAL POVERTY

Almost every outbreak of disease starts in poor countries, or the parts of countries where the poor are concentrated.

Most Americans have no concept of how little the world's poorest scrape by on, because poverty in rich countries like ours bears little resemblance to poverty in poor ones. According to the World Bank, almost 650 million people, 8 percent of the world's population, earn less than $2.15 a day.

In 1996, when I was reporting in Zambia, I had long conversations with the driver I was assigned by Avis Car Rental. His name was Bonaventure Salomo, and he was an educated man, a former English teacher who worked for Avis because the $5 a day they paid him was more than the state paid teachers. (When I initially told Avis I didn't need a driver, I was told the extra insurance would be $15 a day. The driver's main job was to stay with the car to make sure it wasn't stolen.)

At one point he asked me if there were poor people in America. Yes, I said—but probably not what he meant by poor. In America, people could be poor enough to get money from the government every month and still have hot and cold running water. He looked surprised. No one had that in the compounds, he said. (The "compounds," called townships in South Africa, were neighborhoods built for Africans just outside cities when Zambia was white-controlled Northern Rhodesia.) There, each block had one spigot for the homes on it.

An American, I said, could be considered poor and still own a TV set. "But if you own a TV," he said, "you can make money. You invite your friends over to watch, and you sell them beer."

Not only that, I said, but you can be poor enough in America to get a government check and still own a car. "Now I know you're lying," he said. "Because a man who owns a car *is* a rich man. He uses it to give people rides."

To help me report a story about how Zambia's transition from socialism to capitalism was affecting the poorest of its poor, Mr. Salomo introduced me to the women known as "the rock-breakers." (Work for which I additionally paid him what was then the *Times*' rate for a fixer/translator—$100 a day.) On a road running past a defunct limestone quarry, the women spent their days crouched over grapefruit-sized stones, hammering them to break them into gravel. Their babies were strapped on their backs, and their toddlers sat beside them, sometimes banging away with their own smaller hammers to help. A week's work could produce a burlap sack of chips small enough to pave a driveway or finish a concrete floor. Building contractors who drove by would pay about $8 a bag. Most of the women were lucky to sell two bags a month. Out of that, they had to pay the men who lugged stones from the quarry for them, men rich enough to own wheelbarrows.

The switch to capitalism, strongly encouraged by the United States and the International Monetary Fund, meant selling state-owned enterprises, letting the currency float, ending food subsidies, and allowing the market to set prices. As a result, the price of a fifty-pound bag of cornmeal, the staple of the poor, had just shot up from $2 to $7. It was called "structural adjustment shock," and no one was in deeper shock than the women on the rock piles.

Under the socialist former government, they were sometimes whipped by the police when they lined up for subsidized food, Catherine Thembo, one of the rock-breakers, told me. Now there were no lines—but no one had enough money to shop. Most avoided starvation only because mission churches gave food away.

That kind of poverty exists all over the world. I have vivid memories of watching boys fly kites in a slum in Karachi, Pakistan. Their "field"—the only open space around—was an old canal bed so full of plastic bags of garbage that one could run across it—if one was small and light. As my feet squelched into it, I realized that I was wading in a field of raw sewage in one of the last areas of the world where polio was still endemic. When I got back to my hotel, I washed my legs, threw away my socks, and did what I could to disinfect my boots. The kite-flying boys had worn only sandals.

This is not an argument for socialism. It's an argument for doing what we can to alleviate poverty—as much for our own protection as for the sake of the world's poor. Economic development is not my field, and tackling global poverty is way beyond the scope of this book. But I've made a few observations along the way that might be useful to anyone interested in fighting disease at its source. Prevention, as anyone who practices medicine knows, is far easier—and much cheaper—than cure.

It's no accident that most pandemics start in gritty rural areas. Outbreaks may not explode until they reach a city like Wuhan, Monrovia, or Mexico City, but they usually begin somewhere out on the animal-human interface. Poverty forces much of the world to live at that interface, which we, in our air-conditioned bedrooms and cars, plumbed bathrooms, and refrigerated supermarkets, never do.

Poverty forces you to hunt wild game, which contains viruses we have no names for yet. It means entering bat caves to dig guano for fertilizer. It means sleeping with your domestic pigs, chickens, and ducks under your roof in winter or letting them forage in forests and ponds where they might pick up stray viruses from wild relatives. It means subsisting on diets like corn porridge that leave your immune system enfeebled. It means being unable to afford windows or screens that keep insects out, nights so hot that you furl your mosquito net or sleep on your roof to catch a breeze.

It means drinking contaminated pond water or trying to pick your way through a minefield of your neighbors' feces until you find your own place to squat on the railroad tracks running past your slum.

Obviously, we Americans can't solve all those problems. But we can choose policies that don't make them worse. And we can quite cheaply subsidize interventions like food, vitamins, basic drugs, human vaccines, veterinary vaccines, and so on that save lives overseas and prevent the incubation of diseases that will ultimately cross those seas and affect us.

According to the 2022 World Inequality Report, the poorest 50 percent of humanity own a mere 2 percent of the world's wealth, while the richest 10 percent own 76 percent. The speed at which the rich are getting richer is increasing, with the top 0.1 percent—the billionaires—doing the best. The World Bank estimated that Covid, inflation, and the war in Ukraine had pushed between 75 and 95 million people below the $2-a-day poverty line who previously were on track to rise above it.

What does staggering inequality lead to? A world constantly evolving new infectious diseases.

It also means a world in which poor countries become hopelessly reliant on donor aid, which is simply not sustainable. It's not that the money isn't there, it's that international generosity tends to periodically swell and then fade away.

I've read that in history books, and I've seen it during my own career. In the nineteenth century, the United States made itself a refuge for the world's poor, whether they were driven from Ireland and Scandinavia by the potato famine, from central Europe by wars and the tsars, or from China by the Taiping Rebellion. Those workers made this country the agricultural and industrial powerhouse it became. In the wake of World War II, under the Marshall Plan, the United States rebuilt the economies of Western Europe and Japan, while also imposing democracy and market capitalism on them; that led to an era of peace and prosperity unlike any other the world had ever seen—one that, for the West, continues to this day.

What used to be called the Third World was left out of that watershed economic revival because, at the war's end, those countries were still colonies in the disintegrating British, French, Dutch, Portuguese, and Belgian empires. (The Spanish and Portuguese colonies of the Western Hemisphere had freed themselves a century earlier.) The collapse of the colonial era between 1945 and the 1970s produced greater poverty—and more disease—as the capitalist and communist powers financed civil and tribal wars in efforts to drag every newly liberated country into their respective Cold War orbits.

By the 1990s, that dynamic had played itself out to the detriment of the world's poor. The Soviet Union collapsed. Its Eastern European "allies" (which amounted to colonies) defected to the West. The Russian Federation, the exhausted skeleton that remained, had neither the money nor the will to support its former client states in Africa, Asia, and Latin America. But the West had no interest in them, either, because the profit motive was gone. The triumph of capitalism meant private companies could buy their oil, minerals, diamonds, rubber, coffee, cocoa, or bananas at ever-lower prices, but governments would no longer go to war to protect the market share of state-sponsored companies. If one supplier collapsed because of a coup or a drought or a cholera epidemic, there were always others. The poor were on their own—with serious handicaps.

When I began covering global health in 1997, AIDS was killing hundreds of Africans each day and Big Pharma had zero interest in their fate. Over 10 million children died each year before age five, many from easily preventable ills like malaria and measles.

Drug companies shunned diseases of the poor. In the year 2000, according to Doctors Without Borders, of the 1,400 drugs patented during the previous twenty-five years, only 16 were for tropical diseases or tuberculosis. Most of those had been developed by the U.S. military for its troops in Vietnam or by the veterinary industry for livestock. On surveys, pharma scientists said they would willingly tackle such diseases, but were under pressure to cure arthritis, obesity, and erectile dysfunction. The newest blockbuster on the horizon that year was a Novartis drug for separation anxiety—in dogs.

The U.S. government's foreign aid budget then was 0.1 percent of our gross national income, which put us, on a per capita basis, dead last among Western nations, behind even Portugal.

Then, beginning in the early 2000s, remarkable changes occurred. It's hard to say exactly what started it—other than the appalling vista of so many needless deaths. Nonetheless, a syzygy of three great forces emerged, reinforcing each other. First, as I discussed earlier, the Indian generic drug companies entered the market, driving prices down.

Second, global health became briefly fashionable among billionaires, as it had a century before when John D. Rockefeller paid for yellow fever research, fought worm diseases in the American South, and funded modern medical education in China. Bill and Melinda Gates initially signed on to help Rotary International defeat polio, and then broadened their mandate, pouring tens of billions of dollars into the battle against all diseases of poverty. Warren Buffett turned much of his wealth over to them, so that the Gates Foundation became a driving force in setting global health priorities, even for the World Health Organization. Michael Bloomberg targeted health-related causes like tobacco and guns. Foreign billionaires like Carlos Slim Helú of Mexico and Aliko Dangote of Nigeria joined in.

Then, in an even more important change driven by the George W. Bush administration, a rare bipartisan congressional alliance evolved between foreign policy liberals and Christian conservatives whose churches supported missionary hospitals. In 2003, with little fanfare, President Bush announced plans for PEPFAR, the President's Emergency Plan for AIDS Relief, and then the President's Malaria Initiative. Kofi Annan, the former UN secretary-general, organized the Global Fund to Fight AIDS, Tuberculosis and Malaria. Gavi, the Vaccine Alliance supported a basic set of vaccines for almost half of the world's children. Many countries that had previously given very little in foreign aid began ramping up donations.

The next few years were a golden age for foreign aid. Global funding for AIDS went from $5 billion in 2000 to $16 billion by 2010, and funding for vaccines soared as factories in India and Indonesia modernized to meet the demand.

The pharmaceutical industry changed its attitudes, adopting tiered pricing to let poor countries pay pennies on the dollar and sublicensing some patents to generic competitors. The cost of measles shots went down to 25 cents, deworming pills to 30 cents, malaria pills to less than $1, mosquito-repelling nets to $5 each. A year's worth of HIV drugs fell below $100.

Estimates of "lives saved" are inevitably fuzzy but it is probably safe to say that at least 30 million people who would have died of AIDS, malaria, tuberculosis, and vaccine-preventable diseases like measles did not.

The number of children who died before age five dropped by half.

Unfortunately, that golden age was short-lived. The Great Recession of 2008–09 hit the world's new generosity hard. Some countries entirely stopped contributing to the Global Fund. PEPFAR's budget has been essentially flat since 2010. Overall funding for AIDS crept slowly up to $20 billion a year by 2015 but then plateaued. The Trump administration tried to sharply cut it, but Congress resisted.

Goals proved more elusive than expected. Diseases that twenty years ago were hovering on the brink of eradication, including polio, guinea worm, trachoma, elephantiasis, and iodine deficiency, either resisted final elimination or, like measles, made comebacks.

Political shifts in the United States changed the landscape. Christian conservatives were partly edged out by Tea Party conservatives and later by Trump conservatives.

New crises put new demands on the Treasury. The Great Recession's stimulus plan cost more than $800 billion. Stimulus payments during Covid topped $900 billion. The wars in Iraq and Afghanistan ended, but the war in Ukraine is proving costly.

The tastes of billionaires changed. The generation that succeeded Gates and Buffett—Jeff Bezos, MacKenzie Scott, Elon Musk, Sergey Brin, Larry Page, and so on—showed little interest in global health. The Chan

Zuckerberg Initiative, started by the founder of Facebook and his wife, has implications for the poor but is focused on basic science.

And, of course, the Covid pandemic overwhelmed the weak medical systems of many poor countries and consumed the world's resources dedicated to health. Progress was set back by years.

Charity is important but it will not end global poverty. In the last forty years, the biggest gains in life expectancy, infant mortality, and other measures of public health were made in Asia, Eastern Europe, and Latin America. Most gains were not due to Western charity but to growing prosperity. When poor parents earn a few extra dollars, the first thing they spend it on is their children's health.

Much of that progress was made in one country: China. Market capitalism was introduced starting in 1978, but it was preceded and accompanied by decades of brutal social engineering aimed at producing both prosperity and health. In 1950, China's under-five mortality rate was a horrifying 25 percent. Mao's draconian one-child policy meant all the resources of two parents and four grandparents could be focused on protecting and educating one child. His "Patriotic Health Campaign" included immunizations and education, and much of it was compulsory. For example, to eliminate rural worm diseases, the government devised salt laced with deworming drugs. To ensure it was used, health workers would arrive in villages with soldiers and fire trucks. The locals would be ordered to bring all their salt to the central square, where it would be washed away, and the new drug-laden version handed out. Becoming the world's biggest exporter created incentives for millions of villagers to abandon their farms for factory towns that were monotonous but healthier because, instead of shallow wells, outhouses, or open sewers, they had chlorinated water, flush toilets, and central heating. At the same time, restrictive internal movement controls meant cities in China were never allowed to spawn the squalid Dickensian slums where millions live in India, Brazil, Mexico, Pakistan, Kenya, and South Africa.

The most effective kind of charity helps people escape poverty; it also turns them from mendicants into customers. We should not stop at food and medicine. Paved roads, bridges, and airports help economies grow by making it possible to move goods to markets. (Glance at any map of the Roman Empire: The 250,000 miles of roads it built stretched from England to Spain to Turkey to Egypt. The areas left outside that network, from Scotland and Ireland to Scandinavia, Eastern Europe, and central Asia, took centuries longer to prosper.)

The late Paul Polak, the author of *Out of Poverty* (2008), was a genius at inventing simple technologies to empower small entrepreneurs. He came up with $25 foot-powered treadle pumps to irrigate family gardens. Well-digging machines made of bamboo and chains. Ways to make charcoal from invasive plants instead of chopping down trees. Using flashlight batteries and table salt to make chlorine for water purification. More of such work is needed. American companies that buy everything from minerals to coffee should be prodded to get their suppliers to pay living wages to miners and coffee pickers. In some cities, the only consistent source of clean water is the local brewery or Coke or Pepsi plant; they could be encouraged to expand; in many slums and villages, selling clean water in jugs or jerry cans is a thriving business.

Almost any effort that benefits women improves the society they live in. While men often fend for themselves, women tend to help their children, their families, and their neighbors. Numerous studies have shown that, if you educate girls, allow them to have jobs, don't force them into early-teen marriages, protect them against domestic violence, and let them own land, inherit property, and hold elective office, you end up with a healthier society. Everything improves, from children getting enough food to reach their full height and intellectual potential to more doctors and engineers building the economy. It takes time, but the whole country ultimately fares better.

Admittedly, corruption is an enormous problem in foreign aid. It turns eager aid workers cynical and lethargic. It makes a country's young doctors and nurses feel they have no future, so they flee to jobs elsewhere. It scares off donors, who stop giving.

I've seen it eating away at such efforts—it is often thousands of small ten-dollar bites instead of one black hole consuming millions. One day in a dusty rural compound during a polio-eradication drive in Kano, in northern Nigeria, for example, I could see the damage from low-level corruption everywhere: The chief local health official who had a TV and an air conditioner in his office and pictures of himself visiting Geneva while there were too few freezers to store vaccines in. The minibuses that didn't appear because the money for them had been pocketed. The nervous, untrained teenagers who showed up to serve on vaccination teams because their fathers had sent them to collect the $2 paid to "volunteers."

To some extent, that's just a cost of doing business. Bill Gates has said as much about watching some of his money disappear: he can stand it as long as it's a tolerable fraction. But there are also steps that can be taken to reduce it.

One is that it must be called out—and bluntly. It has to be talked about. Aid officials often feel they can't publicly complain, diplomats rarely talk about it on the record, journalists hesitate to cover it—all for fear of being accused of racism. That's not true in-country; African journalists cover corruption arrests and know who is crooked. But their voices are rarely heard outside their countries, and in Washington and New York, it's hard to get anyone to publicly acknowledge the problem.

I have, however, seen a few instances of systemic corruption thwarted. It happens when an insistence on honesty is conveyed from the very top of the donor country to the very top of the recipient country.

Accepting development aid is a wound to national pride. To minimize that, everything must be kept as personal as possible, from one leader to another as equals.

In authoritarian countries, real power rests with the president. The torpid bureaucracy below will respond only if the president insists it be done. And the best way to appeal to a president is to have another president do it.

Former president Jimmy Carter was a master of that. The early success of the campaign he began in 1986 to eradicate guinea worm was amazing.

Cases went down by 99.9 percent from 3.5 million cases in 21 countries to a few hundred. (In recent years, the campaign has struggled. There are now only about a dozen confirmed cases a year, but they pop up unpredictably in the most remote and often war-torn regions of countries like Chad, South Sudan, and Ethiopia.)

Mr. Carter was indefatigable. Well into his nineties, he kept flying to Africa and standing in the sun through endless ceremonies. A big part of his success, as he well knew, was his personal appearance: presidents of poor countries are honored when presidents of rich countries treat them as equals.

His wife, Rosalynn, was a second line of approach. For many years, she accompanied him, meeting the first ladies. First ladies are often even more receptive than their husbands to humanitarian appeals, especially when the health of children is at stake.

Guinea worm is an ancient horror. The worms have been found in Egyptian mummies and may be the "fiery serpents" described in the Old Testament as torturing the Israelites in the desert. They're horrible even to look at; they are microscopic when they are ingested in contaminated drinking water but grow to a yard long beneath the skin. They exit, usually from the foot or leg, by exuding acid to create an excruciatingly painful blister; when the victim puts the limb in water to cool it, the worm spews millions of eggs, starting the cycle anew. But it's now so rare that it is never any president's top priority. It affects the poorest of the poor, in the most remote villages, sometimes in ethnic groups the president doesn't come from and that may oppose him. When he started his campaign, Mr. Carter told me in an interview, many presidents he met—including President Muhammad Zia-ul-Haq of Pakistan—had never even heard of it. However, one of President Zia's top generals hailed from a rural village and volunteered that he knew of it. President Zia—himself a former general—charged that officer with eliminating the disease. By 1993, Pakistan was guinea worm–free. That kind of direct appeal often makes the difference.

Bill Gates is not an ex-president, but the aura of having been the world's richest man made him as famous as one. He also circled the world making direct appeals to leaders.

Presidents can speak bluntly to their peers. In 2008, President George W. Bush made a swing through Tanzania, Benin, Rwanda, Ghana, and Liberia talking up his plans for fighting AIDS and malaria. In each one, he told the president and assembled dignitaries in his basic speech: "The United States wants to partner with leaders and the people, but we're not going to do so with people that steal money—pure and simple."

(None of the reporters accompanying him found this startling language newsworthy—or they did not feel comfortable reporting it. I only learned about it when someone in government told me how relieved he had been to hear it said aloud and looked up the White House transcripts.)

Also, countries that fight corruption can be held up as examples. PEPFAR and the President's Malaria Initiative make grants to local partners that are not in the government and require them to file accounts and submit to audits. If money vanishes, those partners can be dropped, and new ones recruited.

When countries become motivated to fight corruption, the effects can be far-reaching. For example: In 2007, China faced a series of embarrassing export scandals. Chinese cough syrup sweetened with a toxic antifreeze compound had killed 40 people in Panama. Pet food tainted with melamine, an industrial plastic used to fool crude tests for protein, killed American dogs and cats. High levels of antibiotics were detected in farmed seafood, and lead paint was found on toy trains. For years, the government's response had been to issue denials or blame the foreign importers. But President Hu Jintao, fed up, changed direction. The government strengthened regulatory agencies and cracked down viciously. The most shocking result was the example made of the longtime head of the country's Food and Drug Administration, Zheng Xiaoyu, who had personally signed off on 150,000 drugs during his tenure. (Our FDA approves fewer than 200 a year.) Some adulterated ones had caused hundreds of deaths—mostly inside

China. He was convicted of accepting $850,000 in bribes and executed. A year later, 6 babies died and 54,000 were hospitalized with kidney damage after a large dairy company put melamine in its infant formula. Two company officials got death sentences. Chinese companies took notice; the quality of their export products improved.

That's an extreme example, of course, but the point is that prosperity and a population's health go hand in hand, and healthier populations overseas reduce the chances of disease spillovers that affect the whole world.

An obvious target for foreign aid would be to strengthen animal husbandry and veterinary medicine in poor countries. Every dollar that helps them safely raise domestic animals instead of hunting wild ones is a step in the right direction.

The trade in exotic species—both as pets and as food—should be banned. I cannot understand why governments like China's tolerate it. It's a trade that caters to a small number of epicures and believers in folk medicine, but the concomitant risk is incredibly high—and the first wave of victims would be in China itself.

Helping eliminate "wet markets" would also make the world safer. It will be a long, slow process, because habits die hard and live markets do serve a need. Many communities lack the steady electricity supply needed to run refrigerators and freezers. And many countries lack the layers of regulatory agencies needed to guarantee that meat is disease-free when slaughtered and properly chilled when stored. When such safeguards are missing, customers often insist on picking out a healthy-looking live animal and watching as it is killed, and people's eating habits are the hardest to change. But the conditions in live markets are too often filthy: different species penned together; cages piled up so that dung and urine rain down through them; pigeons, rats, cats, and other pests and pest-catchers roaming around; butchers working in a slurry of blood and feces.

"Backyard animals" also must be regulated. Small personal herds and flocks keep outbreaks moving. African swine fever, for example, recently spread all the way from China to Belgium, sometimes via commercial herds, but also often from one backyard sty to another.

Veterinary vaccines, deworming drugs, and farm expertise will help. So will increasing farm biosecurity so that, for example, pigs and camels can't eat fruit that bats have gnawed, rats can't invade food troughs, and wild birds can't shed viruses into farm ponds.

When a dangerous zoonosis is on the move, it's crucial that wealthy countries step in to make sure that poor countries take the right steps to stop it. For a small farmer, seeing a whole flock or herd culled is a financial disaster. If they aren't compensated, they won't do it. During the H5N1 bird flu scare of the early 2000s, some governments refused to reimburse farmers. In others, corrupt officials stole the funds. Cambodia paid farmers nothing; it dispatched soldiers to kill flocks. Vietnam paid only a third of market prices. As a result, desperate farmers would lie about their flocks being diseased—or even truck them to market as fast as possible, hoping to sell them before they all died. That just sped up the spread.

Every dollar that rich nations spend to improve such conditions is a step back from the brink for the whole world.

Chapter Twenty

WE NEED TO BAN RELIGIOUS EXEMPTIONS

A persistent absurdity in public health, in my opinion, is the notion that the law should recognize a "religious exemption" to vaccination.

No major world religion objects to vaccination. They all endorse it. Vaccination exists for only one reason: to save lives. Every major religion regards the preservation of life as sacred.

"Religious exemptions" are red herrings exploited by the anti-vaccine industry. Medical procedures do not challenge religious faith. Cardiac stents, cancer surgery, and root canals are not religious acts; they save lives and reduce pain.

Laws recognizing "philosophical" or "personal belief" exemptions are even more absurd. The First Amendment does not protect freedom of philosophy or personal belief. We don't recognize philosophical exemptions from paying taxes or submitting to a test before receiving a driver's license.

Religious exemptions have consequences. Between 1985 and 1994, measles killed three students in Christian Science schools in St. Louis. In 1987–88, it killed two children in an outbreak that spread through Amish communities in five states. In 1991, hundreds of cases of rubella in Amish communities led to more than a dozen children born with birth defects.

Vaccines are not merely an individual's choice about his or her own body. Individuals may refuse lifesaving medical procedures for themselves, but they do not have the right to deny them to others. American courts have long held, for example, that Jehovah's Witness parents who themselves refuse blood transfusions may not force their children to die for lack of one. If they persist, the court will take the child away and appoint a guardian.

Vaccines affect more than one life: they protect the life of the vaccinated individual *plus* the lives of others whom that individual would have infected.

Courts recognize this. In 1905, when the Supreme Court held in *Jacobson v. Massachusetts* that the state could punish a Lutheran pastor who refused to take a smallpox vaccine, it did not decide the case on religious grounds. In a 7–2 decision, it held that compelling vaccination against a deadly disease was a legitimate exercise of the state's police power. That is, the state can compel you to be vaccinated for the same reason it can take away your gun (despite your Second Amendment right to bear arms) if you are walking down the street shooting people: it has a duty to prevent one citizen from harming others. In 1922, in *Zucht v. King*, the court upheld, 9–0, a San Antonio, Texas, ordinance prohibiting students from attending either public or private school without a certificate of smallpox vaccination. It was permissible for the state to require vaccination, the court held, even in the absence of a smallpox outbreak.

Centuries ago, religious authorities debated whether variolation—using smallpox pus or scabs to protect children during epidemics—was permissible. Dr. Edward Jenner's 1796 experiment added to the controversy. He infected a child—eight-year-old James Phipps, his gardener's son—with cowpox virus and then deliberately exposed him to smallpox to test his theory.

One of the basic religious questions back then was: If illness is sent by God, whether as a punishment or as a test, are vaccines thwarting the will of God? The eventual answer from the high priests of all religions was no. We take many measures to protect ourselves from death. We build fires against the cold, we wear armor into battle. God is not angered.

No major world religion—not Hinduism, Buddhism, Judaism,

Catholic or Orthodox Christianity, Islam, or any modern Protestant denomination—objects to vaccine. They all endorse them. In every denomination, a few clerics oppose them. But they are renegades bucking guidance from above.

In most religions, actions that might otherwise be sinful—such as eating pork or benefiting from the consequences of an abortion—are permissible when a life is at stake.

In Judaism, for example, the principle of *pikuach nefesh* ("saving a life") holds that a devout Jew is not just permitted but *obligated* to break Jewish laws if doing so will save a life. No one may plead, for example, "I let him die because performing CPR would have meant working on the Sabbath." (There are three exceptions: even to save a life, a Jew may not commit murder, incest, or idolatry.)

Even religions like Christian Science and Jehovah's Witnesses that object to some medical procedures do not currently oppose vaccination, according to a study by Dorit R. Reiss, a medical law expert at the University of California College of Law, San Francisco, and a paper in the journal *Vaccine* by John D. Grabenstein, a pharmacist and historian.

Currently, forty-four states have laws on their books allowing "religious exemptions" to vaccines. But the histories of those laws do not go back to the founding of the republic. There is no mention of medical procedures or religious exemptions to them in the Constitution or the Bill of Rights. Instead, they go back to the nineteenth century, when states first passed mandatory vaccination laws. The Industrial Revolution was creating vast urban slums, where epidemics were frequent, and another new set of institutions—public schools—acted as the foci for outbreaks.

Vaccination laws were part of many new compulsory public health measures, including making dairies pasteurize their milk and making urban homeowners hook into the then-new sewer systems. Libertarians who preferred to keep their own cesspools or to drink raw milk objected to such measures, to no avail; the law recognized that the public good should prevail.

The Church of Christ, Scientist, founded by Mary Baker Eddy in 1879 and rejecting medicine in favor of prayer, opposed vaccination laws, arguing that they contravened freedom of religion. By the early twentieth century, it had huge numbers of adherents, despite being repeatedly lampooned by Mark Twain as a belief catering to "the class which is numerically vastly the largest bulk of the human race, i.e. the fools, the idiots, the puddnheads." Starting in the 1960s, as new vaccines were invented in quick succession and as the number of shots mandated for kindergartners grew, forty-eight states passed laws allowing for religious exemptions. Some added philosophical or personal exemptions for people who were not members of a church. The states did so, historians said, to accommodate Christian Scientists and to avoid court fights over what constituted "sincerely held religious beliefs." Two states—Mississippi and West Virginia—never allowed religious or philosophical exemptions, and prior to Covid, Mississippi children were the most consistently vaccinated in the country. (Before the last decade, opposition to vaccines was strongest in left-leaning communities like Berkeley, California. Conservatives were almost uniformly pro-vaccine.)

Because general enthusiasm for vaccines was high in the 1960s while Christian Science membership was steadily shrinking, very few parents ever claimed religious exemptions. Smallpox, polio, and measles disappeared from the United States.

That all changed in 1998 when the spurious possibility of a link between vaccines and autism was raised in a fraudulent paper by the now-disgraced doctor Andrew Wakefield. In states that permitted religious objections, terrified parents began claiming them.

That had predictable results: diseases returned. After California's 2014 "Disneyland measles outbreak," the state passed a law canceling all religious and personal belief exemptions. Vaccination rates among kindergartners rose above 95 percent. After the 2019 measles outbreak in Orthodox Jewish communities, New York and Maine passed similar laws. Connecticut followed suit in 2021.

The anti-vaccine lobby tries to scare devout Jews, Muslims, and Catholics away from vaccines by focusing on their trace ingredients.

Vaccines may contain bits of DNA or proteins in the parts-per-million range from the cell mediums they are grown in: monkey or dog kidneys, moth caterpillars, calf blood, or the immature tissues of human fetuses. (Viruses used for vaccines must be grown in cells; unlike bacteria, which are cells, they can't just be fed sugar water or other nutrients. Ingredients lists are published by the CDC and the Institute for Vaccine Safety at the Johns Hopkins Bloomberg School of Public Health.)

Also, some vaccines contain small amounts of gelatin made from pig skin as a stabilizer to prevent damage from heat or freeze-drying. Older vaccines once contained cow gelatin, but manufacturers changed to pork-derived versions after studies found they triggered fewer dangerous reactions in children with allergies. In a typical vaccine dose, only about three one-hundredths of a teaspoon is gelatin.

Religious authorities, including top Jewish and Islamic scholars and the Vatican, have meticulously studied vaccines and have ruled that they do not violate their respective laws.

"Since it is proven that vaccines are effective to prevent the spread of disease, it is an obligation upon every father to vaccinate his children," Rabbi Moshe Sternbuch, chief rabbi of the Rabbinical Court in Jerusalem, wrote in an open letter to the dean of a major Orthodox yeshiva in the United States during New York's 2019 measles outbreak. Rabbi Sternbuch's opinion was solicited because an anti-vaccine pamphlet called *The Vaccine Safety Handbook*, circulating widely in the Orthodox community, had pages emphasizing pork-based ingredients.

But kosher dietary laws are "just a total nonissue" with vaccines, explained Dr. Naor Bar-Zeev, a professor of international health and vaccine science at the Johns Hopkins Bloomberg School of Public Health. "All these complex laws apply to food ingested by mouth. They are not in any way relevant to injected material."

Observant Jews may inject insulin derived from pig pancreas or have a pig valve implanted in a failing heart, Dr. Bar-Zeev noted. They can also swallow oral vaccines, such as those against rotavirus, polio, and cholera, even if they contain pork gelatin, because they are considered medicine, not food.

During a 1995 meeting, 112 leading Islamic scholars considered many ingested substances, including alcohol, rennet, and even nutmeg, and approved the use of porcine gelatin in medicines.

Like Jewish scholars, the Islamic scholars held that "denatured" substances were not pig meat. "Gelatin formed as a result of the transformation of the bones, skin and tendons of a judicially impure animal is pure, and it is judicially permissible to eat it," the Islamic Organization for Medical Sciences ruled.

More than two hundred years ago, Rabbi Israel Lifschitz, author of a famous commentary on Jewish law, called Edward Jenner a "chasid" (a pious person) and even declared him "one of the righteous among nations" for inventing the vaccine that saved so many lives. Rabbi Nachman of Breslov, founder of a branch of Hasidism, declared that a parent failing to vaccinate infants against smallpox was "like spilling blood"—meaning it was equivalent to murder. He did so even though the vaccines of that era sometimes caused death from sepsis, tetanus, or runaway vaccinia infections.

Vaccines are often grown in broths of cell lines that have been "immortalized" to keep replicating for decades. For example, the MRC-5 and WI-38 cell lines originated in fetal tissues that, had they matured, would have become lungs. (Those tissues were chosen because respiratory diseases like chickenpox and rubella multiply in lung cells.)

Vaccine cell lines must be absolutely free of cancer and stray viruses, which is why they were derived from fetuses removed in sterile surgical environments rather than from stillbirths.

The MRC-5 line originated with a male fetus aborted in Britain in 1964 because the mother suffered psychiatric problems. WI-38 came from a female fetus aborted in Sweden in 1962 because the parents felt they had too many children. (The initials are from "Medical Research Council" and "Wistar Institute.")

In 2005, replying to a request from a Florida-based Catholic group, the Vatican endorsed the use of rubella vaccines grown in cells from aborted fetuses. Catholics, the Vatican said, should press companies to make alternatives because the cell lines did pose ethical problems "even though this evil was carried out 40 years ago." But in the absence of alternatives, vaccination was "morally justified," the Vatican ruled, because it was more important to protect children and pregnant women.

In 2022, Pope Francis described getting Covid vaccine as a "moral obligation." He also called vaccination "an act of love" and "respect for the health of those around us." He called refusal "suicidal" in a religion that forbids suicide. He and his predecessor, Emeritus Pope Benedict XVI, were both vaccinated.

Mormons, Episcopalians, Lutherans, and many other Christian denominations endorse vaccines, require them in their schools, and distribute them at their missionary hospitals.

The Dalai Lama personally gave polio vaccine to children as part of the world's polio-eradication drive. One of the first accounts of variolation was from an eleventh-century Buddhist nun, who blew ground smallpox scabs into the noses of her patients.

Sometimes fringe "religions" are created for one purpose: to give exemptions to people whose churches refuse to grant them.

In 2002, as part of researching articles on the anti-vaccine movement, I joined the Congregation of Universal Wisdom. For $75, I got a membership certificate saying, "This is to certify that the family of Donald McNeil is enrolled as members of this religious order and is subject to the tenets and beliefs of this order. No member of the Congregation shall have injected, ingested or infused into the body any foreign materials of unhealthy or unnatural composition. No member of the Congregation shall have surgical instruments cutting or piercing the tissues of the body."

The church was run out of the house of Dr. Walter P. Schilling, a chiropractor in the Pine Barrens of southern New Jersey. I contacted him because a nurse I had interviewed at a school in Montclair, New Jersey, with more than 150 unvaccinated students said many parents had Dr. Schilling's certificates.

The New Jersey state epidemiologist told me he had to honor them because state law forbade questioning any citizen's religious beliefs.

By contrast, New York City's schools were famous for refusing exemptions, and principals with unvaccinated children enrolled could be fined $2,000 a day per child. Dr. Terry Marx, then the school system's chief medical officer, was notoriously tough. "Nobody can tell me they're Jewish and they want an exemption," she told me. "Because I'd say, 'Oh really? I'm Jewish. Show me in the law where it says "No vaccines."'"

She said she would accept a Schilling certificate "only if somebody really obeyed this," indicating the clauses about foreign materials and surgical instruments. "That means they wouldn't treat their kid for asthma, wouldn't take their kid for an appendectomy."

After I joined the church and requested an interview, Dr. Schilling welcomed me to his home. We went for a walk with one of his skittish rescue greyhounds.

His church, which he said had over 5,500 members in twenty-eight states, had been founded to defend "straight chiropractors" like himself.

Chiropractic emerged in the 1890s and was an offshoot of "magnetic healing," which had been around for two hundred years. Magnetic healers taught that bodies contained a life force flowing up the spine that could be controlled with magnetism. Chiropractic added the notion that diseases could be cured by readjusting bones in the spine. Now most people consult chiropractors for back and neck problems, but "straight chiropractors" believe that all illnesses, including polio and cancer, for example, stem from spinal misalignment.

His own mentor, the congregation's founder, Dr. Schilling said, believed that pharmaceutical drugs and X-rays were witchcraft, that conventional physicians were agents of Satan, and that Western medicine had evolved from worship of the Greek god Hermes. (Hermes, Mercury to the Romans, carried a caduceus—a winged wand entwined with snakes—which is now a medical symbol.)

"What other people see as Western medicine, we see as a state-imposed pagan religion," he said.

The roots of that schism are in the nineteenth century, when modern medical schools were founded and medicine struggled to distinguish itself from faith healing. Like Charles Darwin's theory of evolution, "germ theory"—the belief that disease is caused by invisible particles—was seen as a threat to fundamentalist Christian beliefs that all illness and all healing came from God. The late nineteenth century was an era of religious revivalism. Chiropractic, homeopathy, theosophy, and Christian Science grew out of the struggle between science and religion.

The difference between "conventional" medicine and alternatives is the burden of proof. Faith healing depends on the patient's belief. In other traditions, the test is how closely the practitioner adheres to ancient practices. But in Western medicine, each new proposed treatment must *prove* itself in clinical trials. A scientist is permitted to overthrow received wisdom as long as the new treatment can prevail over the old in clinical trials overseen by independent judges.

There is nothing "religious" about vaccines, any more than there is about seat belts or motorcycle helmets. But most state legislators do understand how belts and helmets work and so don't offer religious exemptions to them. They don't know how vaccines work and therefore treat them as something mysterious or even spiritual. That's a dangerous mistake.

In any case, religious freedoms are not absolute, despite the absolutist-sounding language of the First Amendment.

Archeological digs have shown that numerous religions, from Egypt to the Andes, once practiced human sacrifice. The Abrahamic religions—Judaism, Christianity, and Islam—are founded on Abraham's willingness to prove his faith by sacrificing his son on an altar. In Christianity, Jesus is portrayed as the sacrificial lamb who tells his followers to symbolically eat his body and drink his blood. Nonetheless, we do not permit human sacrifice. We do not offer religious exemptions to those who perform human sacrifices, no matter how sincerely they believe their gods expect them. We arrest them for murder.

Nor do we permit polygamy, even though most marriages in the Old Testament are polygamous, and even though the practice was once a central tenet of Mormonism and even though marriage to four women is permitted in some Muslim countries.

Religious exemptions cost lives. We should end them.

Chapter Twenty-One

WE NEED TO IMPROVE SURVEILLANCE

Nothing makes it easier to contain an outbreak than catching it early.

One of the best efforts at outbreak anticipation was the Pandemic Influenza and Other Emerging Threats program, or PIOET, created by the U.S. Agency for International Development (USAID) in response to the 2003 bird flu scare. It loaned veterinary experts to about fifty nations to help them detect poultry outbreaks and made grants so they could reimburse farmers for culling their flocks—a crucial step, as I described earlier. In 2009, it added four new programs designed to catch other threats: Predict, Prevent, Identify, and Respond.

Predict sent wildlife veterinarians overseas to teach their local counterparts how to trap and sample bats, birds, rodents, monkeys, and other hard-to-catch species. (It also taught esoteric skills such as how to sample a dead gorilla.) Prevent, another program, taught ways to minimize risks to bushmeat hunters and others at the human-animal interface. Identify paid for lab equipment and training. Respond educated veterinarians, public health doctors, environmental specialists, and the like.

Between 2009 and 2019, these programs trained about 5,000 scientists in 30 countries and improved 60 laboratories. They found over 1,000 new viruses, including a new strain of Ebola. They investigated die-offs of wild birds in Mongolian lakes, proved that otters in a Cambodian zoo were killed by eating flu-infected chickens, and identified bat viruses in a Thai cave where a boys' soccer team was trapped. Other teams discovered that bats passed on Nipah virus by urinating in jars tied to trees to collect date palm sap; they invented bamboo skirts that kept bats out of the jars.

Unfortunately, such groundbreaking work was never a good fit for USAID, which is focused on economic development, not exotic diseases. In late 2019, the Trump administration, which was already hostile to foreign aid, quietly allowed Predict to die. Three months later, when a dangerous new bat virus emerged in Wuhan, that decision was criticized as shortsighted.

I think it's crucial to reinvigorate and expand this kind of surveillance. In its decade-long existence, Predict cost less than $300 million. In 2014, the United States spent $5 billion fighting Ebola in West Africa. Various estimates have been made as to how much the Covid pandemic cost; they hover around $16 trillion. It is infinitely cheaper to head off a dozen pandemics than to suffer the consequences of even one.

An even more ambitious vision was the Global Virome Project, which in 2016 proposed to sequence every animal virus in the world. Doubts were raised because it would cost billions and most results would be worthless because most animal viruses are harmless. (Our own bodies play host to billions of viruses, most of which infect the millions of bacteria we harbor.)

As an alternative, some virologists advocate regular sampling of humans in contact with wild animals: to pay hunters, loggers, guano diggers, wet-market workers, park rangers, and even poachers and animal smugglers for blood, nasal, and stool samples and interviews about their recent health. Any viruses found in them would obviously have already begun the process of adapting to humans. Another proposed approach is to screen samples from thousands of people hospitalized for pneumonia, especially in remote areas. Programs like that have already yielded results; for example, doctors at the University of Texas Medical Branch in Galveston, Ohio State University, and the University of Florida discovered that one dog coronavirus had separately infected humans in Malaysia, Haiti, and Arizona.

To test novel pathogens for their potential to infect us, scientists put them through steps that make them more "human-like" with each iteration. First in cultures of human cells, then in mice genetically modified to have "humanized" immune systems, then possibly in ferrets, monkeys, or other mammals.

Even more dangerous is "gain of function" research, in which a virus known to be dangerous to humans is manipulated to make it more so—either more transmissible or more lethal. One way is to "passage" it numerous times through mammals. Another is to tinker with the virus's genes—perhaps to add a surface spike or cleavage site with a known affinity for human cells, for example.

There is always a chance that the virus will infect a researcher, an animal handler, a janitor, or someone else in the building and escape.

The rationale for gain-of-function research is to discover which mutations would be dangerous if they occurred in nature. In theory, vaccines, monoclonal antibodies, or drugs against them could then be stockpiled. I'm not, however, aware of any gain-of-function research that has yet led to that goal.

What it has produced is intense controversy. Some scientists believe the work is inherently too dangerous because the risks of escape are too great. Several limited outbreaks, including a few deaths, have occurred at laboratories storing smallpox and SARS virus. There have also been many close calls, such as vials shipped that were supposed to contain killed organisms that were still alive.

Other scientists argue that it is like nuclear weapons research: inherently dangerous but necessary if you maintain a nuclear arsenal or need to deter a nuclear attack.

My own feeling is that some gain-of-function research is necessary—*if and only if* an imminent threat exists and there is a well-funded plan for the work to lead to a preventive or a cure, rather than just to notoriety and prizes. There also must be far closer oversight than there is now. The riskiest work, I think, should be done far from urban centers, with robots doing high-risk tasks when possible. The scientists involved could work in shifts of a few weeks at a time, then stay quarantined before returning home until it was clear they were uninfected. That would be unpopular among scientists, but far safer.

On much more modest scales, other new technologies abound.

Sewage sampling came into its own in the early 2000s as genetic sequencing became faster and cheaper.

Haiti's devastating 2010 cholera epidemic, which killed more than 10,000 people, was traced to sewage flowing out of a UN peacekeepers camp into the Artibonite River, the source of drinking water for many villages. The peacekeepers were Nepali soldiers and the cholera strain was identical to one circulating in Nepal. Sadly, finding the source had ugly consequences: angry Haitians stoned peacekeeper vehicles and peacekeepers shot at least one Haitian dead in response.

The polio eradication drive, flush with Gates Foundation cash, was an early adopter. In 2013, poliovirus was found in a sewage sample from a Bedouin village in Israel's Negev Desert, near the border with Egypt; it was the same Pakistani strain that had been found earlier in Cairo sewage. Neither Israel nor Egypt had seen a case of polio paralysis for more than a decade, but the discovery of positive samples triggered a drive to vaccinate local children. Presumably it worked, because no paralysis cases occurred and the sewage eventually cleared.

In 2020, in response to Covid, the CDC established the National Wastewater Surveillance System to collect samples across the country. The technique can be used to track any disease. In 2023, New York State announced plans to test sewage for flu, respiratory syncytial virus, hepatitis A, and norovirus, as well as for genes that make pathogens resistant to antimicrobials.

I think it would make sense to rewrite building codes so drainpipes in large buildings eventually all have built-in sampling taps. That would make the process faster and neater, and outbreaks could be narrowed down quickly.

For now, the most intensive sampling should focus on locations with many foreign visitors, such as tourist hotels and theme parks. In December 2021, as soon as the Omicron variant of Covid left South Africa, it was found in samples from Orlando, Florida, home of Walt Disney World, before any human cases were confirmed. A 2023 study in Nevada comparing samples from manholes on the Las Vegas Strip to those from residential neighborhoods found that 60 percent of the viral load came from visitors. Even air passengers can be screened. A study done in late 2022 that tested about a quart of wastewater from each of 88 flights from Europe that landed at New York's John F. Kennedy International Airport found a Covid variant in 81 percent of them.

The value of checking sewage was also reinforced by an incident in the Netherlands: in 2022, live poliovirus was found in sewage flowing out of a polio vaccine factory. Stool samples from more than 50 employees showed that one of them had been silently infected by a live strain used in producing the vaccine. The employee—who was vaccinated and had no symptoms—kept shedding live virus for a month and so had to be kept in isolation until the infection cleared.

For domestic foodborne pathogens, the CDC runs the PulseNet surveillance system. It was created after the 1992–93 Jack in the Box burger crisis, which killed 4 children and left 178 other victims with permanent brain or kidney damage. In that outbreak, 73 different Jack in the Box restaurants had served undercooked beef patties contaminated with a virulent strain of *E. coli* (*Escherichia coli*) bacteria found in cattle manure.

Such contamination usually takes place in careless slaughterhouses. Cattle intestines teem with bacteria, and their hides may be matted with manure. In a typical operation, the animals are stunned and then hoisted into the air with leg chains. Their throats are slit and their bellies cut open to remove the organs. Then the hides are stripped off and the carcasses are hosed with hot water and disinfectant to remove any manure. Then they are rolled into chiller rooms for twenty-four hours because it's easier to saw through carcasses after refrigeration has firmed up the fat and muscle. If any manure is left on the carcass, or if it has splashed around the environment, the greatest danger is that it ends up on beef that is ground into patties at the factory. If they are undercooked, the bacteria deep inside the patty may survive. (*E. coli*, salmonella, and other bacteria also survive freezing.)

PulseNet connects commercial and state laboratories that test stool samples from patients whose doctors suspect they have food poisoning. If pathogens are found, their genes are sequenced and scanned for patterns.

If multiple patients have the same pathogen, investigators contact each one. Since food distribution networks are nationwide, victims may not even live in the same state. Investigators will ask about everything they ate and drank. If a common item—such as meat, or lettuce, or even bean sprouts—is found, the long process of hunting down the source begins. It can prove to be quite obscure. For example, one outbreak of a deadly bacteria on romaine lettuce was tracked to irrigation canals feeding the field sprinklers. The canals themselves were normally safe, but rain had flooded streams on nearby ranches, washing in cattle manure. In norovirus and salmonella outbreaks, big case clusters have been tracked to one sick restaurant employee.

Something like PulseNet should be the model for tracking outbreaks everywhere.

Not every high-tech surveillance plan works out. In 2008, with much fanfare, Google announced a new tool, Flu Trends. In theory it would aggregate flu-related searches (words like *flu*, *fever*, *sinus*, *Theraflu*, and so on) to spot outbreaks early. It became, as one critic said later, "the poster child for Big Data."

A year later, Flu Trends did not spot the 2009 H1N1 swine flu at its source in rural Mexico. Once the flu reached the United States, though, the program was often a week ahead of the CDC in predicting where cases would turn up. After that, however, it fell victim to its own success. At the peak of the 2012–13 flu season, it predicted that far more people would be infected than actually were. Analyses in *Nature* and *Science* said news stories that foretold a bad flu season led to more searches, which led to more stories. The algorithm was fueling itself; its predictions might have been more accurate if it had simply extrapolated from previous years. "In short," said one critic, "you wouldn't have needed big data at all to do better than Google Flu Trends. Ouch." In 2015, Google quietly shut the service down.

One technology I find impressive is Kinsa Health, a network of about two million internet-connected thermometers distributed to families around the country. I started writing about Kinsa after meeting its founder in 2016 and challenging him to prove that he could beat the CDC at predicting the spread of seasonal flu. He agreed, and his maps were consistently at least two weeks ahead of the CDC's weekly FluView. (Disclosure: since I retired from the *Times* in 2021, I have consulted for Kinsa in return for stock options.)

The company sells thermometers and gives thousands more away through school systems that want early warnings of disease outbreaks in their students.

CDC flu surveillance relies on collating weekly reports from hundreds of doctors, emergency rooms, and medical labs. Many patients, of course, never visit a doctor or take a test, and overwhelmed doctors, hospitals, and labs may not make filing CDC paperwork a top priority. Kinsa, by contrast, gets its data on the same morning that people feel sick. When a user takes his or her temperature, it is uploaded to a cell phone app that records the fever and then asks about other symptoms, such as congestion, nausea, and diarrhea and whether anyone in the family has recently tested positive for any related disease. It offers very basic medical advice, such as whether the user should contact a doctor. Each user in a household gets a separate profile with age and sex information.

Kinsa can see when fevers are spiking in a city, and sometimes even in a zip code. By contrasting those spikes with its database of seasonal norms, it can tell when an outbreak is unusual. During Covid, it spotted several trends. In March 2020, it detected fevers rising in small towns in a rough circle from the tip of Long Island to the Berkshires to the Catskills and also in the Miami area. The pattern was clear: New Yorkers who owned vacation homes were fleeing the city, taking the virus with them and infecting the locals.

The United States was winding down from a bad flu season when Covid appeared, and Kinsa could distinguish Covid outbreaks from flu ones because Covid fevers spiked higher and lasted longer. Then, as the country began locking down, Kinsa could tell which lockdown measures worked best: cities that merely banned gatherings did not see cases drop; cities that also closed bars, restaurants, and schools did. During the Omicron variant, Kinsa showed that, within families, the virus typically spread from adults to children, which is the opposite of how flu spreads.

Obviously, a worldwide network of such thermometers would be very useful for detecting disease outbreaks or even bioterrorism events.

Unfortunately, in October 2023, Kinsa's venture capital backing ran out, and it went out of business.

Cell phone tracking is also useful. In August 2020, cell phone data showed where many of the 450,000 bikers who rode to Sturgis, South Dakota, for its annual motorcycle rally had come from, what bars and concerts had been the most crowded, and where they returned to. Because the rally turned into a superspreader event, the cell phone logs predicted where in the country outbreaks would erupt. They were right. Cases soared in South Dakota, and also went noticeably up in counties from northern Minnesota to Southern California from which numerous residents had biked to Sturgis that summer.

Chapter Twenty-Two

WE NEED TO RATIONALIZE "EMERGENCIES"

Once a serious outbreak is under way, what should public health authorities do about it?

The obvious answer is "declare an emergency." But often that just adds to the confusion. Neither the public nor the news media understand the parameters of such declarations. And when emergencies are declared too soon or too often, it becomes a boy-who-cried-wolf situation: officials are accused of overreacting, the media is accused of alarmism, the public becomes cynical. It backfires.

Our domestic process is informal. The secretary of health and human services can unilaterally declare a public health emergency. But that merely authorizes the government to spend money, change Medicare reimbursement rates, and so on. It's often done preemptively simply to head off a potential emergency.

The WHO, by contrast, has a three-step process for declaring a PHEIC, a "public health emergency of international concern." The director-general must convene a committee of outside experts. It usually spends a day hearing the situation described by the health ministries of the affected countries, and then votes on whether to recommend calling it an emergency. The final decision is up to the director-general.

Other than to draw attention to the crisis, a PHEIC has little practical effect. It does not close borders, impose travel restrictions, nor release a pot of money. It does let the director-general issue recommendations, and member countries are in theory obliged to justify any measures they take that go beyond them. But there are no penalties. For example, the WHO generally opposes closing borders and asks countries to share all their data and patient samples. But some countries do close borders or ignore data-sharing requests—with no consequences.

Declaring a PHEIC is different from "declaring a pandemic." Doing that is legally meaningless—it's like declaring a battle instead of declaring war. But the media inevitably focuses on it, constantly asking, "When is the WHO going to declare a pandemic?"

That scenario played itself out with Covid in 2020. On January 23, the expert committee convened by Director-General Tedros Adhanom Ghebreyesus voted to *not* declare a PHEIC because there was no evidence of human-to-human transmission outside China. A week later, when it was clear that it was becoming a global crisis, the committee reversed itself and Dr. Tedros declared a PHEIC. Nonetheless, reporters kept asking when it would declare a pandemic. At first, WHO representatives said they never would, because it was meaningless; under the International Health Regulations, the only thing the agency can declare is a PHEIC.

Also, they had painful memories. In 2009, the agency fumbled the question of whether to declare that year's H1N1 swine flu a pandemic.

At the time, it *did* have an official definition for one: "sustained human-to-human transmission of a novel pathogen in two or more WHO regions." Every few days, as the virus spread to new countries, reporters would ask the midlevel official hosting the agency's regular updates, "Is it a pandemic yet?"

Each time, he would be forced to say no, it had not yet met the definition. Yes, it was a novel pathogen; yes, it had shown sustained human-to-human transmission; yes, it had spread to two continents—North and South America, as well as the Caribbean. But because the Western Hemisphere is all one WHO region, it did not meet the definition.

Then a handful of cases turned up in Britain, in the WHO's Europe region. The press asked again. But there were no links between those early cases, so no sustained transmission *in Europe*, so no pandemic yet. Then there was only "limited" transmission in Europe. Only when there were multiple clearly connected cases in Britain was a pandemic declared.

That made the agency look officious and silly. It resolved to stop declaring pandemics and stick to PHEICs. In 2020, it adhered to that principle for about six weeks. The reluctance, according to Dr. Michael J. Ryan, chief of emergency response, was fear that, if it uttered the word *pandemic*, some countries would just give up. China, Singapore, and South Korea were proving that Covid could be contained, and the WHO was hoping others would follow their example.

But journalists kept asking why the WHO wouldn't pull the trigger. Finally, on March 11, Dr. Tedros reversed himself and announced that the outbreak was, indeed, a pandemic. He admitted that his declaration had no legal meaning, that he was doing it simply to "ring the alarm bell" louder, hoping countries would work harder. In the end, of course, neither declaration made much difference. Each country pursued its own path and suffered its own fate.

In my opinion, the agency should take a completely different tack. Instead of making the Manichean "Yes PHEIC/No PHEIC" or "Yes Pandemic/No Pandemic" choice, it should rate growing epidemics as we do hurricanes: Category 1 to Category 5. The news media and the public find those easy to grasp. They even get excited when a hurricane is upgraded a notch or downgraded to a mere tropical storm.

The WHO, however, should use two scales: one for transmissibility and one for lethality. So, for example, an Ebola epidemic might be a 2/5; a low 2 for transmissibility because it usually requires physical contact, but a 5 for lethality. Covid, by contrast, would be a 5/2. It's almost as infectious as measles but was only rarely lethal, even before vaccines were available.

The 2009 swine flu might have started as a 5/3 but then have been downgraded to 5/1 when it became clear that it was even less lethal than seasonal flu. Monkeypox might have been a 2/3 in Africa but then a 3/1 in Europe when it became known that it was transmitted through sex, which is more common than rodent bites, but it was very seldom fatal when spreading among adults outside Africa.

For fine-tuning, there could be more than five levels. Or it might be sensible to add a third "morbidity" index that would indicate how much misery a disease caused, even if its fatality rate is low. Monkeypox rarely kills, for example, but it can cause suffering in the form of excruciating pain and permanent scars.

But the overall point is that the risk must be conveyed in a measured way that balances legitimate alarm against unnecessary alarmism and that the public and the media can understand.

Chapter Twenty-Three

WE NEED TO RESPECT WITCH DOCTORS

Fighting disease in wealthy countries where almost everyone is connected to the internet or local news and has at least some understanding of modern medicine is one thing. Fighting disease in the dozens of countries where literacy is low and traditionalism is powerful is another.

Those countries, however, usually have at least two groups of health professionals who could be useful both for fighting disease and for spotting new outbreaks. The two were once called "witch doctors" and "lady health workers," but those names are being replaced.

"Witch doctor" was always a misunderstanding, since the doctors—the benign ones, anyway—are not viewed as witches but as healers who lift curses imposed by witches. "Lady health workers"—formerly an official title, abbreviated LHW—are now usually called "community health workers," "health promoters," or "ashas" (for "accredited social health activists").

Westerners tend to laugh off witchcraft, but in much of the world it's still a living reality. Nearly every rural village has someone who practices traditional healing. In many countries they vastly outnumber conventional doctors.

In Africa, according to the WHO, there are about eighty times as many traditional healers as doctors. A 2018 review published in *BMJ Global*

Health concluded that almost 60 percent of all Africans regularly used "traditional, complementary or alternative medicine" for a wide range of conditions from pregnancy to epilepsy. More than 80 percent of them did not disclose this to conventional doctors they consulted, fearing criticism (and, the study noted, because most doctors never asked).

There are good reasons those healers find patients. They live nearby and speak the local language. They charge affordable fees—perhaps a chicken or a basket of garden vegetables. They are often incisive psychologists and know enough about each patient's life to treat him or her with compassion and insight. By contrast, a Western-trained doctor in a far-off city hospital seems terrifying. The proposed cure may be baffling, as in: How can a pill that looks like a bit of candy cost so much? Or frightening, as in: This doctor wants to put me to sleep, cut me open, and remove my insides?

They also often do cure their patients. We're used to getting our medicines out of pill bottles, but plants have many similar bioactive chemicals. Samuel Muriisa, a healer I interviewed in western Uganda, described to me which local plants he used for various ills. When I asked if he knew any of their English or Latin names, he dug beneath some skins in his hut and produced an academic book with pictures. His knowledge of the medicinal effects of their leaves, roots, and seeds appeared to exactly match what the book said.

But mostly, a traditional healer's view of sickness makes more sense. To people with no science background, the notion that you suffer because you've been cursed is more instinctively plausible than the idea that you've been invaded by millions of "animalcules" too tiny to see.

I once asked a woman being treated for sleeping sickness in a Doctors Without Borders hospital in rural Uganda what she thought had made her sick. In Western medicine, the correct answer is "I was bitten by a tsetse fly, which injected parasites that reached my brain." Jovina Oleru's answer, however, was "My husband paid my father only three cattle when he married me, and I have given him three children. So, my family really got nothing for bride-wealth, and they feel bad about me and perhaps wish me to die."

To her, that felt intuitive. I'm sick because my family resents me. I'm sick because I neglected to leave a gift on my ancestors' graves. I'm sick because I offended someone who I didn't know was a witch.

Nonetheless, even if she did not subscribe to Western medicine's diagnosis, she clearly had great faith in its healing power. She had endured torture at its hands. At that time, the only treatment for advanced sleeping sickness was intravenous melarsoprol, which is an arsenic compound that a doctor described to me as "arsenic dissolved in antifreeze." It burned like fire as it dripped in, and each infusion scarred the vein so badly that the next had to be in a different spot.

Unfortunately, we usually hear only about the dark side of the profession. In his memoir about fighting smallpox, Dr. William Foege described a grotesque moment in the struggle. The last smallpox victim in Benin, in West Africa, was visited by several "fetisheurs" who wanted to buy his scabs.

For a fee, fetisheurs would inoculate people against smallpox by making small cuts in their skin and rubbing in powdered scabs. The practice, a form of variolation, had been used in Africa for centuries. The inoculee would usually get a mild infection and then be protected for life. In rare cases, an unlucky one died, but death rates from variolation were far lower than those from smallpox epidemics.

But fetisheurs were not above using the scabs perniciously, Dr. Foege wrote. When there was no smallpox outbreak for them to profit from, they might start one by smearing a paste of scabs on a thorn tree branch and wedging it in a doorway where someone could be scratched.

To my mind, if Western-trained doctors are going to make any progress in the distant countries that act as the nurseries of pandemics, they must embrace and train their traditionalist competitors, not dismiss them.

Yes, some say things that to Western ears sound crazy. Mr. Muriisa said he could predict which patients would live or die based on whether he could balance a stick on a bottle after they left. Another healer told me he could make me bulletproof by brewing a potion from a crocodile skin nailed to his wall. When I asked how he got the skin, he said he had speared the croc. I wanted to point out that the croc was hardly bulletproof, but I didn't want the interview to end.

And yes, there are horrible aspects to witchcraft, such as the "penis riots" that convulsed West Africa in the 1990s or the "albino murders" that were first revealed in the early 2000s and are still haunting eastern and southern Africa. The former were triggered when someone screamed that a stranger had stolen his penis by simply bumping into or looking at him. It may sound comical, but about a dozen accused "witches" were beaten to death by terrified crowds. (Police commanders in Ghana blamed thieves, saying they started the riots to buy time to loot market stalls in the melee.) In the latter, more than 600 albinos, many of them children, have been murdered and chopped up for "medicine" made from their skin, bones, hair, or genitals. Albino "medicine" is supposed to help businessmen make money, politicians win office, or soccer teams win games. The government of Tanzania is fighting the trend by creating guarded "safe villages" for albinos and by imposing the death penalty on sorcerers who buy body parts.

Nonetheless, traditional healers could be the perfect sentinels for the appearance of new diseases in the remote areas where they live. Because they're trusted, they can also convey important health messages, such as that some local practice—like eating bats—is dangerous. Or that something new—like a vaccine—is trustworthy.

Most of the healers I've met have been intelligent, empathic, curious, and open-minded. They're also revered by their patients and often quite influential locally. One I interviewed in Lesotho was consulted by the country's royal family and credited with protecting the royal graveyard from lightning strikes. Many said they were eager to cooperate with Western-trained doctors, as long as they were not mocked or condescended to.

Albert Manqueriapa Vitente, an Amazonian shaman in Peru, told me how he treated his sister while she was hospitalized in Cuzco for uterine cancer. He didn't oppose any of the chemotherapy or radiation she received, but after consultation with her oncologist, he prepared teas—including ayahuasca, a hallucinogen—that helped take away her nausea, pain, and fear. She recovered. If he developed cancer, he added, he would go to the same hospital.

I asked if the government cooperated with him in any way, if it warned him about diseases circulating in his area or asked him to report patients with unusual symptoms. "No," he said bitterly. "The government doesn't help us. They think we're a useless holdover from the old days."

A more productive relationship I once witnessed existed between Dr. Smangaliso Hlengwa, a young doctor in South Africa's KwaZulu-Natal province, and a prominent local healer, Martha Shokwakhe Mtshali. Dr. Hlengwa was putting his HIV patients on the triple-therapy cocktails that were just then becoming available outside the public hospital system. When he asked them what other medicines they used, some admitted to also consulting sangomas, the local healers. Since much of Zulu medicine is based on purging evil influences from the body, they were being given strong emetics and enemas made from herbs and tree bark.

"If I give a patient antiretrovirals, and he sees a sangoma who gives him drugs to throw them up, what's the point?" he said.

So he went to the rural compound of "Mama Mtshali" to pay his respects and ask if they could cooperate.

After much discussion, she agreed to moderate her treatments for the patients they shared. She and the young doctor became friends. "She is one of my patients and I am one of hers," he said.

Dr. Hlengwa, a photographer, and I spent a night in her compound—a ring of thatched huts—to meet several sangomas for a long discussion about AIDS. Like many professionals, they were recognizable by their uniforms: from hair beads to cloaks to sandals, they wore only red, white, and black. Mama Mtshali's apprentice had an inflated goat bladder twisted into her hair to indicate that she was still a student. They showed us how they made diagnoses: as a drummer pounded out a trance-inducing rhythm, they hammered the dirt floor with wooden clubs and chanted. I was mystified, assuming that they were appealing to ancestor spirits, but Dr. Hlengwa explained that they were also calling out various symptoms—which the patient then said he did or did not have. It was a form of differential diagnosis.

They were very eager to know more about HIV transmission. In particular, they wanted to know how long the virus could persist on a razor blade or porcupine quill, since they used those for "injections" by making cuts in a patient's scalp and rubbing in herbs. They couldn't afford a new razor for each patient, but also understood that AIDS was blood-borne, so they used alcohol disinfecting wipes. Mama Mtshali proudly showed me a certificate indicating that she had taken a course from the local hospital in "The Traditional Healer's Role in AIDS."

She was sure she could cure many ills, from hysterical crying to loss of appetite to cancer. "But AIDS," she admitted, "is too difficult to see. And by the time we can see it's AIDS, it's too late." She had learned the early signs of HIV and was referring those patients to Dr. Hlengwa.

To my mind, the bond they had forged was the ideal relationship between two different schools of medical thought: each recognized the limits of his or her powers and agreed to cooperate for the benefit of their patients.

There are hundreds of thousands of such healers in the world. I think public health officials should do what they can to encourage such arrangements, treating the healers with respect, offering them courses in hygiene and medicine, perhaps training them to give vaccines—and paying them to refer patients on to clinics when it will save lives.

The other group—lady health workers, health promoters, ashas—are officially part of government health departments. They have greatly improved public health outcomes in India, Pakistan, Peru, Rwanda, Ethiopia, and a few other countries where the government has trained a dedicated corps of them. In early 2022, India's program—which employs more than 1 million women—won a "Leaders in Global Health" award from the WHO.

The concept is simple: recruit and train local women as intermediaries between their neighbors and the country's formal medical system. (Recruits need not be women, but because the programs were initially launched to help pregnant women and infants, most are.)

They usually work in the village or neighborhood where they live, so they speak the local language, know the customs, and often personally know their patients and family histories. Some are volunteers, some are salaried, some are paid for reaching goals like vaccinating 100 children. In India, the program was originally intended as part-time—a couple of hours a day in return for a small stipend. It proved so essential, however, that tasks were added and some women were working fourteen-hour days, so they struck for full-time salaries and benefits.

An inspiration for the movement was the "barefoot doctors" campaign introduced in Mao's China in the 1950s. Many had little or no training. For example, Chen Zhu, China's health minister from 2007 to 2013, was sent to the countryside in 1969—at age sixteen—simply because his parents were both physicians. He did it for five years until he was allowed to begin medical school. In that era, some new medical graduates were forced to spend years practicing in the countryside. In other cases, local healers were trained to join the program; the one requirement was the ability to read and write.

Nowadays, on a typical home visit, a worker might check a newborn child to see if it is gaining weight and counsel the mother on how to breastfeed and keep the baby warm. She may teach the value of boiling drinking water, and how to make nutritionally balanced food from cheap ingredients.

Some lady health workers can inject vaccines; all will be charged with explaining why they're important. For a sick child, she may take the pulse, temperature, breathing rate, or blood oxygen level and advise the mother on whether to go to a hospital. They teach basic first aid: how to rehydrate a child with diarrhea, how to tie a tourniquet or splint a limb.

In some programs, they help women get birth control (which may mean doing it without the husband knowing). For pregnant women, they may monitor blood pressure to ward off eclampsia or give vitamins and folic acid to prevent birth defects.

Often the most lifesaving intervention they offer is to simply convince a family to let a young woman give birth in a hospital instead of at home. In many societies, new brides live in their husbands' households and are under the thumbs of their mothers-in-law and aunts. Husbands may not want to pay for a hospital birth and the older women may back him up, boasting that they gave birth at home, so anyone can.

Most home births go well, but problems can develop very fast. A clinic is far more likely to have on hand the tools needed in a crisis: a stethoscope, a fetal heart rate monitor, an ultrasound machine, delivery forceps or vacuum cups, oxygen, drugs to stop postpartum hemorrhaging, sutures, surgical kits for Caesareans, and so on. Studies have shown that even the simplest safe-birth kits—those containing just a plastic sheet, soap and antiseptic, and a clean razor and clip for cutting and clamping the umbilical cord—are much more likely to be used correctly when used in a clinic rather than at home.

Health workers can also advise against dangerous traditional practices. For example, at one time in Nepal, it was customary to cut the umbilical cord on an old coin for luck. In the Peruvian Andes, it was customary to daub the stump with llama or goat dung to stop the bleeding. Those customs gave both countries high rates of death from neonatal tetanus.

Local health workers may also be the only people in their village who understand the rudiments of Western medicine. As such, they can be trained to serve as the eyes and ears of a vast human surveillance system, to recognize any unusual new diseases in their area and pass the word up the chain long before government health authorities notice it.

Chapter Twenty-Four

WE NEED TO MAKE MEDICINE CHEAPER

The high price of drugs puts us all in danger. Not just in the obvious way: if a drug is expensive and I lack insurance, I can't afford it and therefore I die. The failure to cure also means a disease stays in circulation. The world's poor are a reservoir for circulating diseases and, once in a while, someone gets on a jet and brings one to a rich country. Untreated diseases are enormous drags on economies. It's not just that people are sick because they are poor. Sickness *keeps* them poor, by sapping their energy for work, by emptying the family's savings, by killing breadwinners in middle age, and so on. Enormous savings are possible.

For example, deworming pills need to be taken only twice a year to make a difference. Children freed of bloodsucking worms gain weight and do measurably better in school. Adults find the strength to work more, which can boost a family's income. In one study in Kenya, women who got deworming drugs worked 17 percent more hours each week and were more likely to plant crops to sell rather than just enough to feed their families. Men were more likely to take on small jobs like repairing bicycle tires or acting as porters. The pills cost just 30 cents each. In other words, for 60 cents a year, one could raise a family's income by many dollars.

The long-term effects of such small victories can be profound. In the

American South in the 1940s, for example, children from communities that had been reached by hookworm-elimination campaigns were more likely to be literate as adults, and to earn almost 50 percent more than their counterparts from areas the campaigns had missed.

Even with a newly patented drug, it's not prohibitively expensive to cure diseases of poverty. An example that worked quite well was the Gilead pharmaceutical company's decision in 2014 to help Egypt tackle its hepatitis C epidemic.

Egypt had the world's highest per capita hep C rate, the legacy of a drive it began in the 1960s to eliminate schistosomiasis from the villages of the Nile Delta. Schisto, also called bilharzia or snail fever, is infestation with flatworms spread by water snails. The first signs are usually abdominal pain and bloody urine. In children, it can cause stunting and learning difficulties; in adults it leads to liver and kidney damage, infertility, and bladder cancer.

Millions of Egyptian schoolchildren in the Delta wetlands got regular injections of antiparasitic drugs. Although that was very effective in curing schisto, it unfortunately vastly multiplied hepatitis cases because poorly trained nurses routinely filled syringes with multiple doses and injected several children in turn.

Abdel Gawad Ellabbad, a fifty-two-year-old air-conditioning repairman when I interviewed him in 2015, remembered marching with his classmates down to a public clinic once a month. He watched the nurse boil a syringe before filling it with five doses. "I didn't want that hot needle touching me," he said, laughing. "So, I thought I'd be smart—I let the other boys go first."

The disease was further spread by poor sanitary practices. Even a tiny smear of blood contains enough hepatitis C virions to start an infection. (Other blood-borne diseases, including AIDS, require more.) Some doctors and dentists in Egypt neglect to sterilize their instruments. A weekly barbershop shave is still common there and some barbers fail to sterilize their razors. The virus also spreads within families when razors or toothbrushes are shared.

Egypt fought its epidemic hard. It has more liver specialists and does more liver transplants per capita than any other country. But until 2013 it was making little headway. Treatment required taking a mix of interferon and ribavirin, which had such harsh side effects that few victims could finish a full course.

Then Gilead invented sofosbuvir, which cured in weeks with very few side effects. In the United States, it charged $84,000 per course.

The company offered it to Egypt for $900, about 1 percent of the American price. But it imposed a set of strict conditions. Patients could get the pills only through designated government clinics. A patient could have only one bottle at a time—no exceptions, even for foreign travel—and had to turn in an empty bottle to receive a full one. Additionally: immediately upon receiving the bottle, the patient had to open it, break the seal, and swallow the first pill under the eyes of the pharmacist.

Gilead imposed those rules to prevent patients from reselling their bottles on the black market. It feared they would quickly flood back into the wealthy countries where it was making billions on sofosbuvir.

Drug-access activists strongly objected, especially to the last condition. Gilead, they argued, was interfering in the doctor-patient relationship by turning pharmacists into enforcers.

But the Egyptian government welcomed the arrangement. And most patients I interviewed were not at all bothered.

"I'm a poor man," Mr. Ellabbad told me. "If I did not have to hand in the bottle each time, I might have sold them to buy my son a house. Before, I felt like I was dying. Now I feel like I'm thirty-five again."

Gilead lowered its own costs even further by licensing its sofosbuvir patents to generic drug companies in Egypt and India. The major pharmaceutical companies have come a long way from the rampant greed and indifference I described earlier in this book. As long as they can protect their profits in rich countries, they often do not object to generic competitors serving poor and lower-middle-income ones. Obviously, Americans need to find ways to lower our own prices—as every other advanced nation has. But that's a matter for another book.

Another move we could make is to lower the barriers to letting companies cooperate to make better drugs.

Pharmaceutical companies love "magic bullets"—a new molecule that cures instantly. During the twenty years that a company has such a drug under patent, it can make tens of billions of dollars.

The best-known magic bullet is penicillin, which changed the course of bacterial diseases and made wounds and surgeries more survivable. But magic bullets inevitably turn to dust because pathogens develop resistance. Cocktails of several drugs that work in different ways do far better in the long run than lone magic bullets.

We've learned this lesson many times, but it never seems to stick. In the 1980s, HIV showed us the folly of the magic-bullet approach. The virus could mutate so fast that AZT, the first bullet, soon failed. That ultimately led to triple-therapy cocktails.

Hepatitis C reinforced the lesson: Since sofosbuvir emerged in 2013, millions of chronic carriers have been cured. But resistance always threatened. There are now eight hep C regimens—all involving cocktails of two, three, or even four antivirals.

We forget that we learned this lesson long ago, back when diseases took longer to cross borders. In the 1940s, tuberculosis could be beaten by streptomycin alone, and many Americans were cured that way. Soon, however, drug-resistant strains proliferated, and by the 1960s, achieving a cure took a mix of four drugs. Until recently, the only hope for someone with a highly resistant strain was to take forty pills a day, sometimes with IV antibiotics as well, for a year or more.

During the Vietnam War, synthetic quinine—chloroquine—stopped working against malaria in Southeast Asia. The world began looking for a magic bullet. With help from the U.S. military, the American drug industry developed mefloquine, sold as Lariam. It worked, but it had such frightening mental side effects, from vivid nightmares to psychotic breaks, that many service members refused to take it. Chinese scientists trying to help the North Vietnamese eventually developed artemisinin—a fast-acting parasite-killer isolated from sweet wormwood, a traditional Asian fever medicine. The discovery eventually won the Nobel Prize. But artemisinin can't work alone because the body quickly eliminates it, so it is always combined with one or two other drugs that linger longer in the blood to mop up survivors.

Why do cocktails work when single therapy fails?

Imagine fighting an opponent who has an ax and can only do one stroke—straight down on your head. If he lands it, you're dead. But if you learn to step aside at the last second, you live, and he's useless. That is the equivalent of a virus evolving resistance to a drug's "mechanism of action."

But suppose you instead face three opponents with three different mechanisms: One has the ax. One has a scimitar and swipes at your neck, which you can dodge by ducking. One has a spear, which he thrusts at your stomach; you can avoid it by jumping back.

But no one can step aside, duck, and jump backward all at the same time. The "cocktail attack" will get you. It's the same for pathogens. Although they constantly mutate, it's very unlikely that mutations will occur simultaneously in three different genes to produce resistance to three different mechanisms of action. As a result, cocktails usually stay effective for many years longer than magic bullets do.

Combining drugs into cocktails would seem like an obvious approach. But companies resist it because it cuts into their magic-bullet profits. And, unfortunately, American laws make cooperation almost impossible.

Patent laws originated in the nineteenth century to protect innovation. Many brilliant inventors were wiped out when competitors stole their ideas and sold cheap copies. In response, new laws granted them a period of exclusivity during which copying was blocked and the patent-holder could sell at any price. Inevitably, however, a downside to those profitable monopolies emerged: when competition was finally allowed, patent-holders would wipe out low-priced rivals by either buying them or combining with them in "trusts" established to fix prices. In the late nineteenth century, trusts stifled competition in virtually everything. There were railroad trusts, oil trusts, coal trusts, even matches trusts, butter trusts, and ice trusts. The Sherman Antitrust Act of 1890 and follow-up laws changed that by making it illegal for companies to collude in any way.

That arrangement works well for inventions like cotton gins, revolvers, toasters, and silicon chips. No one wants a cocktail toaster, they want one that grills bread and is cheap. It does not work well for lifesaving drugs. There are many situations in which cocktails are best.

During Covid, two antiviral drugs were announced almost simultaneously: Pfizer's Paxlovid and Merck's Lagevrio, better known as molnupiravir. They had very different mechanisms of action: Paxlovid is a protease inhibitor—it blocks the enzymes that act like scissors to cut long proteins into useful subunits. Molnupiravir, by contrast, is a nucleoside analog—it slips into replicating RNA by taking the place of the amino acid cytosine, which it closely resembles. As the virus copies itself, the substitution induces errors until it "mutates itself to death," one scientist said.

Paxlovid soon had the upper hand: clinical trials found it was almost 90 percent effective at preventing hospitalization, while molnupiravir was only about 30 percent effective. Also, there were questions as to whether molnupiravir could also cause copying errors in DNA when normal cells copied themselves. That might lead to birth defects or cancer.

Nonetheless, both Merck and Pfizer independently went ahead with their drugs, and Pfizer essentially drove all others out of the field. A better solution might well have been to make cocktails of the various magic bullets then in the works from Merck, Roche, and other companies. Their synergies might cure patients with smaller amounts of each drug and also make it far harder for Covid to evolve resistance. But it never happened.

A similar situation prevailed in monoclonal-antibody therapy. Regeneron, Eli Lilly, Roche, GSK, and others developed antibody infusions that could block the virus. At the outset, they were amazingly effective. President Trump, his lawyer Rudolph Giuliani, his secretary of housing and urban development, Ben Carson, and former New Jersey governor

Chris Christie and others who were seriously ill got monoclonal antibodies and very likely were saved by them.

But, as different variants evolved, most of those antibody monotherapies stopped working and were abandoned. Mixing them in cocktails might have been more protective, but antitrust laws made that impossible. Companies could not run joint clinical trials or discuss how to price a mixed product for fear of being charged with collusion.

I think it would make sense to change the law so that lifesaving drugs are treated differently from toasters. With government oversight, we should encourage pharma companies to create, test, and market multidrug cocktails.

Under unusual circumstances, such cooperation has taken place, and has worked. In 2009, Pfizer and GSK spun off and melded their HIV divisions into a new company, ViiV Healthcare. They assigned it their patents on individual antiretroviral drugs so it could make a three-in-one cocktail to compete with Gilead's popular new three-in-one pill.

Effective cocktails have also been made in countries that do not enforce American patents. Cipla, an Indian company, was making three-in-one pills to fight HIV in Africa almost a decade before anything similar was available in the United States.

The next looming threat to the world may be "superbug" infections. A 2022 *Lancet* study estimated that more than 1 million people die now each year from drug-resistant bacteria and fungi: viral colds that develop secondary bacterial or fungal pneumonia, minor wounds contaminated with flesh-eating bacteria, routine urinary tract infections that kill. The risk is expected to grow rapidly. It might be reduced by ending the practice of putting patients on one magic bullet after another and instead dispensing cocktails.

Before that can happen, however, the laws will have to change. And companies will have to be incentivized—or forced—to cooperate.

Chapter Twenty-Five

LIKE IT OR NOT, WE NEED MANDATES

As I've made clear, I'm very much in favor of mandates. I've seen many countries beat epidemics and save thousands of lives by quickly imposing a firm hand instead of dithering for months—or getting bogged down in protecting the liberties of selfish egomaniacs.

Pandemics are like wars. Innocents die. If officials can save lives, they should.

Yes, that firm hand must be imposed with common sense and judicious scientific guidance, and it should be lifted as soon as possible. But it still should be imposed, because people are not very good at saving their own lives—and they are terrible at saving the lives of others. Along with sheer self-interest, they fall prey to all the forces I've written about: denialism, fatalism, rumors, lying profiteers, and so on.

In 2015, I went to Vietnam to study how it had done so well at fighting tuberculosis. The disease had just surpassed AIDS as the world's leading infectious cause of death. AIDS was then killing about 3,300 people a day; tuberculosis was killing 4,100.

Vietnam, with one of the world's worst epidemics, was doing better than any other country, according to Dr. Mario Raviglione, then WHO's head of TB. Over twenty years, it had cut its caseload by two-thirds and was curing 90 percent of its uncomplicated cases and 75 percent of its drug-resistant ones.

It was succeeding for two reasons, he said. It received substantial foreign aid, including from the United States. (When PEPFAR was created in 2003, it had 14 "focus countries"—12 were in Africa, the other 2 were Haiti and Vietnam. Since Vietnam had a negligible HIV problem, I assumed its mysterious inclusion was an unspoken form of reparations for the Vietnam War.)

But it was also winning, he said, "because it's a communist country." Although its economy was increasingly market-oriented, it was still a highly centralized one-party state. Socialist regimes that care about their people—and not all do—"put a lot of resources into primary care: lots of doctors, lots of clinics," Dr. Raviglione said. "And once central government adopts a thing, they really *do* it. They give orders."

Tuberculosis is a stubborn disease. It demands steadfast pursuit of a regimented response, both by the individual and across society. In 2015, even curing a typical "uncomplicated" infection required taking four different antibiotics every day for six months. Some had unpleasant side effects, including nausea and stomach pain. If that failed and a patient developed a drug-resistant strain, achieving a cure became much harder. The most stubborn XDR strains—the "extensively drug-resistant" ones—required hospitalization for up to two years on a combination of oral and intravenous medicines with severe side effects. They could cause permanent deafness and kidney damage. They could kill nerves in the hands and feet until patients had difficulty walking or even feeding themselves. They could trigger psychotic episodes. Some patients just gave up, choosing to die slowly rather than tolerate the side effects.

The key to being cured was to take *all* the prescribed pills, no matter how unpleasant.

Other countries tried voluntary ways to achieve compliance. In Kenya, for example, a medical charity ran a study in which patients received daily text messages asking them to verify that they had taken their pills. Once they answered, they were shown where they stood in a "compliance contest" against other patients. Those who achieved 90 percent or more were invited into a winner's circle with drawings for prizes.

Patients enrolled in the study did well. But, as is often the case, the techniques worked best when managed by highly motivated study investigators. When they were handed off to the government health ministry, compliance faded away.

Vietnam did not rely on enthusiasm or on lotteries. Its government is used to giving orders; its people are used to taking them. Many poor countries are chaotic and their public spaces dirty. Vietnam is the opposite. Its parks are trimmed and swept. Its public bathrooms are clean. Its police, in peaked caps and sharp dress uniforms, are everywhere and, especially in the north, not to be trifled with.

The country's treatment protocols were set by the National Lung Disease Hospital in Hanoi and followed to the letter by the 64 provincial hospitals, 845 district hospitals, and 11,000 local health clinics. Every neighborhood had a clinic, often in the same cluster of buildings that housed its police station and firehouse, and anyone on outpatient treatment was required to show up in person *every day* to take their pills as a nurse watched, checking off each dose on a big yellow card. Those who proved reliable after a couple of months were allowed a more relaxed regimen: they could take home seven days' worth of pills and report to the clinic only once a week.

Compliance was high, local public health doctors said. In fact, treatment failure was more common among the wealthiest patients who could afford to avoid the regimented public health system and see private practitioners. Those patients were prescribed whatever drugs each doctor favored and took them as they liked. No one chastised a private patient who skipped the pill that triggered vomiting or made his stomach hurt.

The result? About a third of the patients in the public hospitals with drug-resistant strains were those wealthier patients who had formerly dodged the government mandates. They ended up as the ones most likely to die—sometimes after infecting their families with their almost-incurable strains.

Mandates work. Getting the reluctant and the belligerent to protect their own health—sometimes even forcing them to do so—saves their lives. It also saves the lives of their children, their spouses, their parents and grandparents, their coworkers, their classmates, their church congregations, their drinking buddies, and everyone else they might infect.

What people choose to do if they have cancer or heart disease is up to them. But if they have a dangerous *transmissible* disease, how they handle it is no longer merely a personal decision. They are carriers. They have a responsibility to protect others.

Each such decision has a cascading effect. Wearing a mask on the subway is an annoyance, but it's not just a question of whether you personally are protected. You may be the unwitting superspreader, or the person next to you may be. If you won't wear a mask, he or she won't either because the lone mask-wearer is fingered as the carrier. The fewer people wear them, the more end up in the hospital. The more overwhelmed any hospital gets, the more people die needlessly. A study done in U.S. Department of Veterans Affairs hospitals early in the pandemic showed that, when an ICU was over 75 percent of capacity, the risk of death for each Covid patient *doubled*.

I absolutely do not think restrictive measures should last forever. We all go through life accepting some risk. I thought the mask mandates in New York subways, for example, lasted ridiculously long. But I regretted that they were not rigorously enforced in the early days when they would have helped most, when transit workers were dying in droves. I also thought no one who was unvaccinated should have been allowed onto subways or buses. I can't imagine the New York City police finding the political will to enforce that—but other countries did, and I think they were right.

In retrospect, I fault *both* administrations for the deaths of more than a million Americans.

The Trump administration was headed by a president who measured himself by the Dow Jones Industrial Average; he swelled with pride as it rose from 20,000 at his inauguration to almost 30,000 by February 2020. He panicked when Wall Street faced reality in March and drove it down to 18,000. He became a denialist, insisting the virus would "disappear, like a miracle" by April. He grasped at straws, like the notion that a fifteen-day lockdown would stop the spread, or that hydroxychloroquine or convalescent plasma would cure. He blamed governors he disliked and encouraged armed protestors in Michigan, Minnesota, and Virginia to "liberate" themselves from lockdowns that he himself had authorized. He mused cluelessly about injecting people with disinfectants or inserting cell-bursting ultraviolet lights into their lungs. He refused to wear a mask for months. He surrounded himself with lockdown opponents who practiced magical thinking, arguing that all vulnerable Americans could be hidden while the rest developed herd immunity through infection. (Three percent of Americans are immunocompromised, 17 percent are senior citizens, 42 percent are obese. Most of them have jobs, children, or caregivers, so the idea of somehow "hiding" all the vulnerable for months was absurd from the day it was proposed.) He hired scientists who made blatantly false claims, like Dr. Scott Atlas's insistence in the fall of 2020 that the virus was dying out naturally without vaccines because most Americans had "T-cell immunity" from previous bouts with common-cold coronaviruses. (Rather than dying out, the virus went on to kill 900,000 more Americans after Dr. Atlas said that.) When the CDC failed to come up with a test for months, the Trump administration simply lied its way through the crisis, claiming the agency had performed one million tests when it had performed 4,000.

Then, to Mr. Trump's everlasting credit, he launched an $11 billion vaccine program that produced, remarkably, two safe and effective mRNA vaccines in record time. But then he not only failed to encourage his tens of millions of loyalists to accept them, he even concealed for months that he and his wife had been vaccinated. He so twisted up his followers' thinking about vaccines that, one year later, when he realized his voters were dying at more than four times the rate of Biden voters and urged them to get booster shots, they booed him.

But the Biden administration, handed those vaccines as a welcome-to-the-White-House gift from the Trump administration, never did enough to mandate them. When President Biden took office in January 2021, less than 1 percent of all Americans were vaccinated. He waited until July to make vaccines mandatory for federal employees and contractors, and until November to make them mandatory for nurses and doctors in 76,000 hospitals and nursing homes and for employees of companies with more than 100 workers.

His administration never produced a vaccine "passport"—a forgery-proof way to show that the bearer had either been vaccinated or had recovered from an infection, which was also highly protective. In a country with cell phone payments, blockchain technology, and QR codes for restaurant menus, that is a no-brainer. With such passports, it would have been easy to get nearly all Americans vaccinated by simply making it illegal to fly in a plane or enter a restaurant, theater, or grocery story without one. But the Biden administration lacked the courage.

Had it not dithered, had every adult and teenager been given three doses, we could have avoided much of the catastrophic loss of life of the late 2021 Delta wave and the subsequent Omicron waves. Our national epidemic could have been reduced to close to the equivalent of a bad flu season. We could have reopened schools, gone back to work, restarted the economy, and ended the increasingly confusing and unenforceable mask mandates almost a year earlier than we did.

Yes, Americans detest being coerced. And, yes, individualism is part of what makes this country great. But mindless individualism is a destructive force; every mass murderer and terrorist is a driven nonconformist, a hero in his personal fantasies. Medical mandates have been saving American lives since George Washington ordered his troops inoculated against smallpox in 1777. The Continental Army's attack on Quebec had ended in disaster because so many men were down with the pox or deserted for fear of it, and Washington ordered the entire army variolated. Without that order—which was extremely controversial in its day—we might never have become a nation. The British army was largely immune through inoculation or having survived a bout.

Mandates worked for California in 2014, when it got rid of its religious and philosophical vaccine exemptions to defeat the measles threat. Mandates worked during Covid for hospital systems whose nurses resisted Covid vaccines until they were told their jobs were at stake—fewer than 1 percent quit or were fired. They worked for many employers, including for New York City, for United Airlines, and, ironically enough, for Fox News.

Death rates plummeted in every venue where mandates were imposed. There was no epidemic of adverse effects. Thousands of Americans did not die of vaccine-induced blood clots or myocarditis. We were not magnetized; George Soros did not become our overlord; Bill Gates could not read our minds. Nothing bad happened.

If a nationwide one had been enforced, hundreds of thousands of Americans would still be alive.

All of which raises the complex question: How far do you go?

How far would I go, if I weren't just a journalist observing others' actions, if I weren't a CDC official or an American president, required to obey the law and submit to review by fickle courts? If I were, say, the president of a country like Cuba or Vietnam or China. Would I have closed the borders, as President Trump did? Absolutely—and far more harshly, with no exceptions for American citizens, whom I would have quarantined. Would I have shut down travel out of New York, Seattle, and the other cities infected in the first wave? Absolutely. Would I have mandated masks in all enclosed spaces and bans on public gatherings? Absolutely. Would I have mandated daily rapid tests to keep schools open? Absolutely. Once vaccines arrived, would I have mandated them? Absolutely.

What about monkeypox? Would I have delayed Pride events a couple of months until vaccines were available? Absolutely. Would I have offered vaccines to all men who had sex with men? Absolutely. Would I have offered everyone testing positive a month of housing, food, and medical care? Absolutely. Would I have mandated that they accept that housing, food, and medical care? Probably. It's inconvenient and embarrassing to be held in isolation for a month. But is it wrong to inconvenience 1,000 men to keep another 29,000 from suffering? I don't think so.

What about HIV? Would I have done what Cuba initially did—mandate universal testing and then impose an indefinite quarantine on everyone who tested positive?

Well, even if I would have I never could have, of course. In Cuba, most of those initially detained were military members with few rights—and even fewer in Cuba. Here the gay rights movement would never have stood for it; nor would the courts. But if I knew then what I now know: that passivity and silent consent would ultimately cost about 600,000 Americans—most of them gay men—their lives, would I have regretted not trying? Yes, I would.

Cuba did not stick to its policy forever. Even before triple therapy was invented, it began letting people with HIV leave the camps. But it still took seriously the need to contain the epidemic. Testing was still mandatory, and the disease was considered a public health threat, not simply a private matter between doctor and patient. Anyone who tested positive had to leave job and home behind to attend a mandatory two-week workshop on "living responsibly with HIV." Everything about the disease was explained in detail, including how to prevent spreading it. It was made clear that the state traced every case to see who had given it to whom. And it was made clear that controlling one's viral load was not optional: anyone with HIV was expected to take his daily pills. No one could plead "I didn't know."

During Covid, I was shocked at how many times I would explain something fairly mundane about the disease and hear "Oh, really? I didn't know that." I remember one New Mexico fishing guide I spent a day with, for example. It was in late 2021, just before the start of the Omicron wave. His uncle had died of Covid, his father had diabetes and heart failure, his girlfriend was pregnant—and neither he nor any of them were vaccinated.

They weren't staunchly opposed as much as they were just apathetic and unfamiliar. I explained how vaccines worked and why they were important, and how pregnancy suppressed his girlfriend's immune system. "I didn't know that," he said, and then added, rather resentfully, "Why didn't someone tell me?" I wanted to scream, "That's your job! You've got to take some responsibility for your own life! And your girlfriend's! And your kid's! And your father's!" But the truth is, many Americans just don't. They must be helped. And when it's important enough—they must be compelled.

Yes, there is no question it's intrusive. But I don't consider it unreasonable. HIV in the 1980s was an inevitably fatal disease. Covid in 2021 was a sometimes-fatal disease. Monkeypox is not normally fatal, though it can be very painful. Lesser threats require less coercive measures. But we will face other diseases that kill. To my mind, the government has a duty to stop them. That is *why* we form governments—to protect us from existential threats. No right to privacy or freedom should be misconstrued to imply that I have the right to be your executioner because I don't feel like being inconvenienced or embarrassed or ordered about. We need to protect each other. In doing so, we protect ourselves. And with pandemics, we need to protect ourselves in order to protect each other.

EPILOGUE

End of sermon. I feel strongly about such things because I think it's imperative to save lives. To the exclusion of almost every other goal.

There are trade-offs. Mistakes will be made. Feelings will be hurt. Fortunes will be lost. But over time, any of those can be repaired. Needlessly lost lives are gone forever.

I know I'll provoke anger. I don't care. I'm not trying to please anyone. I was never very interested in that anyway—and now in retirement I'm even less so.

I count myself lucky. Twenty-five years is a long time to have a beat, especially at an influential paper. Not many news outlets even bother with science sections—they require relatively rare expertise; their illustrations and data make them expensive to produce, and they sell few ads. I was especially lucky because I almost blundered into the assignment. I had no degree in medicine or biology. (My BA from UC Berkeley is in rhetoric.) I became interested because I was based in Africa in the 1990s and death from AIDS was all around me. After that, I learned on the job—by reading, by interviewing scientists, and by going anywhere I could to see how real people suffered—Zimbabweans, Nepalese, Peruvians, Americans, anyone.

I hope that gave me empathy for the victims—even as I noticed how often they failed to save themselves or to protect those they loved. I had to have some empathy; there were times when I too failed as they had and hated myself for it.

Most of those years, I labored in semi-obscurity. My stories typically had few readers (the *Times*' software lets you know just how few) because many were about poor, nonwhite people in faraway countries. I once covered a pilot project in Zambia in which babies in a village reached only by dirt tracks who were near death from malaria got a suppository containing a new malaria drug and then were raced to a health clinic by bicycle ambulance. Infant death rates dropped by 96 percent. I found it intriguing. Only 35,000 readers did. (The *Times* then had more than 4 million subscribers.)

I didn't really mind. Scientists and science-minded readers respected what I wrote. I tried to focus not just on the misery, but on what helped—new medicines, new devices, new approaches. There was a surprising amount of good news around, even in the killing fields. I also deeply enjoyed covering the doctors I met. Their levels of dedication, the hardships some endured in reaching remote villages, the risks of infection they took, the tenderness they showed toward patients . . . and, on top of that, the hours they spent doing the boring stuff—collating data, writing papers, keeping up in their fields—always impressed me. They actually made the world better. They invented new treatments. They saved lives. Very few were self-promoters. Most, aware that whatever they said could be quoted, were scrupulous about their facts, outlining their data and the exceptions and the caveats until I would lower my notebook and complain: "Look, I need to be able to say this in plain English."

When they made mistakes, or a new study disproved their beliefs, they almost always admitted it. That's good science. It also fit with a *Times* ethic imbued in me since I'd been hired at age twenty-two: if you make an error, you correct it—immediately and publicly.

Then Covid came along. Nothing like it had been seen in a century. My February 2, 2020, story saying experts thought a pandemic was coming got 7 million reads. Suddenly, average Americans cared deeply—because they were terrified. When people are afraid, they lash out, looking for someone to follow—and someone to blame. It happened during the Plague of Athens, it happened during the Black Death, and it happened in 2020.

The next three years changed America—for the worse, which is not what I'd originally expected. I thought we would unite against the common enemy. Instead, once it was within our walls, we disintegrated into a fratricidal brawl. We couldn't agree even on how dangerous it was. Early on, I received emails accusing me of alarmism, with back-of-the-envelope epidemiological math purporting to prove that it was no worse than a bad flu season. "I've been covering flu for twenty years," I would reply. "I've never seen a season so bad that hospitals had to rent trucks to hold the dead bodies."

What I found the most discouraging was that science was suddenly treated as just another manifestation of liberal elitism.

I understand the urge to despise elites. Even though, as a Berkeley graduate and *Times* reporter, I'm pegged as a de facto member of that sect, I often feel it myself, especially when it comes from out-of-touch snobs trying to dictate what opinions or vocabularies they find acceptable. But seeing anti-elitism metamorphose into something much bigger—a rejection of data, of science, of facts themselves—was something else. Seeing scientists I had long respected pilloried as liars and targeted by death threats was disturbing. Seeing phony "dissident scientists" trotted out to confront them as if they were equals was infuriating. Seeing that done by politicians was doubly so. My nightmare had always been to be assigned to Washington, Albany, or city hall. To spend my life covering politicians, transcribing and seeking comment on their lies felt like an utter waste.

I hope that, with the passage of time, we get past this crisis in belief. I've seen politics undermine science before, and I notice that denialists reject only the fields that disturb the one notion they hold dearest. Many of those who doubt global warming still accept evolution. Those who reject evolution still accept gravity and thermodynamics. Those who embrace snake-healing still understand auto repair. In the end, people are practical. In extremis, they want to be rescued rather than to die. There were many deathbed conversions to vaccine acceptance, though all, sadly, came too late. The blunt truths that science produces—and that good journalism defends—do tend to win out . . . albeit slowly. I'll wait.

ACKNOWLEDGMENTS

Because this book covers twenty-five years of my career and life, I cannot thank everyone who was kind to me, and I dare not try for fear of offending those I forget. But I must thank Andy and Linda Ach. Andy and I have been friends since we were teenagers and I've relied on Linda's advice for decades. I was fishing with them in early 2020 when I began to sense how bad an obscure outbreak in Wuhan would become, and much of this book was written in the study of their San Francisco home or on the couch of their fishing cabin. Thank you.

NOTES

Chapter 1: Covid as a Nervous Condition

3 *I helped our Beijing and Hong Kong bureaus*: Sui-Lee Wee and Donald G. McNeil Jr., “China Identifies New Virus Causing Pneumonialike Illness,” *New York Times*, January 8, 2020.

4 *January 19 potluck dinner*: “Coronavirus: Wuhan Community Identifies ‘Fever Buildings’ after 40,000 Families Gather for Potluck,” *Straits Times,* February 6, 2020.

4 *local party congress*: James Griffiths, “Is Wuhan’s Mayor Being Set Up to Be the Fall Guy for the Virus Outbreak?” CNN, January 29, 2020, https://www.cnn.com/asia/live-news/coronavirus-outbreak-01-29-20-intl-hnk/h_6d8cf9d5c0b2cf01447dd24325ed6dd3.

5 *Dr. Zhong said on national TV*: China Global Television Network, January 20, 2020, https://news.cgtn.com/news/2020-01-20/Chinese-experts-express-confidence-in-controlling-new-coronavirus--NpKofFhlza/index.html.

5 *not as contagious*: Gong Zhe, Guo Meiping, and Bu Shi, “New Coronavirus Update: Human-to-Human Infection Confirmed,” China Global Television Network, March 20, 2020, https://news.cgtn.com/news/2020-01-20/Chinese-experts-express-confidence-in-controlling-new-coronavirus--NpKofFhlza/index.html.

5 *the WHO did declare one*: Sui-Lee Wee, Donald G. McNeil Jr., and Javier C. Hernandez, “W.H.O. Declares Global Emergency as Wuhan Coronavirus Spreads,” *New York Times*, January 30, 2020.

5 *Mayor Zhou apologized*: Sarah Zheng, “Wuhan Mayor under Pressure to Resign over Response to Coronavirus Outbreak,” *South China Morning Post*, January 23, 2020.

6 *nearly 10,000 cases*: “China Reports Nearly 10,000 Coronavirus Cases,” *VOA News*, January 31, 2020.

6 *On February 2*: Donald G. McNeil Jr., "Wuhan Coronavirus Looks Increasingly Like a Pandemic, Experts Say," *New York Times*, February 2, 2020.

7 *I wrote an article*: Donald G. McNeil Jr., "Mask Hoarders May Raise Risk of a Coronavirus Outbreak in the U.S.," *New York Times*, January 29, 2020.

8 *The stock market*: Matt Phillips, Jason Horowitz, and Choe Sang-Hun, "U.S. Stocks Plunge as Coronavirus Crisis Spreads," *New York Times,* February 24, 2020.

8 "*not so much a question of if*": Transcript for the CDC Telebriefing Update on COVID-19, https://www.cdc.gov/media/releases/2020/t0225-cdc-telebriefing-covid-19.html, February 26, 2020.

9 *On February 27*: Donald G. McNeil Jr., "The Coronavirus Goes Global," *The Daily* podcast, *New York Times*, February 27, 2020.

9 *China's study*: Novel Coronavirus Pneumonia Emergency Response Epidemiology Team, "Vital Surveillances: The Epidemiological Characteristics of an Outbreak of 2019 Novel Coronavirus Diseases (COVID-19)—China, 2020," *China CDC Weekly* 2, no. 8 (2020): 113–22.

13 *My April 18 piece*: Donald G. McNeil Jr., "The Coronavirus in America: The Year Ahead," *New York Times*, April 18, 2020.

14 *Tomas Pueyo's seminal Medium essay*: Tomas Pueyo, "Coronavirus: The Hammer and the Dance," Medium.com, March 19, 2020.

14 *He was proven right*: Daniel Wood and Geoff Brumfiel, "Pro-Trump Counties Now Have Far Higher COVID Death Rates. Misinformation Is to Blame," NPR, December 5, 2021.

15 *On* The Daily: Donald G. McNeil Jr., "The Next Year (or Two) of the Pandemic," *The Daily* podcast, *New York Times,* April 20, 2020.

Chapter 2: How I Got Here

20 *Even with such a blatant blackmail threat*: Donald G. McNeil Jr., "South Africa's Bitter Pill for World's Drug Makers," *New York Times*, March 29, 1998.

21 *In 1917, when the military*: "The Wright/Smithsonian Controversy: The Patent Pool," https://www.wright-brothers.org/History_Wing/History_of_the_Airplane/Doers_and_Dreamers/Wright_Smithsonian_Controversy/08_The_Patent_Pool.htm.

21 *To force Bayer to lower its prices*: Keith Bradsher with Edmund L. Andrews, "A Nation Challenged: Cipro; U.S. Says Bayer Will Cut Cost of Its Anthrax Drug," *New York Times*, October 24, 2001.

22 *On December 1, 2000*: Donald G. McNeil Jr., "Selling Cheap 'Generic' Drugs, India's Copycats Irk Industry," *New York Times*, December 1, 2000.
23 *In part because my last story*: Donald G. McNeil Jr., "Indian Company Offers to Supply AIDS Drugs at Low Cost in Africa," *New York Times*, February 7, 2001.

Chapter 3: What I Learned on the Way

26 *It was under the headline*: Donald G. McNeil Jr., "News Analysis: To Take On the Coronavirus, Go Medieval on It," *New York Times*, February 28, 2020.
26 *Every three days*: Ma Yujie, Yue Wenwan, Yu Pei, and Wang Zuokui, "Wuhan Reopens after 76-Day Life-or-death Battle against Novel Coronavirus," Xinhuanet, April 8, 2020, http://www.xinhuanet.com/english/2020-04/08/c_138958718.htm.
27 *Freezing everyone in place*: Huaiyu Tian, Yonghong Liu, et al., "An Investigation of Transmission Control Measures during the First 50 Days of the COVID-19 Epidemic in China," *Science* 368, no. 6491 (March 31, 2020): 638–42, https://www.science.org/doi/10.1126/science.abb6105.
27 *Everyone testing positive*: Simiao Chen, Zongjiu Zhang, Juntao Yang, Jian Wang, Xiaohui Zhai, and Till Bärnighausen, "Fangcang Shelter Hospitals: A Novel Concept for Responding to Public Health Emergencies," *Lancet Health Policy* 395, no. 10232 (April 18, 2020): 1305–14.
27 *Local hospitals were staffed*: "The Lockdown: One Month in Wuhan," China Global Television Network, February 28, 2020, https://news.cgtn.com/news/2020-02-28/The-lockdown-One-month-in-Wuhan-OsaehknbVu/index.html.
29 *Cuba's response to its AIDS epidemic*: Donald G. McNeil Jr., "A Regime's Tight Grip on AIDS," *New York Times,* May 7, 2012.
30 *Far more controversial*: Donald G. McNeil Jr., "Cuba's Fortresses Against a Viral Foe" *New York Times,* May 7, 2012.
30 *Late in life*: Carmen Lira Saade, "I Am Responsible for the Persecution of Homosexuals That Took Place in Cuba: Fidel Castro," *La Journada*, August 31, 2010.
30 *The amount of sex*: Vivian Kouri, Ricardo Khouri, et al., "CRF19_cpx Is an Evolutionary Fit HIV-1 Variant Strongly Associated with Rapid Progression to AIDS in Cuba," *EBio Medicine* 2, no. 3 (March 2015): 244–54.
30 *While the American epidemic*: Liuber Y. Machado-Zaldivar, Héctor M. Diaz-Torres, Madeline Blance-de Armas, Dania Romay-Franchy, and

Marta Dubed-Echevarría, "Origin and Evolutionary History of HIV-1 Subtype B in Cuba," *International Journal of Cuban Health and Medicine* 19, nos. 2–3 (April–July 2017).

33 *His autobiographical essay*: Jeffrey Schmalz, "Covering AIDS and Living It: A Reporter's Testimony," *New York Times*, December 20, 1992.

Chapter 4: What If We'd Handled Covid Differently?

39 *Total excess mortality*: Matt McGough, Edouard Long, Krutika Amin and Cynthia Cox, "Premature Mortality During Covid-19 in the U.S. and Peer Countries," KFF.org, April 24, 2023, https://www.kff.org/coronavirus-covid-19/issue-brief/premature-mortality-during-covid-19-in-the-u-s-and-peer-countries/.

39 *A study in*: Alyssa Bilinski, Kathryn Thompson, and Ezekiel Emanuel, "COVID-19 and Excess All-Cause Mortality in the US and 20 Comparison Countries, June 2021–March 2022," *Journal of the American Medical Association* 329, no. 1 (November 18, 2022): 92–94.

40 *A study from Brown*: Brown School of Public Health and Microsoft AI for Health, "New Analysis Shows Vaccines Could Have Prevented 318,000 Deaths," May 13, 2022, https://globalepidemics.org/2022/05/13/new-analysis-shows-vaccines-could-have-prevented-318000-deaths.

40 *But by early 2023*: https://www.worldometers.info/coronavirus/.

42 *In Wuhan alone*: World Health Organization, "Report of the WHO-China Joint Mission on Coronavirus Disease 2019 (COVID-19)," February 16–24, 2020, 8.

42 *Few New Yorkers cooperated*: Sharon Otterman, "City Praises Contact-Tracing Program. Workers Call Rollout a 'Disaster,'" *New York Times*, July 29, 2020.

42 *Early studies suggested*: Luis Rajmil, "Role of Children in the Transmission of the COVID-19 Pandemic: A Rapid Scoping Review," *BMJ Paediatrics Open 2020,* 4:e000722, June 21, 2020.

43 *Germany reported its first case*: Euractiv.com with Reuters, "Pass the Salt: How Coronavirus Came to Germany, and How It Was Traced," April 10, 2020, https://www.euractiv.com/section/coronavirus/news/pass-the-salt-how-coronavirus-came-to-germany-and-how-it-was-traced/.

44 *It even had a fatal shooting*: "German Gas Station Worker Killed over Face Mask," DW, September 20, 2021.

44 *Nonetheless, the United States would*: https://www.worldometers.info/coronavirus/.

45 *The first case in the United States*: Michelle L. Holshue, Chas De Bolt, et al., "First Case of 2019 Novel Coronavirus in the United States," *New England Journal of Medicine* 382 (March 5, 2020): 929–36.

45 *Assuming no one else*: Sheri Fink and Mike Baker, "'It's Just Everywhere Already': How Delays in Testing Set Back the U.S. Coronavirus Response," *New York Times*, March 10, 2020.

45 *By mid-February*: Temet M. McMichael, Shauna Clark, et al., "COVID-19 in a Long-Term Care Facility—King County Washington, February 27–March 9, 2020," *Morbidity and Mortality Weekly Report* 69, no. 12 (March 27, 2020): 339–42.

45 *The first confirmed case*: Joseph Goldstein and Jesse McKinley, "Coronavirus in N.Y.: Manhattan Woman Is First Confirmed Case in State," *New York Times*, March 1, 2020.

45 *But genetic testing*: Ana S. Gonzalez-Reiche, Matthew M. Hernandez, et al., "Introductions and Early Spread of SARS-CoV-2 in the New York City Area," *Science* 369, no. 6501 (May 29, 2020): 297–301.

45 *But because it took*: Michael D. Shear, Abby Goodnough, Sheila Kaplan, Sheri Fink, Katie Thomas, and Noah Weiland, "The Lost Month: How a Failure to Test Blinded the U.S. to Covid-19," *New York Times*, March 28, 2020.

45 *Ultimately, Canada had*: Bernd Debusmann Jr., "Why Is Canada's Covid Death Rate So Much Lower than US?" BBC News, February 15, 2022.

46 *For months he even kept secret*: Maggie Haberman, "Trump and His Wife Received Coronavirus Vaccine before Leaving the White House," *New York Times*, March 1, 2021.

46 *The toll of 1.1 million*: Benjamin Mueller and Eleanor Lutz, "U.S. Has Far Higher Covid Death Rate Than Other Wealthy Countries," *New York Times*, February 1, 2022.

47 *Its economy had reopened*: Ma Yujie, Yue Wenwan, Yu Pei, and Wang Zuokui, "Wuhan Reopens after 76-Day Life-or-death Battle against Novel Coronavirus," Xinhuanet, April 8, 2020, http://www.xinhuanet.com/english/2020-04/08/c_138958718.htm.

47 *His scientists had made*: Smriti Mallapaty, "China's COVID Vaccines Have Been Crucial—Now Immunity Is Waning," *Nature*, October 14, 2021.

48 *But there was no way to know*: Wendy Wu, "China Stops Declaring Daily Covid Cases as Wave Strains Hospitals, Funeral Services," *South China Morning Post*, December 25, 2022.

48 *In mid-February, the Communist Party leadership*: Staff reporters, "China Achieves a Major, Decisive Victory against COVID Epidemic," *Global Times,* February 16, 2023.

48 *Various outside epidemiologists*: James Glanz, Mara Hvistendahl, and Agnes Chang, "How Deadly Was China's Covid Wave?" *New York Times*, February 15, 2023.

48 The New York Times: Pablo Robles, Vivian Wang, and Joy Dong, "In China's Covid Fog, Deaths of Scholars Offer a Clue," *New York Times*, February 5, 2023.

Chapter 5: What If We'd Handled Monkeypox Differently?

50 *For a generation of gay men*: Centers for Disease Control and Prevention, "2022 Mpox Outbreak Global Map," https://www.cdc.gov/poxvirus/monkeypox/response/2022/world-map.html.

51 *In 2003, we had lived through*: Centers for Disease Control and Prevention, "Update: Multistate Outbreak of Monkeypox—Illinois, Indiana, Kansas, Missouri, Ohio, and Wisconsin, 2003," *Morbidity and Mortality Weekly Report* 52, no. 27 (July 11, 2003): 642–46, https://www.cdc.gov/mmwr/preview/mmwrhtml/mm5227a5.htm.

52 *It got the name*: Preben von Magnus, Else Krag Andersen, Knud Birkum Petersen, and Aksel Birch-Andersen, "A Pox-like Disease in Cynomolgus Monkeys," *Acta Pathologica Microbiologica Scandinavica*, September 1959.

52 *How those Asian monkeys got it*: Shin Jie Yong, "Monkeypox's Biggest Mystery: It Suddenly Appeared in Labs from 1958 Onwards without Explanation," Medium, September 19, 2022.

52 *After elimination*: Centers for Disease Control and Prevention, "Side Effects of Smallpox Vaccination," https://www.cdc.gov/smallpox/vaccine-basics/vaccination-effects.html.

52 *Then, in 2017*: Dimie Ogoina, James Hendris Izibewule, et al., "The 2017 Human Monkeypox Outbreak in Nigeria—Report of Outbreak Experience and Response in the Niger Delta University Teaching Hospital, Bayelsa State, Nigeria," *PLOS ONE*, April 17, 2019.

52 *But when he tried*: Michaeleen Doucleff, "He Discovered the Origin of the Monkeypox Outbreak—and Tried to Warn the World," *Goats and Soda* blog, NPR, July 29, 2022.

53 *Starting on May 23, 2022*: Donald G. McNeil Jr., "Let's Take Monkey-

pox Seriously," Medium, May 23, 2022, https://donaldgmcneiljr1954.medium.com/lets-take-monkeypox-seriously-8dd585a57624.

54 *That paragraph was quietly removed*: CDC Travel Notices, "Monkeypox in Multiple Countries," https://web.archive.org/web/20220606212334/https://wwwnc.cdc.gov/travel/notices/alert/monkeypox.

54 *To its credit, the CDC*: Centers for Disease Control and Prevention, "Safer Sex, Social Gatherings, and Mpox," https://www.cdc.gov/poxvirus/monkeypox/prevention/sexual-health.html.

55 *"Why don't we offer"*: McNeil, "Let's Take Monkeypox Seriously."

56 *Now more than 100 other countries*: Stephanie Nolen, "Monkeypox Shots, Treatments and Tests Are Unavailable in Much of the World," *New York Times*, September 12, 2022.

56 *It slowly dawned*: New York City Health Department, "Health Department Launches Monkeypox Vaccine Clinic for People Who May Have Been Exposed to Monkeypox," June 23, 2022, https://www.nyc.gov/site/doh/about/press/pr2022/monkeypox-vaccine-clinic.page.

57 *Five days later*: Apoorva Mandavilli, "As Monkeypox Spreads, U.S. Plans a Vaccination Campaign," *New York Times*, June 28, 2022.

57 *Given the combination*: Donald G. McNeil Jr., "We Are Already Blowing Our Monkeypox Response," Medium, June 11, 2022, https://donaldgmcneiljr1954.medium.com/we-are-already-blowing-our-monkeypox-response-2b86a8980e90.

57 *It was not until*: Rob Masson, WVUE, "Health Officials Vaccinate Nearly 700 around Southern Decadence Festivities," KALB, September 5, 2022, https://www.kalb.com/2022/09/06/health-officials-vaccinate-nearly-700-around-southern-decadence-festivities/.

57 *I also argued*: Donald G. McNeil Jr., "Let's Offer Housing to Men with Monkeypox," Medium, July 11, 2022, https://donaldgmcneiljr1954.medium.com/lets-offer-housing-to-men-with-monkeypox-666c3b4ef1fe.

58 *Finally, on July 23*: World Health Organization, "WHO Director-General Declares the Ongoing Monkeypox Outbreak a Public Health Emergency of International Concern," July 23, 2022, https://www.who.int/europe/news/item/23-07-2022-who-director-general-declares-the-ongoing-monkeypox-outbreak-a-public-health-event-of-international-concern.

58 *It was not until August 2*: Sheryl Gay Stolberg and Apoorva Mandavilli, "As Monkeypox Spreads, U.S. Declares a Health Emergency," *New York Times*, August 4, 2022.

58 *But to my mind*: Donald G. McNeil Jr., "Stop Saying Monkeypox Is 'Almost Over,'" Medium, November 14, 2022, https://donaldgmcneiljr1954.medium.com/stop-saying-monkeypox-is-almost-over-f0b8c6e58b8f.

58 *Case clusters:* Lisa Schnirring, "Recent French Mpox Cluster Includes Fully Vaccinated Patients," CIDRAP News, April 6, 2023, https://www.cidrap.umn.edu/mpox/recent-french-mpox-cluster-includes-fully-vaccinated-patients; Lisa Schnirring, "CDC warns of possible mpox resurgence," CIDRAP News, May 15, 2023, https://www.cidrap.umn.edu/mpox/cdc-warns-possible-mpox-resurgence.

58 *It was already known*: Stephanie Soucheray, "Studies Show Jynneos Protection Against Mpox Ranges from 66% to 89%," CIDRAP News, May 18, 2023, https://www.cidrap.umn.edu/mpox/studies-show-jynneos-protection-against-mpox-ranges-66-89.

58 *A British study*: Thomas Ward, Rachel Christie, et al., "Transmission Dynamics of Monkeypox in the United Kingdom," *BMJ*, 2022;379:e073153, November 2, 2022, https://www.bmj.com/content/379/bmj-2022-073153; Soucheray, "Before-symptom spread of monkeypox."

58 *In mid-May*: CDC Health Alert Network, "Potential Risk for New Mpox Cases," cdc.gov, May 15, 2023, https://emergency.cdc.gov/han/2023/han00490.asp.

59 *A CDC study*: Lisa P. Oakley, Kaitlin Hufstetler, et al., "Mpox Cases Among Cisgender Women and Pregnant Persons—United States, May 11–November 7, 2022," *Morbidity and Mortality Weekly Report* 72, no. 1 (January 6, 2023): 9–14, https://www.cdc.gov/mmwr/volumes/72/wr/mm7201a2.htm.

60 *Another worrying trend*: Lisa P. Oakley, Kaitlin Hufstetler, et al., "Epidemiological and Clinical Features of Children and Adolescents Aged <18 Years with Monkeypox—United States, May 17–September 24, 2022," *Morbidity and Mortality Weekly Report* 71, no. 44 (November 4, 2022): 1407–11, https://www.cdc.gov/mmwr/volumes/71/wr/mm7144a4.htm.

60 *He was reassigned*: Carl Campanile, "NYC Infection Control Specialist Claims 'Retaliation' in Monkeypox Dispute," *New York Post*, July 28, 2022.

60 *Internal emails*: Joseph Goldstein, "Debate over Monkeypox Messaging Divides N.Y.C. Health Department," *New York Times*, July 18, 2022.

Chapter 6: Where Pandemics Came From, and How They Changed Us

65 *"We could but surmise"*: John M. Barry, *The Great Influenza: The Story of the Deadliest Pandemic in History* (New York: Viking Press, 2004), 385.

67 *I took a weeklong trek*: Donald G. McNeil Jr., "The Great Ape Massacre," *New York Times Magazine*, May 9, 1999, https://www.nytimes.com/1999/05/09/magazine/the-great-ape-massacre.html.

73 *For example, in the 1990s*: Donald G. McNeil Jr., "Predators Get More Than They Bargained For: Tuberculosis," *New York Times*, April 15, 1997.

76 *The huge 2014 outbreak*: Gretchen Vogel, "Bat-Filled Tree May Have Been Ground Zero for the Ebola Epidemic," *Science*, December 30, 2014.

77 *What was suddenly and unexpectedly added*: Centers for Disease Control and Prevention, "Origins of 2009 H1N1 Flu (Swine Flu): Questions and Answers," November 25, 2009, https://www.cdc.gov/h1n1flu/information_h1n1_virus_qa.htm.

77 *It is illegal*: Donald G. McNeil Jr., "Virus's Tangled Genes Straddle Continents, Raising a Mystery About Its Origins," *New York Times*, April 30, 2009.

77 *Although it was impossible to prove*: Donald G. McNeil Jr., "In New Theory, Swine Flu Started in Asia, Not Mexico," *New York Times*, June 23, 2009.

78 *Global meat consumption*: Hannah Ritchie, Pablo Rosado, and Max Roser, "Meat and Dairy Production," Our World in Data, August 2017, https://ourworldindata.org/meat-production.

79 *Another in 1822*: Ephemeral New York, "A Yellow Fever Outbreak Made Greenwich Village," April 6, 2020, https://ephemeralnewyork.wordpress.com/2020/04/06/a-yellow-fever-outbreak-made-greenwich-village/.

79 *In the nineteenth*: Centers for Disease Control and Prevention, "Elimination of Malaria in the United States (1947–1951)," https://www.cdc.gov/malaria/about/history/elimination_us.html.

79 *Dengue virus*: Germán Añez and Maria Rios, "Dengue in the United States of America: A Worsening Scenario?" *BioMed Research International* (2013): 678645, https://www.ncbi.nlm.nih.gov/pmc/articles/PMC3705843.

80 *In the continental*: Aneri Pattani, "It's High Time for Ticks, Which Are Spreading Diseases Farther," *New York Times*, July 24, 2017.

80 *The Asian long-horned tick*: Donald G. McNeil Jr., "An Invasive New Tick Is Spreading in the U.S.," *New York Times*, August 6, 2018.

80 *Even the magnificent American moose*: Jess Bidgood, "Ticks, Thriving in Warm Weather, Take a Ghastly Toll on New England Moose," *New York Times*, January 19, 2017.

Chapter 7: Why No Pandemic Will Be Our Last

82 *A 2008 study*: Kate E. Jones, Nikita G. Patel, et al., "Global Trends in Emerging Infectious Diseases," *Nature* 451 (February 21, 2008): 990–93, https://www.nature.com/articles/nature06536.

82 *A 2016 report*: United Nations Environment Programme, "Frontiers 2016: Emerging Issues of Environmental Concern," 2016, https://www.unep.org/resources/frontiers-2016-emerging-issues-environmen tal-concern.

83 *A 2022 WHO analysis*: WHO Africa, "In Africa, 63% Jump in Diseases Spread from Animals to People Seen in Last Decade," July 14, 2022, https://www.afro.who.int/news/africa-63-jump-diseases-spread-ani mals-people-seen-last-decade.

83 *Given the dates*: Tom Schnabel, "Coughing During Concerts and Recordings," KCRW Music News, January 19, 2015, https://www.kcrw .com/music/articles/coughing-during-concerts-and-recordings.

83 *In 2015, genetic sequencing revealed*: Michelle Rozo and Gigi Kwik Gronval, "The Reemergent 1977 H1N1 Strain and the Gain-of-Function Debate," *mBio* 6, no. 4 (July–August 2015): e01013-15, https://www.ncbi.nlm.nih.gov/pmc/articles/PMC4542197/.

84 *Ten years after it ended*: Centers for Disease Control and Prevention, "2009 H1N1 Pandemic (H1N1pdm09 virus)," https://www.cdc.gov /flu/pandemic-resources/2009-h1n1-pandemic.html.

84 *A concept in virology*: Various editors, "Original Antigenic Sin," Wikipedia, https://en.wikipedia.org/wiki/Original_antigenic_sin.

86 *Since the mid-1980s*: Adrian R. Marques, Franc Strle, and Gary P. Wormser, "Comparison of Lyme Disease in the United States and Europe," *Emerging Infectious Disease* 27, no. 8 (August 2021): 2017–24, https://www.ncbi.nlm.nih.gov/pmc/articles/PMC8314816/.

86 *Odd symptoms*: Willy Burgdorfer, "The Historical Road to the Discovery of *Borrelia burgdorferi*," in *Aspects of Lyme Borreliosis* (Berlin: Springer, 1993), 21–28, https://link.springer.com/chapter/10.1007/97 8-3-642-77614-4_2.

86 *Since 2011*: Johns Hopkins Bloomberg School of Public Health, "Lyme Disease Overview," https://www.hopkinslymetracker.org/overview/.

87 *In 2009, two prominent virologists*: Scott C. Weaver and William K. Reisen, "Present and Future Arboviral Threats," *Antiviral Research* 85, no. 2 (February 2010): 328, https://www.ncbi.nlm.nih.gov/pmc/arti cles/PMC2815176/.

90 *But Covid's Delta variant*: American Society for Microbiology, "How Dangerous Is the Delta Variant (B.1.617.2)?" July 30, 2021, https://asm.org/Articles/2021/July/How-Dangerous-is-the-Delta-Variant-B-1-617-2.

90 *Admittedly, Delta was later chased out*: Donald G. McNeil Jr., "Here in New York, the Omicron Variant Is Getting Weird," Medium, December 24, 2021, https://donaldgmcneiljr1954.medium.com/here-in-new-york-the-omicron-variant-is-getting-weird-db6d39058b18.

Chapter 8: The Networks That Trigger Blame

94 *No one knew where it had come from*: Charles Q. Choi, "Case Closed? Columbus Introduced Syphilis to Europe," *Scientific American*, December 27, 2011.

95 *The French called it*: John Frith, "Syphilis, Its Early History of Treatment Before Penicillin and the Debate on Its Origins," *Journal of Military and Veterans' Health* 20, no. 4 (2012), https://jmvh.org/article/syphilis-its-early-history-and-treatment-until-penicillin-and-the-debate-on-its-origins/.

95 *In 2009, the Yeshiva University Museum*: Donald G. McNeil Jr., "Finding a Scapegoat When Epidemics Strike," *New York Times*, August 31, 2009.

96 *In 1892*: Howard Markel, *Quarantine! East European Jewish Immigrants and the New York City Epidemics of 1892* (Baltimore: Johns Hopkins University Press, 1997).

96 *In 2019, New York suffered*: Sharon Otterman, "New York Confronts Its Worst Measles Outbreak in Decades," *New York Times*, January 17, 2019.

96 *The cases in both*: Stephanie Soucheray, "US Measles Cases Hit 1,234 as Brooklyn Outbreak Called Over," CIDRAP News, September 3, 2019.

96 *In 2018, measles spread*: Donald G. McNeil Jr., "Scientists Thought They Had Measles Cornered. They Were Wrong," *New York Times*, April 3, 2019.

97 *It was the first case*: Vincent Racaniello, "Polio among the Amish," *Virology Blog*, March 9, 2009.

97 *Health officials estimated*: Ari Daniel, "New York Counties Gear Up to Fight a Polio Outbreak among the Unvaccinated," *Shots* blog, NPR, August 24, 2022.

98 *In the 1990s*: Mireya Navarro, "Confining Tuberculosis Patients:

Weighing Rights vs. Health Risks," *New York Times*, November 21, 1993.

98 *Boston and Denver*: Mireya Navarro, "Grappling with the Care of Problem TB Patients," *New York Times*, April 14, 1992.

99 *That reversal was largely triggered*: Amy Harmon, Frances Robles, Alan Blinder, and Thomas Fuller, "'Frats Are Being Frats': Greek Life Is Stoking the Virus on Some Campuses," *New York Times*, August 18, 2020.

99 *It then reached Iran*: Robin Wright, "How Iran Became a New Epicenter of the Coronavirus Outbreak," *New Yorker*, February 28, 2020.

99 *Or perhaps via*: Zulqarnain Baloch, Zhongren Ma, et al., "Unique Challenges to Control the Spread of COVID-19 in the Middle East," *Journal of Infection and Public Health* 13, no. 9 (September 2020): 1247–50.

99 *It's not entirely clear why*: Jason Horowitz, "Behind the Curve: The Lost Days That Made Bergamo a Coronavirus Tragedy," *New York Times*, November 29, 2020.

99 *Once there, the virus spread*: Selam Gebrekidan, Katrin Bennhold, Matt Apuzzo, and David D. Kirkpatrick, "Behind the Curve: Ski, Party, Seed a Pandemic: The Travel Rules That Let COVID-19 Take Flight," *New York Times*, September 30, 2020.

99 *From there it*: Gabriel Felbermayr, Julian Hinz, and Sonali Chowdhry, "Après-ski: The Spread of Coronavirus from Ischgl through Germany," *German Economic Review*, June 22, 2021.

99 *Skiers may also*: "Coronavirus, Five Britons in French Ski Chalet Catch Virus," BBC News, February 8, 2020.

100 *Skiers and workers*: Katie Kerwin McCrimmon, "Novel Coronavirus Outbreak in Colorado's Ski Communities 'Very Serious,' UCHealth Expert Warns," UCHealth News, March 17, 2020.

100 *On a per capita basis*: Deni Hawkins, "Sun Valley and COVID-19: One Year Later in Idaho's Coronavirus 'Ground Zero,'" CBS2 Idaho News, February 15, 2021.

100 *Those were the home counties*: Donald G. McNeil Jr., "Once Again, the Virus Is Being Spread by an Unusual Vector: Skiers," Medium, January 8, 2022, https://donaldgmcneiljr1954.medium.com/once-again-the-virus-is-being-spread-by-an-unusual-vector-skiers-403d4c8af7ee.

100 *Resorts in the Italian Alps*: Eric Sylvers, "Europe's Ski Slopes Are Open Despite Omicron, at Least for Now," *Wall Street Journal*, December 18, 2021.

101 *The hajj also played a role*: "Europe's Last Smallpox Epidemic," BBC

News: Witness History, November 23, 2021, https://www.bbc.co.uk/programmes/w3ct1x69.

101 *Because he was vaccinated*: Suzana Vuljevic, "Vaccinating Yugoslavia: When Communism Beat Smallpox," Eurozine, April 25, 2022, https://www.eurozine.com/vaccinating-yugoslavia-when-communism-beat-smallpox/.

102 *In 2020, fearing a repeat of earlier disasters*: Ben Hubbard and Declan Walsh, "The Hajj Pilgrimage Is Canceled, and Grief Rocks the Muslim World," *New York Times*, June 23, 2020.

102 *The 2013 Kumbh Mela*: S. Sridhar, P. Gautret, and P. Brouqui, "A Comprehensive Review of the Kumbh Mela: Identifying Risks for Spread of Infectious Diseases," *Clinical Microbiology and Infection* 21, no. 2 (February 2015): 128–33.

102 *In 2008, World Youth Day*: Christopher C. Blyth, Hong Foo, Sebastiaan J. van Hal, et al.,"Influenza Outbreaks during World Youth Day 2008 Mass Gathering," *Emerging Infectious Diseases* 16, no. 5 (May 2010): 809–15.

103 *How it spread from a few apes*: Jacques Pépin, *The Origins of AIDS* (Cambridge: Cambridge University Press, 2011).

103 *That virus was itself*: Donald G. McNeil Jr., "Precursor to H.I.V. Was in Monkeys for Millenniums," *New York Times*, September 16, 2010.

105 *Before HIV tests were developed*: Gilbert C. White II, "Hemophilia: An Amazing 35-Year Journey from the Depths of HIV to the Threshold of Cure," *Transactions of the American Clinical and Climatological Association* 121 (2010): 61–75.

Chapter 9: The Missed Opportunities

109 *For more than twenty years*: Grant Robertson, "What Happened with Canada's Pandemic Alert System? The GHPIN Controversy Explained," *Globe and Mail*, October 5, 2020.

109 *But it went dark*: Grant Robertson, "'Without Early Warning You Can't Have Early Response': How Canada's World-class Pandemic Alert System Failed," *Globe and Mail*, July 25, 2020.

109 *According to a study*: Michael Worobey, "Dissecting the Early COVID-19 Cases in Wuhan," *Science* 374, no. 6572 (November 18, 2021): 1202–4.

111 *With my deadline rapidly approaching*: Donald G. McNeil Jr., "Zika Virus, a Mosquito-Borne Infection, May Threaten Brazil's Newborns," *New York Times*, December 28, 2015.

112 *Simon's story*: Simon Romero, "Alarm Spreads in Brazil Over a Virus and a Surge in Malformed Infants," *New York Times*, December 30, 2015.

112 *To prod the agency*: Donald G. McNeil Jr., "C.D.C. May Warn Pregnant Women Against Travel to Countries with Zika Virus," *New York Times*, January 13, 2016.

113 *The one that first raised the alarm*: "The Doctor Whose Gut Instinct Beat AI in Spotting the Coronavirus," Oliver Wyman Forum, March 5, 2020, https://www.oliverwymanforum.com/city-readiness/2020/mar/the-doctor-whose-gut-instinct-beat-ai-in-spotting-the-coronavirus.html.

113 *ProMED was created in 1994*: Larry Madoff, "Rapid Reporting of Emerging Disease Outbreaks Using Unofficial Sources: Lessons from ProMED," lecture, Eurosurveillance twentieth anniversary seminar, Stockholm, Sweden, November 30, 2016, https://www.eurosurveillance.org/upload/site-assets/imgs/Larry%20Madoff%20presentation.pdf.

114 *The media paid little attention*: Donald G. McNeil Jr. with Lawrence K. Altman, "As SARS Outbreak Took Shape, Health Agency Took Fast Action," *New York Times*, May 4, 2003.

115 *On November 27*: David L. Heymann and Guénaël Rodier, "Global Surveillance, National Surveillance, and SARS," *Emerging Infectious Disease* 10, no. 2 (February 2004): 173–75.

116 *Dr. Malik Peiris*: Apoorva Mandavilli, "Profile: Malik Peiris," *Nature Medicine* 10, no. 9 (2004): 886.

118 *"This is an alarming systemic failure"*: Editorial, "Killer Virus Demands Open Accounting," *Washington Post*, June 15, 2014.

Chapter 10: The "Not Me" Denialism

119 *Even experts took a wait-and-see attitude*: Novel Coronavirus Pneumonia Emergency Response Epidemiology Team, "Vital Surveillances: The Epidemiological Characteristics of an Outbreak of 2019 Novel Coronavirus Diseases (COVID-19)—China, 2020, *China CDC Weekly* 2, no. 8 (2020): 113–22.

119 *On March 11*: Donald G. McNeil Jr., "Confronting a Pandemic," *The Daily* podcast, *New York Times*, March 12, 2020.

120 *By 1985, it was killing*: Boyce Rensberger, "AIDS Cases in 1985 Exceed Total of All Previous Years," *Washington Post*, January 17, 1986.

122 *In 1990, Dr. Nthato Motlana*: Christopher S. Wren, "AIDS Rising Fast Among Black South Africans," *New York Times*, September 27, 1990.

123 *a 2008 study*: "Securing Our Future: Final Report from Commission on HIV/AIDS and Governance in Africa," UNAIDS, June 9, 2008, https://www.unaids.org/en/resources/presscentre/featurestories/2008/june/20080609securingourfuture.

123 *By 1985, after HIV tests were developed*: D. Serwadda, N. K. Sewankambo, et al., "Slim Disease: A New Disease in Uganda and Its Association with HTLV-III Infection," *Lancet*, October 19, 1985, 849–52.

124 *In 2008, soon after Mr. Mbeki*: Pride Chigwedere, George R. Seage 3d, et al., "Estimating the Lost Benefits of Antiretroviral Drug Use in South Africa," *Journal of Acquired Immune Deficiency Syndrome* 49, no. 4 (December 1, 2008): 410–15.

126 *Newspaper editors agonized*: Pat Sidley, "Rumors Suggest Mbeki's Spokesman Died of AIDS Related Disease," *BMJ* 321, no. 7269 (November 4, 2000): 1100.

126 *The African potato*: Celia M. J. Matyanga, Gene D. Morse, et al., "African Potato (*Hypoxis hemerocallidea*): A Systematic Review of Its Chemistry, Pharmacology and Ethno Medicinal Properties," *BMC Complementary Medicine and Therapies*, June 11, 2020.

127 *Mr. Mbeki was ultimately*: Katie Cooksey and agencies, "Thabo Mbeki to Step Down as South African President after ANC Request," *Guardian*, September 20, 2008.

129 *When I wrote*: Donald G. McNeil Jr., "New Concern on Polio Among Mecca Pilgrims," *New York Times*, February 11, 2005.

Chapter 11: The Toxic Fatalism

132 *By August*: Shoshana Kedem, "30 Million Johnson & Johnson Vaccines Destroyed in South Africa," *African Business*, September 23, 2021, https://african.business/2021/09/technology-information/30-million-contaminated-jj-vaccines-destroyed-in-south-africa/.

132 *"Let's pause and avoid the risk"*: Daniel Payne, "Africa CDC to Ask World to Pause Covid-19 Vaccine Donations," *Politico*, February 22, 2022, https://www.politico.com/news/2022/02/22/africa-asks-covid-vaccine-donation-pause-00010667.

132 *Some countries lacked syringes*: Stephanie Nolen and Rebecca Robbins, "In Africa, a Mix of Shots Drives an Uncertain Covid Vaccination Push," *New York Times*, March 15, 2022.

133 *I remember an exchange*: Gary Tuchman, "Despite Warnings, Churchgoers Explain Why They're Still Going to Services," CNN, April 4,

2020, https://www.cnn.com/videos/us/2020/04/04/ohio-church-service-covid-19-pandemic-tuchman-pkg-ac360-vpx.cnn.

133 *Fatalism is "one of the greatest challenges"*: William H. Foege, *House on Fire: The Fight to Eradicate Smallpox* (Berkeley: University of California Press, 2011).

134 *"Because if you are a man"*: Donald G. McNeil Jr., "AIDS and Death Hold No Sting for Fatalistic Men at African Bar," *New York Times*, November 29, 2001.

135 *That echoed something*: Randy Shilts, *And the Band Played On: Politics, People, and the AIDS Epidemic* (New York: St. Martin's Press, 1987).

135 *In 2016, genetic testing*: Michael Worobey, Thomas D. Watts, et al., "1970s and 'Patient 0': HIV-1 Genomes Illuminate Early HIV/AIDS History in North America," *Nature* 539 (October 26, 2016): 98–101.

Chapter 12: The Failures to Understand Culture

137 *More than 60 percent*: UNAIDS, "Fact Sheet 2022: Global HIV Statistics," 2022, https://www.unaids.org/sites/default/files/media_asset/UNAIDS_FactSheet_en.pdf.

137 *The latest failure*: Tim Murphy, "The Latest Big HIV Vaccine Disappointment Means We Must Double Down on Other Prevention Methods," TheBody, September 9, 2021, https://www.thebody.com/article/hiv-vaccine-trial-disappointment.

139 *Then difficulties arose*: Donald G. McNeil Jr., "Faulty Condoms Thwart AIDS Fight in Africa," *New York Times*, December 27, 1998.

140 *The first was that, initially*: Donald G. McNeil Jr., "Aw, C'mon, You Don't Really Believe Those AIDS Myths?" *Mail & Guardian*, June 11, 1999, https://mg.co.za/article/1999-06-11-aw-cmon-you-dont-really-believe-those/.

140 *A woman who asked a man to wear one*: Donald G. McNeil Jr., "AIDS and Death Hold No Sting for Fatalistic Men at African Bar," *New York Times*, November 29, 2001.

141 *When I interviewed African sex workers*: Donald G. McNeil Jr, "Rare Condoms, Deadly Odds for Truck-Stop Prostitutes," *New York Times*, November 29, 2001.

141 *But it had serious drawbacks*: Donald G. McNeil Jr., "Condoms for Women Gain Approval Among Africans," *New York Times*, July 24, 1999.

142 *In 2007, the WHO endorsed*: Donald G. McNeil Jr., "W.H.O. Urges Circumcision to Reduce Spread of AIDS," *New York Times*, March 29, 2007.

142 *Three clinical trials*: Donald G. McNeil Jr., "Circumcision Halves HIV Risk, U.S. Agency Finds," *New York Times*, December 14, 2006.

142 *Nonetheless, as rumors slowly grew*: N. Westercamp and R. C. Bailey, "Acceptability of Male Circumcision for Prevention of HIV/AIDS in Sub-Saharan Africa: A Review," *AIDS and Behavior* 11, no. 3 (May 2007): 341–55.

142 *Between 2015 and 2022*: USAID, "Voluntary Male Medical Circumcision," https://www.usaid.gov/global-health/health-areas/hiv-and-aids/technical-areas/accelerating-scale-voluntary-medical-male.

142 *In 2010, a huge breakthrough*: Centers for Disease Control and Prevention, "HIV: PrEP Effectiveness," https://www.cdc.gov/hiv/basics/prep/prep-effectiveness.html.

143 *The worldwide iPrEx study*: Robert M. Grant, Javier R. Lama, et al., "Preexposure Chemoprophylaxis for HIV Prevention in Men Who Have Sex with Men," *New England Journal of Medicine* 363 (December 30, 2010): 2587–99.

143 *Partners in PrEP*: Jared M. Baeten, Deborah Donnell, et al., "Antiretroviral Prophylaxis for HIV Prevention in Heterosexual Men and Women," *New England Journal of Medicine* 367 (August 2, 2012): 399–410.

143 *One by one*: Donald G. McNeil Jr., "AIDS Prevention Gel Fails in Trial, Researchers Say," *New York Times*, December 14, 2009.

143 *Clinical trials*: Donald G. McNeil Jr., "Advance on AIDS Raises Questions as Well as Joy," *New York Times*, July 26, 2010.

143 *Dr. Ariane van der Straten*: Donald G. McNeil Jr., "A Failed Trial in Africa Raises Questions About How to Test H.I.V. Drugs," *New York Times*, February 4, 2015.

144 *Similar patterns*: Denise Grady, "Vaginal Ring with Drug Lowers H.I.V. Rates in African Women," *New York Times*, February 22, 2016.

144 *Older women*: Jared M. Baeten, Thesla Palanee-Phillips, et al., "Use of a Vaginal Ring Containing Dapivirine for HIV-1 Prevention in Women," *New England Journal of Medicine* 375 (December 1, 2016): 2121–32.

145 *It also prevented genital herpes*: Donald G. McNeil Jr., "Gel Cuts Women's Risk of Herpes, Study Finds," *New York Times*, October 20, 2011.

145 *The WHO endorsed*: "WHO Recommends the Dapivirine Vaginal Ring as a New Choice for HIV Prevention for Women at Substantial Risk of HIV Infection," WHO departmental news, January 26, 2021.

145 *"In the communities"*: Catherine Tomlinson, "In-depth: What Will It

Take to Bring HIV Prevention Injections to SA's Clinics?" Spotlight, September 1, 2021, https://www.spotlightnsp.co.za/2021/09/01/in-depth-what-will-it-take-to-bring-hiv-prevention-injections-to-sas-clinics/.

146 *They dismissed Truvada*: David Tuller, "A Resisted Pill to Prevent H.I.V.," *New York Times*, December 30, 2013.

146 *A drug named Enovid*: Donald G. McNeil Jr., "News Analysis: Are We Ready for H.I.V.'s Sexual Revolution?" *New York Times*, May 23, 2014.

146 *As of this writing*: Apoorva Mandavilli, "Shot to Prevent H.I.V. Works Better Than Daily Pill in Women," *New York Times*, November 9, 2020.

147 *The fact that women prefer*: Donald G. McNeil Jr., "Depo-Provera, an Injectable Contraceptive, Does Not Raise H.I.V. Risk," *New York Times*, June 13, 2019.

147 *In early 2022, my successor*: Stephanie Nolen, "Yes, a Raging Pandemic Can Be Quelled. Recent History Shows How," *New York Times*, January 11, 2022.

147 *By mid-2022*: UNAIDS, "Fact Sheet 2022: Global HIV Statistics," 2022, https://www.unaids.org/en/resources/documents/2022/UNAIDS_FactSheet.

Chapter 13: The Cancer of Rumors

149 *A 2007 outbreak on Yap Island*: Mark R. Duffy, Tai-Ho Chen, et al., "Zika Virus Outbreak on Yap Island, Federated States of Micronesia," *New England Journal of Medicine* 360 (June 11, 2009): 2536–43.

149 *In 2013, it hit French Polynesia*: Didier Musso, Hervé Bossin, et al., "Zika Virus in French Polynesia, 2013–2014: Anatomy of a Completed Outbreak," *Lancet Infectious Diseases* 18, no. 5 (May 2018): E172–E182.

150 *There were so many that*: Donald G. McNeil Jr., "Zika Virus Rumors and Theories That You Should Doubt," *New York Times*, February 18, 2016.

152 *More to the point, multiple reporters*: Donald G. McNeil Jr., Simon Romero, and Sabrina Tavernise, "How a Medical Mystery in Brazil Led Doctors to Zika," *New York Times*, February 7, 2016.

153 *Ultimately, months of work*: Donald G. McNeil Jr., "6 Reasons to Think the Zika Virus Causes Microcephaly," *New York Times*, April 1, 2016, updated May 3, 2016.

153 *Epidemiological studies*: World Health Organization, "Zika Virus, Mi-

crocephaly and Guillain-Barré Syndrome Situation Report," April 14, 2016, https://apps.who.int/iris/bitstream/handle/10665/205189/zikasitrep_14Apr2016_eng.pdf?sequence=1.

153 *Autopsies on miscarried and aborted fetuses*: Roosecelis Brasil Martines, Julu Bhatnagar, et al., "Notes from the Field: Evidence of Zika Virus Infection in Brain and Placental Tissues from Two Congenitally Infected Newborns and Two Fetal Losses—Brazil, 2015," *Morbidity and Mortality Weekly Report* 65, no. 06 (February 19, 2016): 159–60; Jernej Mlakar, Misa Korva, et al., "Zika Virus Associated with Microcephaly," *New England Journal of Medicine* 374 (March 10, 2016): 951–58.

153 *Studies in which pregnant mice or monkeys*: Kristina M. Adams Waldorf, Jennifer E Stencel-Baerenwald, et al., "Fetal Brain Lesions after Subcutaneous Inoculation of Zika Virus in a Pregnant Nonhuman Primate," *Nature Medicine* 22 (September 12, 2016): 1256–59; Kong-Yan Wu, Guo-Long Zuo, et al., "Vertical Transmission of Zika Virus Targeting the Radial Glial Cells Affects Cortex Development of Offspring Mice," *Cell Research* 26 (May 13, 2016): 645–54.

154 *In her book*: Heidi J. Larson, *Stuck: How Vaccine Rumors Start—and Why They Don't Go Away* (New York: Oxford University Press, 2020).

154 *There were rumors*: Janelle Ross, "Coronavirus Outbreak Revives Dangerous Race Myths and Pseudoscience," NBC News, March 19, 2020; Tom Kertscher, "Melanin Doesn't Protect against Coronavirus," PolitiFact, March 10, 2020, https://www.politifact.com/factchecks/2020/mar/10/facebook-posts/melanin-doesnt-protect-against-coronavirus/.

154 *Poison control centers*: Vanessa Romo, "Poison Control Centers Are Fielding a Surge of Ivermectin Overdose Calls," NPR, September 4, 2021, https://www.npr.org/sections/coronavirus-live-updates/2021/09/04/1034217306/ivermectin-overdose-exposure-cases-poison-control-centers.

154 *Doctors were threatened*: Matt Volz, "Hospitals Refused to Give Patients lvermectin. Lockdowns and Political Pressure Followed," *Kaiser Health News*, December 2, 2021, https://khn.org/news/article/ivermectin-covid-treatment-hospital-threats-political-pressure/.

155 *By as early as May 2021*: Carla K. Johnson and Mike Stobbe, "Nearly All COVID Deaths in US Are Now among Unvaccinated," Associated Press, June 29, 2021, https://apnews.com/article/coronavirus-pandemic-health-941fcf43d9731c76c16e7354f5d5e187.

155 *The worm enters*: James I. Robertson, Jr., "Civil War Series: The Civil War's Common Soldier: Prisoners of War," National Park Service,

History E-Library, https://www.nps.gov/parkhistory/online_books /civil_war_series/3/sec4.htm.

156 *A 2022 article*: Sam Husseini and Jonathan Latham, "Did West Africa's Ebola Outbreak of 2014 Have a Lab Origin?" *Independent Science News*, October 25, 2022, https://www.independentsciencenews.org /health/did-west-africas-ebola-outbreak-of-2014-have-a-lab-origin/.

156 *In 2009, the WHO debunked*: A. J. Gibbs, J. S. Armstrong, and J. C. Downie, "From Where Did the 2009 'Swine-Origin' Influenza A Virus (H1N1) Emerge?" *Virology Journal* 6, no. 207 (November 24, 2009), https://link.springer.com/article/10.1186/1743-422X-6-207; Donald G. McNeil Jr., "Swine Flu Not an Accident From a Lab, W.H.O. Says," *New York Times*, May 14, 2009.

156 *In 2011, a paper*: H. V. Wyatt, "The 1916 New York City Epidemic of Poliomyelitis: Where Did the Virus Come From?" *Open Vaccine Journal* 4 (2011): 13–17, https://benthamopen.com/contents/pdf/TOVACJ /TOVACJ-4-13.pdf.

157 *By 2003, as described by*: Ayodele Samuel Jegede, "What Led to the Nigerian Boycott of the Polio Vaccination Campaign?" *PLOS Medicine* 4, no. 3 (March 2007): e73, https://www.ncbi.nlm.nih.gov/pmc /articles/PMC1831725/; Maryam Yahya, "Polio Vaccines—'No Thank You!' Barriers to Polio Eradication in Northern Nigeria," *African Affairs* 106, no. 423 (April 2007): 185–204, https://academic.oup.com/ afraf/article/106/423/185/50647; Maryam Yahya, "Polio Vaccines—Difficult to Swallow: The Story of a Controversy in Northern Nigeria," Institute of Development Studies Working Paper 261, March 2006, https://core.ac.uk/download/pdf/29134939.pdf.

158 *Some rural West Africans*: Yahya, "Polio Vaccines—'No Thank You!'"

159 *It sprang from the controversial 1999 book*: Edward Hooper, *The River: A Journey Back to the Source of HIV and AIDS* (Boston: Little, Brown, 1999).

162 *The hepatitis B vaccination campaign*: Saeed Shah, "CIA Organized Fake Vaccination Drive to Get Osama bin Laden's Family DNA," *Guardian*, July 11, 2011, https://www.theguardian.com/world/2011/jul/11/cia -fake-vaccinations-osama-bin-ladens-dna.

162 *Doctors Without Borders*: "Alleged Fake CIA Vaccination Campaign Undermines Medical Care," July 14, 2011, https://www.doctorswithoutbor ders.org/latest/alleged-fake-cia-vaccination-campaign-undermines-med ical-care; Saeed Shah, "CIA Tactics to Trap Bin Laden Linked with Polio Crisis, Say Aid Groups," *Guardian*, March 2, 2012, https://www .theguardian.com/world/2012/mar/02/aid-groups-cia-osama-bin-laden

-polio-crisis; Donald G. McNeil Jr., "Deans Condemn Vaccine Ruse Used in Bin Laden Hunt," *New York Times*, January 7, 2013.

162 *When I wrote about it*: Donald G. McNeil Jr., "Pakistan Battles Polio, and Its People's Mistrust," *New York Times*, July 21, 2013.

162 *Then Taliban leaders*: Declan Walsh, "Taliban Block Vaccinations in Pakistan," *New York Times*, June 8, 2012.

162 *In late 2012, the killings began*: Jason Burke, "Polio Vaccination Workers Shot Dead in Pakistan," *Guardian*, December 18, 2012.

163 *President Asif Ali Zardari*: Heather Clark, "Killings Will Not Halt Vaccinations, Vows Bhutto's Daughter," *Independent*, December 23, 2012.

164 *The latest five-year plan*: Global Polio Eradication Initiative, "Polio Eradication Strategy 2022–2026: Delivering on a Promise," https://polioeradication.org/gpei-strategy-2022-2026/.

164 *In the early 2000s*: Gina Samaan, Mahomed Patel, et al., "Rumor Surveillance and Avian Influenza H5N1," *Emerging Infectious Disease* 11, no. 3 (March 2005): 463–66, https://www.ncbi.nlm.nih.gov/pmc/articles/PMC3298271/.

164 *Soviet and Russian disinformation*: Linda Qiu, "Fingerprints of Russian Disinformation: From AIDS to Fake News," *New York Times*, December 12, 2017.

165 *Russia's intelligence services*: Steven Lee Myers, "Russia's Unfounded Claims of Secret U.S. Bioweapons Linger On and On," *New York Times*, September 4, 2022.

166 *The idea that*: Glenn Kessler, Salvador Rizzo, and Meg Kelly, "Trump's False or Misleading Claims Total 30,573 over 4 Years," *Washington Post*, January 24, 2021.

Chapter 14: The Despicable Profiteers

169 *Because vitamins*: U.S. Food and Drug Administration, "FDA 101: Dietary Supplements," June 6, 2022, https://www.fda.gov/consumers/consumer-updates/fda-101-dietary-supplements.

169 *In the rare cases*: U.S. Food and Drug Administration Safety Recalls, "Shopaax.com Issues Voluntary Recall of Kingdom Honey Royal Honey VIP Due to Presence of Undeclared Sildenafil," July 13, 2022, https://www.fda.gov/safety/recalls-market-withdrawals-safety-alerts/shopaaxcom-issues-voluntary-recall-kingdom-honey-royal-honey-vip-due-presence-undeclared-sildenafil.

170 *The subsequent "Virodene scandal"*: James Myburgh, "The Virodene

Affair: The Secret History of the ANC's Response to the HIV/AIDS Epidemic," Politicsweb, September 17, 2007, https://www.politicsweb.co.za/news-and-analysis/the-virodene-affair-i; Stefaans Brümmer, Sam Sole, "The ANC's Virodene Backers," *Mail & Guardian,* July 5, 2002, https://mg.co.za/article/2002-07-05-the-ancs-virodene-backers/.

170 *She was a cryonics specialist*: Charles Platt, "Hearts, Brains, and Minds," CryoCare, http://www.cryocare.org/index.cgi?subdir=ccrpt10&url=visser.html; Lizeka Mda, "Who Is . . . Olga Visser?" *Mail & Guardian*, December 12, 1997, https://mg.co.za/article/1997-1212-who-is-olga-visser/.

171 *Who paid for the trials*: Sam Sole and Stefaans Brümmer, "Who's Bankrolling Virodene?" *Mail & Guardian*, June 28, 2002, https://web.archive.org/web/20081030063327/http://www.aegis.com/news/dmg/2002/MG020610.html.

172 *A close parallel*: "The Angry Politics of Kemron," *Newsweek*, January 3, 1993, https://www.newsweek.com/angry-politics-kemron-192118; Jane Perlez, "In Kenya, a New AIDS Drug Gets Mired in Politics and Financial Disputes," *New York Times*, October 3, 1990.

172 *Starting in 1990*: D. K. Koech and A. O. Obel, "Efficacy of Kemron (Low Dose Oral Natural Human Interferon Alpha) in the Management of HIV-1 Infection and Acquired Immune Deficiency Syndrome (AIDS)," *East African Medical Journal* 67 (July 1990) (7 Suppl 2): SS64–70, https://pubmed.ncbi.nlm.nih.gov/2226235/.

173 *Kemron and Pearl Omega*: Rebecca Dodd, "Patients Sue 'AIDS-Cure' Kenyan Scientist," *Lancet* 347, no. 9016 (June 1996): 1688.

173 *The South African government wasted*: Celia W. Dugger, "Study Cites Toll of AIDS Policy in South Africa," *New York Times*, November 25, 2008.

174 *An iconoclastic French doctor*: Scott Sayare, "He Was a Science Star. Then He Promoted a Questionable Cure for Covid-19," *New York Times Magazine*, May 12, 2020.

174 *Everyone who has studied medicine*: Dr. Howard Markel, "In 1850, Ignaz Semmelweis Saved Lives with Three Words: Wash Your Hands," *PBS NewsHour*, May 15, 2015, https://www.pbs.org/newshour/health/ignaz-semmelweis-doctor-prescribed-hand-washing.

176 *Dr. Immanuel*: Will Sommer, "Trump's New Favorite COVID Doctor Believes in Alien DNA, Demon Sperm and Hydroxychloroquine," Daily Beast, July 28, 2020.

176 *In March 2023*: Amanda D'Ambrosio, "Stella Immanuel Highest U.S.

Prescriber of Ivermectin and HCQ," MedPage Today, March 2, 2023, https://www.medpagetoday.com/special-reports/exclusives/103353.

176 *The founder of*: Spencer S. Hsu, "Anti-Vaccine Doctor Sentenced to Prison for Jan. 6 Trespassing," *Washington Post*, June 16, 2022.

176 *After her release*: Cheryl Clark, "Internal Strife at America's Frontline Doctors: Simone Gold Accused of Misusing $$$," MedPage Today, November 7, 2022, https://www.medpagetoday.com/special-reports/exclusives/101640.

176 *In 1918, as flu began killing*: Howard Markel, Harvey B. Lipman, et al., "Nonpharmaceutical Interventions Implemented by US Cities During the 1918–1919 Influenza Pandemic," *Journal of the American Medical Association* 298, no. 6 (2007): 644–54, August 8, 2007, https://jamanetwork.com/journals/jama/fullarticle/208354; Nina Strochlic and Riley D. Champine, "How Some Cities 'Flattened the Curve' during the 1918 Flu Pandemic," *National Geographic*, March 27, 2020.

177 *Dr. Bayer called Mr. Shilts*: Ronald Bayer, *Private Acts, Social Consequences: AIDS and the Politics of Public Health* (New York: Free Press, 1989), 29.

178 *"I used to live in the Portrero District"*: Dr. Dean F. Echenberg, interview with the author, October 2021.

178 *Diagnoses of rectal gonorrhea*: San Francisco Department of Health, *City Clinic AIDS/Hepatitis Cohort Study*, as described in testimony of Dr. Dean Echenberg in *State of California v. Ima Jean Owen et al.*, October 29, 1984, 22.

179 *In a 1984 survey*: San Francisco Department of Health, *City Clinic AIDS/Hepatitis Cohort Study*, as described in testimony of Dr. Dean Echenberg in *State of California v. Ima Jean Owen et al.*, October 29, 1984, 13.

179 *Later tests*: San Francisco Department of Health, *City Clinic AIDS/Hepatitis Cohort Study*, as described in testimony of Dr. Dean Echenberg in *State of California v. Ima Jean Owen et al.*, October 29, 1984, 18; Bruce Lambert, "10 Years Later, Hepatitis Study Still Yields Critical Data on AIDS," *New York Times*, July 17, 1990.

179 *"It was as if"*: Dr. Dean F. Echenberg, interview with the author, October 2021.

180 *"So, we didn't close them"*: Dr. Dean F. Echenberg, interview with the author, April 18, 2022.

180 *In Britain*: Elizabeth Earl, "The Victorian Anti-Vaccination Movement," *Atlantic*, July 15, 2015.

180 *In the 1950s*: Paul A. Offit, *The Cutter Incident: How America's First Polio Vaccine Led to the Growing Vaccine Crisis* (New Haven, CT: Yale University Press, 2005).

181 *In 2010, Dr. Wakefield's*: Sarah Boseley, "Andrew Wakefield Found 'Irresponsible' by GMC over MMR Vaccine Scare," *Guardian*, January 28, 2010.

181 *Mr. Wakefield moved*: Brian Deer, *The Doctor Who Fooled the World: Science, Deception, and the War on Vaccines* (Baltimore: Johns Hopkins University Press, 2020).

181 *Science reporters*: Anna Merlan, "Everything I Learned While Getting Kicked Out of America's Biggest Anti-Vaccine Conference," Jezebel, June 20, 2019, https://jezebel.com/everything-i-learned-while-getting-kicked-out-of-americ-1834992879.

181 *Anti-vaccine "charities"*: Michelle R. Smith, "How a Kennedy Built an Anti-Vaccine Juggernaut Amid COVID-19," NBC10 Boston, December 15, 2021, https://www.nbcboston.com/news/local/how-a-kennedy-built-an-anti-vaccine-juggernaut-amid-covid-19/2590911/.

182 *When autism appeared to be on the rise there*: Donald G. McNeil Jr., "An Outbreak of Autism, or a Statistical Fluke?" *New York Times*, March 16, 2009.

182 *Two years later*: Owen Dyer, "Measles Outbreak in Somali American Community Follows Anti-Vaccine Talks," *BMJ* 357 (May 16, 2017).

182 *In 2022, vaccination rejection*: Ruth Link-Gelles, Emily Lutterloh, et al., "Public Health Response to a Case of Paralytic Polio in an Unvaccinated Person and Detection of Poliovirus in Wastewater—New York, June–August 2022," *Morbidity and Mortality Weekly Report* 71, no. 33 (August 19, 2022):1065–68.

183 *In 2021, Kennedy, Dr. Joseph Mercola*: "The Disinformation Dozen: Why Platforms Must Act on Twelve Leading Online Anti-Vaxxers," Center for Countering Digital Hate, March 24, 2021, https://counterhate.com/research/the-disinformation-dozen/; Sheera Frenkel, "The Most Influential Spreader of Coronavirus Misinformation Online," *New York Times*, July 24, 2021.

184 *There is precedent for this*: Alan Taylor, "American Nazis in the 1930s—The German American Bund," *Atlantic*, June 5, 2017, https://www.theatlantic.com/photo/2017/06/american-nazis-in-the-1930sthe-german-american-bund/529185/; Jason Daley, "The Screenwriting Mystic Who Wanted to Be the American Führer," *Smithsonian*, October 3,

2018, https://www.smithsonianmag.com/history/meet-screenwriting-mystic-who-wanted-be-american-fuhrer-180970449/.

Chapter 15: The Rare Politicians Who Outwit Scientists

186 *I remember watching*: "Watch China Use 'Talking Drones' to Warn Citizens," CNN, February 2, 2020, https://www.youtube.com/watch?v=QPw6xjwAlHc; Chas Danner, "Watch Drones Scold Civilians for Not Wearing Masks in China," *New York*, January 31, 2020, https://nymag.com/intelligencer/2020/01/coronavirus-watch-drones-scold-maskless-civilians-in-china.html.

187 *On March 13*: "Learning to Live with the Coronavirus," *The Daily* podcast, *New York Times*, March 13, 2020.

189 *Dr. George Gao*: Jon Cohen, "Not Wearing Masks to Protect against Coronavirus Is a 'Big Mistake,' Top Chinese Scientist Says," *Science*, March 27, 2020, https://www.science.org/content/article/not-wearing-masks-protect-against-coronavirus-big-mistake-top-chinese-scientist-says.

189 *On March 28*: World Health Organization, "Fact Check: Covid-19 Is NOT Airborne," @WHO, Twitter, March 28, 2020, https://twitter.com/WHO/status/1243972193169616898?lang=en.

189 *Also, the virus's mutability*: Katy Katella, "Omicron, Delta, Alpha, and More: What to Know About the Coronavirus Variants," Yale Medicine, February 3, 2023, https://www.yalemedicine.org/news/covid-19-variants-of-concern-omicron; Chris Kay and Dhwani Pandya, "How Errors, Inaction Sent a Deadly Covid Variant Around the World," Bloomberg News, December 29, 2021, https://www.bloomberg.com/news/features/2021-12-29/how-delta-variant-spread-in-india-deadly-errors-inaction-covid-crisis; Smriti Mallapaty, "Where Did Omicron Come From? Three Key Theories," *Nature,* January 28, 2022, https://www.nature.com/articles/d41586-022-04357-1.

190 *Physicists in Japan*: Douglas Broom, "This Japanese Experiment Shows How Easily Coronavirus Can Spread—and What You Can Do about It," World Economic Forum, April 14, 2020, https://www.weforum.org/agenda/2020/04/coronavirus-microdroplets-talking-breathing-spread-covid-19/.

190 *The Czech Republic*: Steven Kashkett, "Czech Republic Has Lifesaving COVID-19 Lesson for America: Wear a Face Mask," *USA Today*, July 14, 2020.

190 *Eventually, epidemiological studies*: Timo Mitze, Reinhold Kosfeld, Johannes Rode, and Klaus Wälde, "Face Masks Considerably Reduce COVID-19 Cases in Germany," *PNAS* 117, no. 51 (December 3, 2020): 32293–301, https://www.pnas.org/doi/10.1073/pnas.2015954117; M. Shane Gallaway, Jessica Rigler, et al., "Trends in COVID-19 Incidence After Implementation of Mitigation Measures—Arizona, January 22–August 7, 2020," *Morbidity and Mortality Weekly Report* 69, no. 40 (October 9, 2020): 1460–63, https://www.cdc.gov/mmwr/volumes/69/wr/mm6940e3.htm; Carlos Zambrana, Donna K. Ginther, and Roy A. Roberts, "Do Masks Matter in Kansas?" University of Kansas Institute for Policy and Social Research, October 25, 2020, https://mediahub.ku.edu/media/Masks/1_49bb9aid.

191 *Cashiers and security guards*: Jemima McEvoy, "Killing of Georgia Cashier Is Latest in a String of Fatal Shootings Over Mask-Wearing: Here Are the Rest," *Forbes*, June 15, 2021, https://www.forbes.com/sites/jemimamcevoy/2021/06/15/killing-of-georgia-cashier-is-latest-in-a-string-of-fatal-shootings-over-mask-wearing-here-are-the-rest.

191 *Interestingly, New York City*: "Tracking Coronavirus in New York City, N.Y.: Latest Map and Case Count," *New York Times*, https://www.nytimes.com/interactive/2021/us/new-york-city-new-york-covid-cases.html.

192 *The pandemic "ended" for me*: Donald G. McNeil Jr., "The End IS Near. No, Seriously," Medium, May 24, 2021, https://donaldgmcneiljr1954.medium.com/the-end-is-near-no-seriously-142683fb085e.

192 *Israel and then Britain*: Hadas Gold, "What the World Could Learn from Israel's Covid-19 Vaccine Booster Rollout," CNN, November 24, 2021, https://www.cnn.com/2021/11/24/health/israel-covid-boosterlessons-intl-cmd/index.html; Jacqui Wise, "Covid-19: Booster Doses to Be Offered to 30 Million People in UK," *BMJ* 374, no. 2261 (September 14, 2021), https://www.bmj.com/content/374/bmj.n2261.

193 *Dr. Michael J. Ryan*: Kevin Dunleavy, "Biden Administration's Push for Covid Boosters Raises Concern about the Science and Morality of the Plan," Fierce Pharma, August 19, 2021, https://www.fiercepharma.com/pharma/u-s-rush-to-endorse-covid-boosters-raises-concerns-about-process-and-morality.

193 *That was untrue*: U.S. Food and Drug Administration, "Coronavirus (COVID-19) Update: FDA Takes Action to Help Facilitate Timely Development of Safe, Effective COVID-19 Vaccines," press release, June 30, 2020, https://www.fda.gov/news-events/press-an

nouncements/coronavirus-covid-19-update-fda-takes-action-help-facilitate-timely-development-safe-effective-covid; Alison Aubrey, "A COVID-19 Vaccine May Be Only 50% Effective. Is That Good Enough?" *Shots* blog, NPR, September 12, 2020, https://www.npr.org/sections/health-shots/2020/09/12/911987987/a-covid-19-vaccine-may-be-only-50-effective-is-that-good-enough.

193 *Deaths, which had dropped*: "Coronavirus in the U.S.: Latest Map and Case Count," *New York Times*, https://www.nytimes.com/interactive/2021/us/covid-cases.html.

194 *That rage was visible*: Lili Loofbourow, "The Unbelievable Grimness of HermanCainAward, the Subreddit That Catalogs Anti-Vaxxer COVID Deaths," Slate, September 21, 2021, https://slate.com/technology/2021/09/hermancainaward-subreddit-antivaxxer-deaths-cataloged.html; https://www.sorryantivaxxer.com/.

194 *The rage grew even greater*: Lenny Bernstein, "Biden Administration Moves to Stave Off Shortages of Monoclonal Antibodies," *Washington Post*, September 14, 2021.

195 *President Biden said he would do both*: "President Biden Announces New Actions to Protect Americans Against the Delta and Omicron Variants as We Battle COVID-19 this Winter," White House press release, December 2, 2021, https://www.whitehouse.gov/briefing-room/statements-releases/2021/12/02/fact-sheet-president-biden-announces-new-actions-to-protect-americans-against-the-delta-and-omicron-variants-as-we-battle-covid-19-this-winter/.

195 *Simultaneously, the unexpected happened*: Stephanie Nolen, "As Vaccines Trickle into Africa, Zambia's Challenges Highlight Obstacles," *New York Times*, December 11, 2021.

195 *The Africa CDC*: Daniel Payne, "Africa CDC to Ask World to Pause Covid-19 Vaccine Donations," *Politico*, February 22, 2022, https://www.politico.com/news/2022/02/22/africa-asks-covid-vaccine-donation-pause-00010667.

195 *Very quickly, what had been*: Donald G. McNeil Jr., "It's No Longer the 'Pandemic of the Unvaccinated,'" Medium, December 15, 2021, https://donaldgmcneiljr1954.medium.com/its-no-longer-the-pandemic-of-the-unvaccinated-a0451d1ebdec; Aaron Blake, "Yes, It's Still a Pandemic of the Unvaccinated—Arguably Even More So Now," *Washington Post*, February 3, 2022; David Leonhardt, "The Power of Boosters," *New York Times*, January 31, 2022.

195 *Scientists began saying*: Ralph Ellis, "Fauci: 'Fully Vaccinated' Will

Eventually Mean 3 Doses," WebMD, December 10, 2021, https://www.webmd.com/vaccines/covid-19-vaccine/news/20211210/fauci-says-fully-vaccinated-will-eventually-mean-three-doses.

Chapter 16: The Media's Forced Errors

198 *The virus reached*: Anemona Hartocollis, "School Nurse's Response to Flu Virus Wins Applause," *New York Times*, April 28, 2009.

198 *On April 24*: Marc Lacey and Donald G. McNeil Jr., "Fighting Deadly Flu, Mexico Shuts Schools," *New York Times*, April 24, 2009.

198 *Perhaps prompted by that*: Donald G. McNeil Jr., "U.S. Declares Public Health Emergency Over Swine Flu," *New York Times*, April 26, 2009.

198 *Most subsequent flu cases*: Denise Grady and Liz Robbins, "Outbreak in Mexico May Be Smaller Than Feared," *New York Times*, May 1, 2009.

198 *The rest of the media*: Anemona Hartocollis, "New York Reports Its First Swine Flu Death," *New York Times*, May 17, 2009.

199 *Its conclusion was alarming*: President's Council of Advisors on Science and Technology, *Report to the President on U.S. Preparations for 2009 H1N1 Influenza*, August 7, 2009, https://www.globalsecurity.org/security/library/report/2009/pcast_h1n1-report_090807.htm.

200 *Their front pages*: Rob Stein, "Swine Flu Could Infect Half of U.S., Panel Estimates," *Washington Post*, August 25, 2009; Steve Sternberg, "U.S. Report Predicts 30,000 to 90,000 H1N1 Deaths," *USA Today*, August 24, 2009.

201 *I really detest*: Jennifer Rubin, "The Obama White House and the Media," *Washington Post*, February 28, 2013.

202 *The headline on my story*: Donald G. McNeil Jr., "Agency Urges Caution on Estimates of Swine Flu," *New York Times*, August 25, 2009.

202 *One day later, the* Columbia Journalism Review: Curtis Brainard, "Media Hype Swine Flu Report," *Columbia Journalism Review*, August 26, 2009, https://archives.cjr.org/the_observatory/media_hypes_swine_flu_report.php.

202 *In late July 2023*: Alex Gutentag, Leighton Woodhouse, Michael Shellenberger, and Matt Taibbi, "Top Scientists Misled Congress About Covid Origins, Newly Released Emails and Messages Show," *Public/Substack*, July 18, 2023; Gutentag, et al., "Covid Origins Scientist Denounces Reporting on His Messages as a 'Conspiracy Theory,'" *Public/Substack*, July 20, 2023.

203 *The first such article*: Bill Gertz, "Coronavirus Link to China Biowarfare Program Possible, Analyst Says," *Washington Times*, January 26, 2020, https://www.washingtontimes.com/news/2020/jan/26/coronavirus-link-to-china-biowarfare-program-possi/.

203 *As the comedian Jon Stewart*: *The Late Show with Stephen Colbert*, "Jon Stewart on Vaccine Science and the Wuhan Lab Theory," YouTube, June 15, 2021, https://www.youtube.com/watch?v=sSfejgwbDQ8.

203 *Meanwhile, other rumors*: Prashant Pradhan, Ashutosh Kumar Pandey, et al., "Uncanny Similarity of Unique Inserts in the 2019-nCoV Spike Protein to HIV-1 gp120 and Gag," bioRxiv, January 31, 2020, https://www.biorxiv.org/content/10.1101/2020.01.30.927871v1.

203 *Chinese labs were accused*: Liu Caiyu and Leng Shumei, "Biosafety Guideline Issued to Fix Chronic Management Loopholes at Virus Labs," *Global Times*, February 16, 2020, https://www.globaltimes.cn/content/1179747.shtml.

203 *We science reporters*: Victoria Forster, "No, the Coronavirus Was Not Genetically Engineered to Put Pieces of HIV in It," *Forbes*, February 2, 2020; Megan Molteni, "Snakes?! The Slippery Truth of a Flawed Wuhan Virus Theory," *Wired*, January 23, 2020, https://www.wired.com/story/wuhan-coronavirus-snake-flu-theory/.

204 *That conference call and the emails*: Emily Kopp, "Francis Collins and Anthony Fauci Emailed about Whether NIH Funded Wuhan Lab before Secret Call," U.S. Right to Know, September 7, 2022, https://usrtk.org/covid-19-origins/francis-collins-and-anthony-fauci-worried-about-nih-funding-wuhan-lab/; Jimmy Tobias, "Evolution of a Theory: Unredacted NIH Emails Show Efforts to Rule Out Lab Origin of Covid," Intercept, January 19, 2023, https://theintercept.com/2023/01/19/covid-origin-nih-emails/.

204 *On February 3*: P. Zhou, X. L. Yang, X. G. Wang, et al., "A Pneumonia Outbreak Associated with a New Coronavirus of Probable Bat Origin," *Nature* 579 (2020): 270–73, https://www.nature.com/articles/s41586-020-2012-7.

204 *Virologists publicly pooh-poohed*: Maciej F. Boni, Philippe Lemey, Xiaowei Jiang, et al., "Evolutionary Origins of the SARS-CoV-2 Sarbecovirus Lineage Responsible for the COVID-19 Pandemic," *Nature Microbiology* 5 (July 28, 2020): 1408–17, https://www.nature.com/articles/s41564-020-0771-4.

205 *On February 16*: Kristian G. Andersen, Andrew Rambaut, W. Ian Lipkin, Edward C. Holmes, and Robert F. Garry, "The Proximal Origin of

SARS-CoV-2," virological.org, February16, 2020, https://virological.org/t/the-proximal-origin-of-sars-cov-2/398.

207 *Coronaviruses with furin cleavage sites and pangolin viruses*: T. TY. Lam, N. Jia, Y. W. Zhang, et al., "Identifying SARS-CoV-2-Related Coronaviruses in Malayan Pangolins," *Nature* 583 (February 7, 2020): 282–85, https://www.nature.com/articles/s41586-020-2169-0; David Cyranoski, "Did Pangolins Spread the China Coronavirus to People?" *Nature*, February 7, 2020, https://www.nature.com/articles/d41586-020-00364-2.

207 *After the market was hosed down*: Xinhua, "China Detects Large Quantity of Novel Coronavirus at Wuhan Seafood Market," Xinhua News, January 27, 2020, https://www.xinhuanet.com/english/2020-01/27/c_138735677.htm; George Gao, William Liu, Peipei Liu, et al., "Surveillance of SARS-CoV-2 in the Environment and Animal Samples of the Huanan Seafood Market," Research Square, February 25, 2022, https://www.researchsquare.com/article/rs-1370392/v1.

207 *My story never ran, for two reasons*: Alex Isenstadt, "GOP Memo Urges Anti-China Assault over Coronavirus," *Politico*, April 24, 2020, https://www.politico.com/news/2020/04/24/gop-memo-anti-china-coronavirus-207244; David E. Sanger, "For Trump, a New Crisis and a Familiar Response: It's China's Fault, and Europe's," *New York Times*, March 12, 2020; Eric Lipton, David E. Sanger, Maggie Haberman, Michael D. Shear, Mark Mazzetti, and Julian E. Barnes, "He Could Have Seen What Was Coming: Behind Trump's Failure on the Virus," *New York Times*, April 11, 2020.

208 *I can only surmise that their sources*: Bret Baier and Gregg Re, "Sources Believe Coronavirus Outbreak Originated in Wuhan Lab as Part of China's Efforts to Compete with US," Fox News, April 15, 2020.

208 *Other scientists noted what the "Proximal Origins" authors*: Shing Hei Zhan, Benjamin E. Deverman, and Yujia Alina Chan, "SARS CoV-2 Is Well Adapted for Humans. What Does This Mean for Re-emergence?" bioRxiv, May 2, 2020, https://www.biorxiv.org/content/10.1101/2020.05.01.073262v1.

208 The Wall Street Journal: Michael R. Gordon, Warren P. Strobel, and Drew Hinshaw, "Intelligence on Sick Staff at Wuhan Lab Fuels Debate on Covid-19 Origin," *Wall Street Journal*, May 23, 2021.

208 *It later turned out, however*: Office of the Spokesperson, "Fact Sheet: Activity at the Wuhan Institute of Virology," U.S. Department of State, January 15, 2021, https:/2017-2021.state.gov/fact-sheet-activity-at-the-wuhan-institute-of-virology/index.html.

209 *In June 2023*: Michael Shellenberger, Matt Taibbi, and Alex Gutentag, "First People Sickened by Covid-19 Were Chinese Scientists at Wuhan Institute of Virology, Say U.S. Government Sources," *Public/Substack*, June 13, 2023, https://public.substack.com/p/first-people-sickened-by-covid-19.

209 *They denied having been sick*: Jon Cohen, "'Ridiculous,' Says Chinese Scientist Accused of Being Pandemic's Patient Zero," *Science*, June 23, 2023, https://www.science.org/content/article/ridiculous-says-chinese-scientist-accused-being-pandemic-s-patient-zero.

209 *Bizarrely, China repeatedly behaved*: Associated Press, "China Has Rejected a WHO Plan for Further Investigation into the Origins of COVID-19," NPR, July 22, 2022, https://www.npr.org/sections/coronavirus-live-updates/2021/07/22/1019244601/china-who-coronavirus-lab-leak-theory; Benjamin Mueller, "W.H.O. Accuses China of Hiding Data That May Link Covid's Origins to Animals," *New York Times*, March 17, 2023; Jennifer Rigby, "Pandemic's Origins Obscured by Lack of Chinese Data—WHO Panel," Reuters, June 9, 2022, https://www.reuters.com/business/healthcare-pharmaceuticals/pandemics-origins-obscured-by-lack-chinese-data-who-panel-2022-06-09/.

209 *It also raised silly red herrings*: Jiahui Wang, Fengqin Li, Zhaoping Liu, and Ning Li, "Perspectives: COVID-19 Outbreaks Linked to imported Frozen Food in China: Status and Challege [*sic*]," *China CDC Weekly* 4, no. 22 (2022): 483–87, https://weekly.chinacdc.cn/en/article/doi/10.46234/ccdcw2022.072; Ryan Pickrell, "Chinese Foreign Ministry Spokesman Pushes Coronavirus Conspiracy Theory That the US Army 'Brought the Epidemic to Wuhan,'" Business Insider, March 14, 2020, https://www.businessinsider.com/chinese-official-says-us-army-maybe-brought-coronavirus-to-wuhan-2020-3.

209 *Most important in my eyes*: Jonathan Latham and Allison Wilson, "A Proposed Origin for SARS-CoV-2 and the COVID-19 Pandemic," *Independent Science News*, July 15, 2020, https://www.independentsciencenews.org/commentaries/a-proposed-origin-for-sars-cov-2-and-the-covid-19-pandemic/; Monali C. Rahalkar and Rahul A. Bahulikar, "Understanding the Origin of 'BatCoVRaTG13,' a Virus Closest to SARS-CoV-2," Preprints.org, May 20, 2020, https://www.preprints.org/manuscript/202005.0322/v2; X. Y. Ge, N. Wang, W. Zhang, et al., "Coexistence of Multiple Coronaviruses in Several Bat Colonies in an Abandoned Mineshaft," *Virologica Sinica* 31 (2016): 31–40, https://link.springer.com

/article/10.1007/s12250-016-3713-9; Monali C. Rahalkar and Rahul A Bahulikar, “Lethal Pneumonia Cases in Mojian Miners (2012) and the Mineshaft Could Provide Important Clues to the Origin of SARS-CoV-2,” *Frontiers in Public Health* 8 (October 20, 2020), https://www.frontiersin.org/articles/10.3389/fpubh.2020.581569/full#B12; Rossana Segreto and Yuri Deigin, “The Genetic Structure of SARS-CoV-2 Does Not Rule Out a Laboratory Origin,” *BioEssays*, November 17, 2020, https://onlinelibrary.wiley.com/doi/10.1002/bies.202000240.

209 *It was also revealed that*: P. Zhou, X. L. Yang, X. G. Wang, et al., “Addendum: A Pneumonia Outbreak Associated with a New Coronavirus of Probable Bat Origin,” *Nature* 588, E6 (November 17, 2020), https://www.nature.com/articles/s41586-020-2951-z; Jon Cohen, “Wuhan Coronavirus Hunter Shi Zhengli Speaks Out,” *Science* 369, no. 6503 (July 31, 2020): 487–88, https://www.science.org/doi/10.1126/science.369.6503.487; V. Menachery, B. Yount, K. Debbink, et al., “A SARS-like Cluster of Circulating Bat Coronaviruses Shows Potential for Human Emergence,” *Nature Medicine* 21 (2015): 1508–13, https://www.nature.com/articles/nm.3985.

210 *In an interview with* Scientific American: Jane Qiu, “How China’s ‘Bat Woman’ Hunted Down Viruses from SARS to the New Coronavirus,” *Scientific American*, June 1, 2020, https://www.scientificamerican.com/article/how-chinas-bat-woman-hunted-down-viruses-from-sars-to-the-new-coronavirus1/.

210 *In a June 2021 interview*: Amy Qin and Chris Buckley, “A Top Virologist in China, at Center of a Pandemic Storm, Speaks Out,” *New York Times*, June 14, 2021.

210 *In a 2022 article*: Jane Qiu, “Meet the Scientist at the Center of the Covid Lab Leak Controversy,” *MIT Technology Review*, February 9, 2022, https://www.technologyreview.com/2022/02/09/1044985/shi-zhengli-covid-lab-leak-wuhan/.

210 *Wang Linfa*: John Sudworth and Simon Maybin, “Covid: Top Chinese Scientist Says Don’t Rule Out Lab Leak,” BBC News, May 30, 2023, https://www.bbc.com/news/world-asia-65708746.

210 *On May 17, 2021*: Donald G. McNeil Jr., “How I Learned to Stop Worrying and Love the Lab Leak Theory,” Medium, May 17, 2021, https://donaldgmcneiljr1954.medium.com/how-i-learned-to-stop-worrying-and-love-the-lab-leak-theory-f4f88446b04d.

210 *In September 2021*: Sarah Temmam, Khamsing Vongphayloth, et al., “Coronaviruses with a SARS-CoV-2-like Receptor-Binding Domain

Allowing ACE2-Mediated Entry into Human Cells Isolated from Bats of Indochinese Peninsula," Research Square preprint, September 17, 2021, https://www.researchsquare.com/article/rs-871965/v1; Carl Zimmer, "Newly Discovered Bat Viruses Give Hints to Covid's Origins," *New York Times*, October 14, 2021.

211 *Since then, scientific detective work*: Carl Zimmer and Benjamin Mueller, "New Research Points to Wuhan Market as Pandemic Origin," *New York Times*, February 26, 2022.

211 *He debunked reports*: Carl Zimmer, Benjamin Mueller, and Chris Buckley, "First Known Covid Case Was Vendor at Wuhan Market, Scientist Says," *New York Times*, November 18, 2021.

211 *Dr. Worobey and his collaborators*: Michael Worobey, Joshua I. Levy, Lorena Malpica Serrano, et al., "The Huanan Seafood Wholesale Market in Wuhan was the Early Epicenter of the COVID-19 Pandemic," *Science* 377, no. 6609 (July 26, 2022): 951–59, https://www.science.org/doi/10.1126/science.abp8715.

211 *Photographs taken in 2014*: Carl Zimmer, "He Goes Where the Fire Is: A Virus Hunter in the Wuhan Market," *New York Times*, March 21, 2022.

211 *They further argued that*: Jonathan E. Pekar, Andrew Magee, Edyth Parker, et al., "The Molecular Epidemiology of Multiple Zoonotic Origins of SARS-CoV-2," *Science* 377, no. 6609 (July 26, 2022): 960–66, https://www.science.org/doi/10.1126/science.abp8337.

211 *In March 2023*: Katherine J. Wu, "The Strongest Evidence Yet That an Animal Started the Pandemic," *Atlantic*, March 16, 2023; Benjamin Mueller, "New Data Links Pandemic's Origins to Raccoon Dogs at Wuhan Market," *New York Times*, March 16, 2023.

Chapter 17: The Crises of Trust and Fetishization of Science

213 *On the March 12, 2020, episode*: "Confronting a Pandemic," *The Daily* podcast, *New York Times*, March 12, 2020.

214 *In a study of 7,324 early cases*: Hua Qian, Te Miao, et al., "Indoor Transmission of SARS-CoV-2," *Indoor Air*, October 31, 2020, https://onlinelibrary.wiley.com/doi/10.1111/ina.12766.

214 *Later studies*: Ronan McGreevy, "Outdoor Transmission Accounts for 0.1% of State's Covid-19 Cases," *Irish Times*, April 5, 2021, https://www.irishtimes.com/news/ireland/irish-news/outdoor-transmission-accounts-for-0-1-of-state-s-covid-19-cases-1.4529036; Canterbury Christ

Church University, "Rapid Scoping Review of Evidence of Outdoor Transmission of Covid-19," September 2020, https://www.canterbury.ac.uk/science-engineering-and-social-sciences/spear/research-projects/rapid-scoping-review-COVID-19.aspx.

214 *In 2020 and 2021*: Joal Ryan and Carolin Lehmann, "Counterfeit N95 and KN95 Face Masks: How Can You Spot Fakes?" CBS News, updated March 10, 2022, https://www.cbsnews.com/essentials/n95-kn95-masks-counterfeit-fake; CDC National Personal Protective Technology Laboratory, "Counterfeit Respirators/Misrepresentation of NIOSH Approval," Respirator User Notices, https://www.cdc.gov/niosh/npptl/usernotices/counterfeitResp.html.

215 *On March 20, 2020*: Press release, "Governor Cuomo Signs the 'New York State on PAUSE' Executive Order," New York State Office of the Governor, March 20, 2020, https://www.governor.ny.gov/news/governor-cuomo-signs-new-york-state-pause-executive-order.

216 *Germany used*: Christoper F. Schuetze and Melissa Eddy, "Germany Makes Rapid Virus Tests a Key to Everyday Freedoms," *New York Times*, June 9, 2021.

217 *The most infamous*: Centers for Disease Control and Prevention, "The U.S. Public Health Service Study at Tuskegee: The Timeline," https://www.cdc.gov/tuskegee/timeline.htm.

218 *Only in 1972*: Jean Heller, "AP WAS THERE: Black men untreated in Tuskegee Syphilis Study," AP News, May 10, 2017, https://apnews.com/article/business-science-health-race-and-ethnicity-syphilis-e9dd07eaa4e74052878a68132cd3803a.

218 *Children were immobilized*: H. V. Wyatt, "Before the Vaccines: Medical Treatments of Acute Paralysis in the 1916 New York Epidemic of Poliomyelitis," *Open Microbiology Journal* 8 (December 12, 2014): 144–47, https://www.ncbi.nlm.nih.gov/pmc/articles/PMC4293735/; Tony Gould, *A Summer Plague: Polio and Its Survivors* (New Haven, CT: Yale University Press, 1995), 23.

219 *In the end*: "39 Die of Paralysis, Highest Day's Toll," *New York Times,* July 23, 1916, 7, https://timesmachine.nytimes.com/timesmachine/1916/07/23/104237561.html?zoom=15&pageNumber=7.

219 *But the economic crisis*: Centers for Disease Control and Prevention, "Public Health Assessment: Russian Federation, 1992," *Morbidity and Mortality Weekly Report* 41, no. 06 (February 14, 1992): 89–91, https://www.cdc.gov/mmwr/preview/mmwrhtml/00016056.htm; Centers for Disease Control and Prevention, "Diphtheria Outbreak:

Russian Federation 1990–1993," *Morbidity and Mortality Weekly Report* 42, no. 43 (November 5, 1993): 840–41, 847, https://www.cdc.gov/mmwr/preview/mmwrhtml/00022128.htm#.

220 *Polio immunization*: World Health Organization, Global Health Observatory data repository, "Polio [Pol3] Immunization Coverage Estimates by Country (Through 2021)," https://apps.who.int/gho/data/node.main.A831?lang=en.

220 *Since the disease was discovered*: Wikipedia, "List of Ebola Outbreaks," https://en.wikipedia.org/wiki/List_of_Ebola_outbreaks.

221 *ALIMA*: Sharmila Devi, "Frontline: A New Treatment Facility for Ebola Virus Disease," *Lancet* 392, no. 10163 (December 8, 2018): 2428, https://www.thelancet.com/journals/lancet/article/PIIS0140 6736(18)33118-0/fulltext.

221 *Burial practices also changed*: Mosoka P. Fallah, "To Beat Ebola in Uganda, Fund What Worked in Liberia," *Nature* 611, no. 427 (November 15, 2022), https://www.nature.com/articles/d41586-022-03695-4.

221 *In 2019, two successful treatments*: Donald G. McNeil Jr., "A Cure for Ebola? Two New Treatments Prove Highly Effective in Congo," *New York Times*, August 12, 2019.

222 *"I'm a little sentimental"*: Donald G. McNeil Jr., "A Cure for Ebola? Two New Treatments Prove Highly Effective in Congo," *New York Times*, August 12, 2019.

222 *For example, in Los Angeles*: Donald G. McNeil Jr., "Unlikely Model in H.I.V. Efforts: Sex Film Industry," *New York Times*, November 5, 2012.

223 *In 2003, Vancouver*: Donald G. McNeil Jr., "An H.I.V. Strategy Invites Addicts In," *New York Times*, February 7, 2011.

223 *In Johannesburg*: Jonathan Stadler and Sinead Delany, "The 'Healthy Brothel': The Context of Clinical Services for Sex Workers in Hillbrow, South Africa," *Culture Health and Sexuality* 8, no. 5 (September 2006): 451–64, https://www.tandfonline.com/doi/full/10.1080/13691050600872107; Donald G. McNeil Jr., "Three Approaches to Beating the AIDS Epidemic in South Africa," *New York Times*, August 25, 2014.

223 *In San Francisco*: Donald G. McNeil Jr., "San Francisco Is Changing Face of AIDS Treatment," *New York Times*, October 5, 2015.

Chapter 18: We Need a Pentagon for Disease

228 *Although the first alarms*: Sheryl Gay Stolberg and Peter Baker, "Biden Names White House Coordinator for Monkeypox," *New York Times*, August 2, 2022.

229 *Previously, the White House said*: "FACT SHEET: Biden-Harris Administration's Monkeypox Outbreak Response," White House Briefing Room Statements and Releases, June 28, 2022, https://www.whitehouse.gov/briefing-room/statements-releases/2022/06/28/fact-sheet-biden-harris-administrations-monkeypox-outbreak-response/.

229 *At Mr. Fenton's first news conference*: Matthew Perrone, "WATCH: White House Monkeypox Response Team Says U.S. Will Stretch Vaccine Supply with Smaller Doses," AP News and *PBS NewsHour*, August 9, 2022, https://www.pbs.org/newshour/health/watch-live-white-house-monkeypox-response-team-and-public-health-officials-hold-news-briefing.

232 *As we learned*: Nathaniel Weixel, "Trump Officials Interfered with CDC Guidance for Political Purposes, House Panel Finds," *The Hill*, October 17, 2022, https://thehill.com/policy/healthcare/3693002-trump-white-house-officials-interfered-with-cdc-guidance-for-political-purposes/.

233 *During the Korean War*: "Doctors' Draft," *CQ Almanac*, 1953, CQ Press Online editions, https://library.cqpress.com/cqalmanac/document.php?id=cqal53-1364043; Dwight Jon Zimmerman, "Battlefield Medicine in the Korean War," Defense Media Network, May 14, 2021, https://www.defensemedianetwork.com/stories/battlefield-medicine-in-the-korean-war/.

234 *Since 1986, the Selective Service*: Med School Insiders, "Can Doctors Get Drafted Into the Military?" MedPage Today, March 17, 2022, https://www.medpagetoday.com/reading-room/popmedicine/popmedicine/97727.

234 *We already face a shortage*: IHS Markit Ltd., "The Complexities of Physician Supply and Demand: Projections from 2019 to 2034," AAMC Report, June 11, 2021, https://www.aamc.org/news-insights/press-releases/aamc-report-reinforces-mounting-physician-shortage.

234 *In a 2023 op-ed piece*: Bill Gates, "I Worry We're Making the Same Mistakes Again," *New York Times*, March 19, 2023.

Chapter 19: We Need to Fight Global Poverty

236 *According to the World Bank*: Marta Schoch, Samuel Kofi Tetteh Baah, et al., "Half the Global Population Lives on Less than US$6.85 per Person per Day," *Let's Talk Development* blog, World Bank, December 8, 2022, https://blogs.worldbank.org/developmenttalk/half-global-population-lives-less-us685-person-day.

237 *To help me report a story*: Donald G. McNeil Jr., "Zambian Women, Doomed to Life on a Rock Pile," *New York Times*, August 2, 1996.

239 *According to the 2022 World Inequality Report*: World Inequality Lab, "World Inequality Report 2022," December 7, 2021, https://wir2022.wid.world/.

239 *The World Bank estimated*: Daniel Gerszon Mahler, Nishant Yonzan, et al., "Pandemic, Prices and Poverty," *Data Blog*, World Bank, April 13, 2022, https://blogs.worldbank.org/opendata/pandemic-prices-and-poverty.

240 *Over 10 million children*: UNICEF, "Under 5 Mortality," January 2023, https://data.unicef.org/topic/child-survival/under-five-mortality/.

240 *In the year 2000*: Patrice Trouiller, Piero Olliaro, et al., "Drug Development for Neglected Diseases: A Deficient Market and a Public-Health Policy Failure," *Lancet* 359, no. 9324 (June 22, 2002): 2188–94, https://www.thelancet.com/journals/lancet/article/PIIS0140673602090967/fulltext.

240 *The newest blockbuster*: Denise Grady, "Human Drugs Approved for Mental Problems in Dogs," *New York Times*, January 6, 1999.

241 *Global funding for AIDS*: UNAIDS, "Fact Sheet Global AIDS 2022," https://www.unaids.org/sites/default/files/media_asset/UNAIDS_FactSheet_en.pdf.

242 *The number of children who died*: Donald G. McNeil Jr., "Child Mortality at Record Low; Further Drop Seen," *New York Times*, September 13, 2007; Josh Katz, Alicia Parlapiano, and Margo Sanger-Katz, "Almost Everywhere, Fewer Children Are Dying," *New York Times*, September 17, 2019.

242 *PEPFAR's budget*: Kaiser Family Foundation, "Global Health Policy: The U.S. President's Emergency Plan for AIDS Relief (PEPFAR)," July 12, 2022, https://www.kff.org/global-health-policy/fact-sheet/the-u-s-presidents-emergency-plan-for-aids-relief-pepfar/.

243 *Much of that progress*: Kimberly Singer Babiarz, Karen Eggleston, Grant Miller, and Qiong Zhang, "An Exploration of China's Mortality

Decline under Mao: A Provincial Analysis, 1950–1980," *Population Studies* 69, no. 1 (March 2015): 39–56, https://www.ncbi.nlm.nih.gov/pmc/articles/PMC4331212/.

244 *The late Paul Polak*: Paul Polak, *Out of Poverty: What Works When Traditional Approaches Fail* (San Francisco: Berrett-Koehler, 2008).

244 *He came up with*: Donald G. McNeil Jr., "Paul Polak, Entrepreneur for Those Living on $2 a Day, Dies at 86," *New York Times*, October 20, 2019.

245 *Former president Jimmy Carter*: "Guinea Worm Disease Reaches All-Time Low: Only 13* Human Cases Reported in 2022," Carter Center, January 24, 2023, https://www.cartercenter.org/news/pr/2023/2022-guinea-worm-worldwide-cases-announcement.html.

246 *Guinea worm*: Donald G. McNeil Jr., "Dose of Tenacity Wears Down a Horrific Disease," *New York Times*, March 26, 2006.

247 *Presidents can speak bluntly*: "President Bush Participates in Joint Press Availability with President Yayi of Benin," White House press release, February 16, 2008, https://georgewbush-whitehouse.archives.gov/news/releases/2008/02/text/20080216-2.html.

247 *The most shocking result*: "Former SFDA Chief Executed for Corruption," *China Daily*, July 10, 2007, https://www.chinadaily.com.cn/china/2007-07/10/content_5424937.htm; David Barboza, "A Chinese Reformer Betrays His Cause, and Pays," *New York Times*, July 13, 2007.

248 *A year later, 6 babies died*: "2008 Chinese Milk Scandal," Wikipedia, https://en.wikipedia.org/wiki/2008_Chinese_milk_scandal.

Chapter 20: We Need to Ban Religious Exemptions

251 *American courts have long held*: S. Woolley, "Children of Jehovah's Witnesses and Adolescent Jehovah's Witnesses: What Are Their Rights?" *Archives of Diseases in Childhood* 90, no. 7 (July 2005): 715–19, https://www.ncbi.nlm.nih.gov/pmc/articles/PMC1720472/.

251 *Courts recognize this*: Wendy K. Mariner, George J. Annas, and Leonard H. Glantz, "Jacobson v. Massachusetts: It's Not Your Great-Great-Grandfather's Public Health Law," *American Journal of Public Health* 95, no. 4 (April 2005): 581–90, https://www.ncbi.nlm.nih.gov/pmc/articles/PMC1449224/#r47.

251 *In 1922, in* Zucht v. King: Law School Case Brief, "Zucht v. King—260 U.S. 174 43 S. Ct. 24 (1922)," Lexis-Nexis, https://www.lexisnexis.com/community/casebrief/p/casebrief-zucht-v-king.

252 *Even religions like*: Dorit Rubinstein Reiss, "Thou Shalt Not Take the Name of the Lord Thy God in Vain: Use and Abuse of Religious Exemptions from School Immunization Requirements," *Hastings Law Journal* 65 (2014): 1551–1602, https://www.hastingslawjournal.org/wp-content/uploads/Reiss-65.6.pdf; John D. Grabenstein, "What the World's Religions Teach, Applied to Vaccines and Immune Globulins," *Vaccine* 31, no. 16 (April 12, 2013): 2011–23, https://www.immunize.org/talking-about-vaccines/pdf/religion-vaccines-antibodies-grabenstein-2011.pdf.

252 *Currently, forty-four states*: Douglas S. Diekema, "Personal Belief Exemptions from School Vaccination Requirements," *Annual Review of Public Health* 35 (March 2014): 275–92, https://www.annualreviews.org/doi/full/10.1146/annurev-publhealth-032013-182452.

253 *Mark Twain*: Mark Twain letter to Joseph Twichell, January 8, 1900, cited at www.twainquotes.com/ChristianScience.html.

253 *Starting in the 1960s*: National Conference of State Legislatures, "States with Religious and Philosophical Exemptions from School Immunization Requirements Title," updated May 25, 2022, https://www.ncsl.org/health/states-with-religious-and-philosophical-exemptions-from-school-immunization-requirements.

253 *That had predictable results*: Jennifer Zipprich, Katleen Winter, et al., "Measles Outbreak: California, December 2014–February 2015," *Morbidity and Mortality Weekly Report* 64, no. 06 (February 20, 2015): 153–54, https://www.cdc.gov/mmwr/preview/mmwrhtml/mm6406a5.htm.

253 *Vaccination rates among kindergartners*: Sindiso Nyathi, Hannah C. Karpel, et al., "The 2016 California Policy to Eliminate Nonmedical Vaccine Exemptions and Changes in Vaccine Coverage: An Empirical Policy Analysis," *PLOS Medicine*, February 23, 2019, https://journals.plos.org/plosmedicine/article?id=10.1371/journal.pmed.1002994.

254 *The anti-vaccine lobby tries*: Tyler Pager, "'Monkey, Rat and Pig DNA': How Misinformation Is Driving the Measles Outbreak Among Ultra-Orthodox Jews," *New York Times*, April 9, 2019.

254 *Vaccines may contain*: Centers for Disease Control and Prevention, "Appendix B: Vaccine Excipient Summary," *Epidemiology and Prevention of Vaccine-Preventable Diseases* ("Pink Book"), 2021 edition, https://www.cdc.gov/vaccines/pubs/pinkbook/downloads/appendices/B/excipient-table-2.pdf; Johns Hopkins Bloomberg School of Public Health, Institute for Vaccine Safety, "Components of Vaccines," https://www.vaccinesafety.edu/components-of-vaccines/.

254 *Also, some vaccines contain*: Tetsuo Nakayama and Chikara Aizawa, "Changes in Gelatin Content of Vaccines Associated with Reduction in Reports of Allergic Reactions," *Journal of Allergy and Clinical Immunology* 106, no. 3 (September 2000): 591–92, https://www.jacionline.org/article/S0091-6749(00)68940-6/fulltext.

254 *"Since it is proven"*: "Rav Moshe Sternbuch Writes Letter to Rav Malkiel Kotler About the Halachic Requirement to Vaccinate," Yeshiva World, November 27, 2018, https://www.theyeshivaworld.com/news/general/1631188/rav-moshe-sternbuch-writes-letter-to-rav-malkiel-kotler-about-the-halachic-requirement-to-vaccinate.html.

254 *Rabbi Sternbuch's opinion*: Parents Educating and Advocating for Children's Health (PEACH), *The Vaccine Safety Handbook*, December 1, 2017, https://issuu.com/peachmoms/docs/the_vaccine_safety_handbook_a4.

254 *But kosher dietary laws*: Donald G. McNeil Jr., "Religious Objections to the Measles Vaccine? Get the Shots, Faith Leaders Say," *New York Times*, April 26, 2019.

255 *During a 1995 meeting*: Hussein A. Gezairy, letter from the director of the WHO Eastern Mediterranean Region, July 17, 2001, https://www.immunize.org/talking-about-vaccines/porcine.pdf.

255 *More than two hundred years ago*: Rabbi Mark Glass, "A Historical, Jewish Perspective on Vaccinations," *Kansas City Jewish Chronicle*, July 29, 2021, https://www.kcjc.com/opinions/speaker-s-corner/7211-a-historical-jewish-perspective-on-vaccinations; Rav Asher Weiss, "Is It Permissible to Refrain from Vaccinating Children?" Baltimore Jewish Life, January 3, 2019, https://baltimorejewishlife.com/news/news-detail.php?SECTION_ID=1&ARTICLE_ID=112570.

255 *Rabbi Nachman of Breslov*: Rabbi Dr. Goldie Milgram, "Regarding Immunizations for Children Who Will Be Attending Day (Jewish or Parochial) Schools: What Is the Jewish View on Whether This Is Obligatory or Optional? What Jewish Values or Ethics Are Involved in this Question?" Jewish Values Online, http://www.jewishvaluesonline.org/question.php?id=566.

255 *The MRC-5 line*: Coriell Institute for Medical Research, "MRC-5: Normal Human Fetal Lung Fibroblast," https://www.coriell.org/0/Sections/Search/Sample_Detail.aspx?Ref=AG05965-C&PgId=166; Meredith Wadman, "Medical Research: Cell Division," *Nature* 498 (June 26, 2013): 422–26, https://www.nature.com/articles/498422a.

256 *In 2005, replying to a request*: E. Sgreccia, president, Pontificia Academia Pro Vita, "Letter to Mrs. Debra L. Vinnedge, Executive Direc-

tor, Children of God for Life," June 9, 2005, https://www.immunize.org/talking-about-vaccines/vaticandocument.htm.

256 *In 2022, Pope Francis*: Joshua J. McElwee, "Pope Francis Suggests People Have Moral Obligation to Take Coronavirus Vaccine," *National Catholic Reporter*, January 11, 2022, https://www.ncronline.org/vatican/pope-francis-suggests-people-have-moral-obligation-take-coronavirus-vaccine.

256 *In 2002, as part of researching*: Donald G. McNeil Jr., "Worship Optional: Joining a Church to Avoid Vaccines," *New York Times*, January 14, 2003.

Chapter 21: We Need to Improve Surveillance

260 *One of the best efforts*: "Emerging Pandemic Threats," USAID, 2012–17, https:/2012-2017.usaid.gov/news-information/fact-sheets/emerging-pandemic-threats-program.

260 *Predict sent wildlife veterinarians*: Donald G. McNeil Jr., "You're Swabbing a Dead Gorilla for Ebola. Then It Gets Worse," *New York Times*, October 14, 2019.

261 *In late 2019*: Donald G. McNeil Jr., "Scientists Were Hunting for the Next Ebola. Now the U.S. Has Cut Off Their Funding," *New York Times*, October 25, 2019.

261 *Various estimates*: David M. Cutler and Lawrence H. Summers, "The COVID-19 Pandemic and the $16 Trillion Virus," *JAMA* 324, no. 15 (October 12, 2020): 1495–96, https://jamanetwork.com/journals/jama/article-abstract/2771764; Richard Bruns and Nikki Teran, "Weighing the Cost of the Pandemic," Institute for Progress, April 21, 2022, https://progress.institute/weighing-the-cost-of-the-pandemic/.

261 *An even more ambitious vision*: Global Virome Project, "Our History," https://www.globalviromeproject.org/our-history.

261 *Programs like that*: Michaeleen Doucleff, "How Do Pandemics Begin? There's a New Theory—and a New Strategy to Thwart Them," *Goats and Soda* blog, NPR, February 15, 2023, https://www.npr.org/sections/goatsandsoda/2023/02/15/1152892721/how-to-stop-pandemics.

263 *Haiti's devastating 2010 cholera epidemic*: Jonathan M. Katz, "U.N. Admits Role in Cholera Epidemic in Haiti," *New York Times*, August 17, 2016.

263 *In 2013, poliovirus*: Donald G. McNeil Jr., "Polio Virus Discovered in Sewage from Israel," *New York Times,* June 3, 2013; Donald G. McNeil Jr., "Egypt: Polio Virus Is Found in Cairo's Sewers," *New York Times*, January 23, 2013.

263 *In 2020, in response to Covid*: Centers for Disease Control and Prevention, "National Wastewater Surveillance System (NWSS)," September 2020, https://www.cdc.gov/nwss/wastewater-surveillance/index.html.

263 *In 2023, New York State*: Chris Dall, "New York to Expand Its Wastewater Surveillance Network," CIDRAP News, January 26, 2023, https://www.cidrap.umn.edu/influenza-general/new-york-expand-its-wastewater-surveillance-network.

264 *A 2023 study in Nevada*: Mary Van Beusekom, "What Stays in Vegas: Tourist Sewage May Inflate Community COVID Prevalence," CIDRAP News, February 24, 2023, https://www.cidrap.umn.edu/covid-19/what-stays-vegas-tourist-sewage-may-inflate-community-covid-prevalence.

264 *A study done in late 2022*: Robert C. Morfino, Stephen M. Bart, et al., "Notes from the Field: Aircraft Wastewater Surveillance for Early Detection of SARS-CoV-2 Variants—John F. Kennedy International Airport, New York City, August–September 2022," *Morbidity and Mortality Weekly Report* 72, no. 8 (February 23, 2023): 210–11.

264 *The value of checking sewage*: Erwin Duizer, Wilhemin LM Ruijs, et al., "Wild Poliovirus Type 3 (WPV3)-Shedding Event Following Detection in Environmental Surveillance of Poliovirus Essential Facilities, the Netherlands, November 2022 to January 2023," *Eurosurveillance* 28, no. 5 (February 2, 2023).

264 *It was created after*: "1992–1993 Jack in the Box *E. coli* Outbreak," Wikipedia, https://en.wikipedia.org/wiki/1992%E2%80%931993_Jack_in_the_Box_E._coli_outbreak.

265 *Not every high-tech surveillance plan*: Miguel Helft, "Using the Internet to Track Flu's Spread," *New York Times*, October 11, 2008; Gary Marcus and Ernest Davis, "Eight (No, Nine!) Problems with Big Data," *New York Times*, April 6, 2014.

265 *A year later, Flu Trends*: Nick Bilton, "Disruptions: Data without Context Tells a Misleading Story," *New York Times*, February 24, 2013.

266 *Analyses in* Nature *and* Science: Declan Butler, "When Google Got Flu Wrong," *Nature* 494 (February 13, 2013): 155–56, https://www.nature.com/articles/494155a; David Lazer, Ryan Kennedy, Gary King, and Alessandro Vespignani, "The Parable of Google Flu: Traps in Big Data Analysis," *Science* 343, no. 6176 (March 14, 2014): 1203–05, March 14, 2014, https://www.science.org/doi/10.1126/science.1248506.

266 *"In short," said one critic*: Kaiser Fung, "Google Flu Trends' Failure

Shows Good Data > Big Data," *Harvard Business Review*, March 25, 2014, https://hbr.org/2014/03/google-flu-trends-failure-shows-good-data-big-data.

266 *One technology*: Donald G. McNeil Jr., "'Smart Thermometers' Track Flu Season in Real Time," *New York Times*, January 16, 2018.

267 *The United States was winding down*: Donald G. McNeil Jr., "Can Smart Thermometers Track the Spread of the Coronavirus?" *New York Times*, March 18, 2020.

267 *Then, as the country began locking down*: Donald G. McNeil Jr., "Restrictions Are Slowing Coronavirus Infections, New Data Suggest," *New York Times*, March 30, 2020.

267 *Cell phone tracking is also useful*: Dhaval Dave, Drew McNichols, and Joseph J. Sabia, "The Contagion Externality of a Superspreading Event: The Sturgis Motorcycle Rally and COVID-19," *Southern Economic Journal* 87, no. 3 (January 2021): 769–807, https://www.ncbi.nlm.nih.gov/pmc/articles/PMC7753804/.

Chapter 22: We Need to Rationalize "Emergencies"

268 *The secretary of health and human services*: Department of Health and Human Services, Administration for Strategic Preparedness and Response, "A Public Health Emergency Declaration," https://aspr.hhs.gov/legal/PHE/Pages/Public-Health-Emergency-Declaration.aspx.

268 *The WHO, by contrast*: World Health Organization, "Emergencies: International Health Regulations and Emergency Committees Q&A," December 19, 2019, https://www.who.int/news-room/questions-and-answers/item/emergencies-international-health-regulations-and-emergency-committees.

269 *On January 23*: Denise Grady, "Coronavirus Is Spreading, but W.H.O. Says It's Not a Global Emergency," *New York Times*, January 23, 2020.

269 *A week later*: Sui-Lee Wee, Donald G. McNeil Jr., and Javier C. Hernandez, "W.H.O. Declares Global Emergency as Wuhan Coronavirus Spreads," *New York Times*, January 30, 2020.

269 *In 2009, the agency fumbled*: Donald G. McNeil Jr., "Technically, Monkeypox Already IS a Pandemic," Medium, May 31, 2022, https://donaldgmcneiljr1954.medium.com/technically-monkeypox-already-is-a-pandemic-dd88eda08562.

270 *The reluctance, according to Dr. Michael J. Ryan*: "Coronavirus Outbreak: WHO Official Says Virus Not at Stage to Declare Pandemic,"

Global News, February 28, 2020, https://www.youtube.com/watch?v=XQChCZWmkK.

270 *But journalists kept asking why*: Debora Mackenzie, "Covid-19: Why Won't the WHO Officially Declare a Coronavirus Pandemic?" *New Scientist*, February 26, 2020, https://www.newscientist.com/article/2235342-covid-19-why-wont-the-who-officially-declare-a-coronavirus-pandemic/.

270 *Finally, on March 11*: Donald G. McNeil Jr., "Coronavirus Has Become a Pandemic, W.H.O. Says," *New York Times*, March 11, 2020.

Chapter 23: We Need to Respect Witch Doctors

272 *In Africa, according to the WHO*: World Health Organization, *WHO Traditional Medicine Strategy, 2014–2023* (Geneva: WHO Press, 2013), 28, https://apps.who.int/iris/bitstream/handle/10665/92455/9789241506090_eng.pdf?sequence=1#page=28.

272 *A 2018 review published*: Peter Bai James, Jon Wardle, Amie Steel, and Jon Adams, "Traditional, Complementary and Alternative Medicine Use in Sub-Saharan Africa: A Systematic Review," *BMJ Global Health* 3, no. 5 (October 31, 2018), https://gh.bmj.com/content/3/5.

273 *Samuel Muriisa*: Donald G. McNeil Jr., "Diagnoses by Horn, Payment in Goats: An African Healer at Work," *New York Times*, March 4, 2019.

273 *To people with no science background*: Andy Coghlan, "Leeuwenhoek's 'Animalcules,' Just as He Saw Them 340 Years Ago," *New Scientist*, May 20, 2015, https://www.newscientist.com/article/dn27563-leeuwenhoeks-animalcules-just-as-he-saw-them-340-years-ago/.

273 *I once asked a woman*: Donald G. McNeil Jr., "Drug Makers and 3rd World: A Study in Neglect," *New York Times*, May 21, 2000.

274 *At that time, the only treatment*: Donald G. McNeil Jr., "Jump-Start on Slow Trek to Treatment for a Disease," *New York Times*, January 8, 2008.

274 *In his memoir*: William H. Foege, *House on Fire: The Fight to Eradicate Smallpox* (Berkeley: University of California Press, 2011).

275 *And yes, there are horrible aspects*: "7 Killed in Ghana over 'Penis-Snatching' Episodes," CNN, January 7, 1997, http://www.cnn.com/WORLD/9701/18/briefs/ghana.penis.html; Ellen Wulfhorst, "Long Persecuted, Tanzanian Albinos Find Acceptance Growing Slowly," Reuters, February 1, 2019, https://www.reuters.com/article/us-usa

-tanzania-albinism/long-persecuted-tanzanian-albinos-find-acceptance-growing-slowly-idUSKCN1PQ5KJ.

275 *In the latter*: Jeffrey Gettleman, "Albinos in Tanzania Face Deadly Threat," *New York Times*, June 8, 2008; "Pictures: Inside the Lives of Albinos in Tanzania," *National Geographic*, January 27, 2013, https://www.nationalgeographic.com/culture/article/130125-albino-albinism-tanzania-witch-doctors.

276 *Dr. Hlengwa, a photographer, and I*: Donald G. McNeil Jr., "AIDS Crisis Leaves Africa's Oldest Ways at a Loss," *New York Times*, November 27, 2001.

277 *In early 2022*: Sushmita Pathak, "These Female Health-Care Workers Won a Huge WHO Honor. They'd Like a Raise Too," *Goats and Soda* blog, NPR, June 2, 2022.

278 *For example, Chen Zhu*: Jonathan Watts, "Chen Zhu: From Barefoot Doctor to China's Minister of Health," *Lancet* 372, no. 9648 (October 25, 2008): 1455, https://www.thelancet.com/journals/lancet/article/PIIS0140-6736(08)61561-5/fulltext.

279 *Studies have shown*: Jessica Leight, Vandana Sharma, and Martina Björkman Nyqvist, "Safe Birth Kits—A Promise Unfulfilled? Evidence from a Randomized Trial in Northern Nigeria," *Healthy Newborn Network* blog, February 1, 2019, https://www.healthynewbornnetwork.org/blog/safe-birth-kits-a-promise-unfulfilled-evidence-from-a-randomized-trial-in-northern-nigeria/.

Chapter 24: We Need to Make Medicine Cheaper

280 *For example, deworming pills*: Amitra Ahuja, Sarah Baird et al., "Economics of Mass Deworming Programs," in *Child and Adolescent Health and Development*, 3d ed. (Washington, DC: International Bank for Reconstruction and Development/World Bank, 2017), https://www.ncbi.nlm.nih.gov/books/NBK525237/.

280 *The long-term effects of such small victories*: Hoyt Bleakley, "Disease and Development: Evidence from Hookworm Eradication in the American South," *Quarterly Journal of Economics* 122, no. 1 (2007): 73–117, https://www.ncbi.nlm.nih.gov/pmc/articles/PMC3800113/.

281 *An example that worked quite well*: Donald G. McNeil Jr., "Curing Hepatitis C, in an Experiment the Size of Egypt," *New York Times*, December 15, 2015.

283 *Soon, however, drug-resistant strains*: Giovanni Sotgiu, Rosella Centis,

et al., "Tuberculosis Treatment and Drug Regimens," *Cold Spring Harbor Perspectives on Medicine* 5, no. 5 (May 2015): a017822, https://www.ncbi.nlm.nih.gov/pmc/articles/PMC4448591/.

283 *Until recently, the only hope*: Donald G. McNeil Jr., "Scientists Discover New Cure for the Deadliest Strain of Tuberculosis," *New York Times*, August 14, 2019.

283 *Chinese scientists*: Donald G. McNeil Jr., "New Drug for Malaria Pits U.S. Against Africa," *New York Times*, May 28, 2002; Donald G. McNeil Jr., "For Intrigue, Malaria Drug Gets the Prize," *New York Times*, January 16, 2012.

284 *The discovery eventually*: Lawrence K. Altman, "Nobel Prize in Medicine Awarded to 3 Scientists for Parasite-Fighting Therapies," *New York Times*, October 5, 2015.

285 *As the virus copies itself*: Cassandra Willyard, "How Antiviral Pill Molnupiravir Shot Ahead in the COVID Drug Hunt," *Scientific American*, October 12, 2021, https://www.scientificamerican.com/article/how-antiviral-pill-molnupiravir-shot-ahead-in-the-covid-drug-hunt/.

285 *President Trump*: Sheryl Gay Stolberg, "Trump and Friends Got Coronavirus Care Many Others Couldn't," *New York Times*, December 9, 2020.

286 *Under unusual circumstances*: ViiV Healthcare, "GlaxoSmithKline and Pfizer Announce Innovative Agreement to Create a New World-Leading, Specialist HIV Company," press release, April 16, 2009, https://viivhealthcare.com/hiv-news-and-media/news/press-releases/2009/april/glaxosmithkline-and-pfizer-announce-innovative-agreement-to-create-a-new-world-leading-specialist-hiv-company/.

286 *Cipla, an Indian company*: M. Villar Garcia, D. Mukeba-Tshialala, et al., "A Fixed Dose anti-HIV Combination for the Poor? Triomune," *Réview Medical du Liège* 64, no. 1 (January 2009): 32–36, https://pubmed.ncbi.nlm.nih.gov/19317099/.

286 *A 2022* Lancet *study*: Antimicrobial Resistance Collaborators, "Global Burden of Bacterial Antimicrobial Resistance in 2019, a Systematic Analysis," *Lancet* 399, no. 10325 (February 12, 2022): 629–55, https://www.thelancet.com/journals/lancet/article/PIIS0140-6736(21)02724-0/fulltext.

Chapter 25: Like It or Not, We Need Mandates

287 *In 2015, I went to Vietnam*: Donald G. McNeil Jr., "Vietnam's Battle with Tuberculosis," *New York Times*, March 28, 2016.

288 *When PEPFAR was created*: Kaiser Family Foundation, Global Health Policy, "The U.S. President's Emergency Plan for AIDS Relief (PEPFAR): Key Facts," July 12, 2022, https://www.kff.org/global-health-policy/fact-sheet/the-u-s-presidents-emergency-plan-for-aids-relief-pepfar.

288 *In Kenya, for example*: Donald G. McNeil Jr., "How to Get TB Patients to Take Their Pills? Persistent Texting and a 'Winners Circle,'" *New York Times*, September 4, 2019.

290 *The more overwhelmed*: Dawn M. Bravata, Anthony J. Perkins, et al., "Association of Intensive Care Unit Patient Load and Demand with Mortality Rates in US Department of Veterans Affairs Hospitals During the COVID-19 Pandemic," *JAMA Network Open* 4, no. 1 (2021): e2034266, https://jamanetwork.com/journals/jamanetworkopen/fullarticle/2775236.

291 *Three percent*: Rafael Harpaz, Rebecca M. Dahl, and Kathleen L. Dooling, "Prevalence of Immunosuppression Among US Adults, 2013," *Journal of the American Medical Association* 316, no. 23 (December 20, 2016), https://jamanetwork.com/journals/jama/fullarticle/2572798.

291 *17 percent*: Jonathan Vespa, Lauren Medina, and David M. Armstrong, "Demographic Turning Points for the United States: Population Projections for 2020 to 2060," U.S. Census Bureau Current Population Reports, February 2020, 25–1144, https://www.census.gov/content/dam/Census/library/publications/2020/demo/p25-1144.pdf.

291 *42 percent*: "Adult Obesity Facts," CDC Overweight and Obesity Data and Statistics, March 2020, https://www.cdc.gov/obesity/data/adult.html.

291 *He hired scientists*: Yasmeen Abutaleb, Philip Rucker, Josh Dawsey, and Robert Costa, "Trump's Den of Dissent: Inside the White House Task Force as Coronavirus Surges," *Washington Post*, October 19, 2020.

291 *He so twisted up*: David Leonhardt, "Red Covid," *New York Times*, September 27, 2021; Rebecca Shabad and Marc Caputo, "Trump Calls Politicians Who Refuse to Say They Received Covid Boosters 'Gutless,'" NBC News, January 12, 2022; Brigid Kennedy, "Tough Crowd: Trump Waves Off Boos after He, Bill O'Reilly Reveal They've Received the COVID Booster," *The Week*, December 20, 2021.

292 *He waited until*: "Fact Sheet: Biden Administration Announces Details of Two Major Vaccination Policies," White House press release, November 4, 2021, https://www.whitehouse.gov/briefing-room/statements-releases/2021/11/04/fact-sheet-biden-administration-announces-details-of-two-major-vaccination-policies/; Annie Lin-

skey, John Wagner, and Seung Min Kim, "Biden to Federal Workers: Get Vaccinated or Face Restrictions," *Washington Post*, July 29, 2021.

292 *Medical mandates have been saving*: George Washington, letter to the New York Convention, February 10, 1777, Founders Online, National Archives, https://founders.archives.gov/documents/Washington/03-08-02-0320.

293 *Without that order*: "Smallpox, Inoculation, and the Revolutionary War," National Park Service, https://www.nps.gov/articles/000/smallpox-inoculation-revolutionary-war.htm.

293 *Mandates worked for California*: Sindiso Nyathi, Hannah C. Karpel, et al., "The 2016 California Policy to Eliminate Nonmedical Vaccine Exemptions and Changes in Vaccine Coverage: An Empirical Policy Analysis," *PLOS Medicine*, February 23, 2019, https://journals.plos.org/plosmedicine/article?id=10.1371/journal.pmed.1002994.

293 *Mandates worked during Covid*: Dave Muoio, "How Many Employees Have Hospitals Lost to Vaccine Mandates? Here Are the Numbers So Far," Fierce Health Care, February 22, 2022, https://www.fiercehealthcare.com/hospitals/how-many-employees-have-hospitals-lost-to-vaccine-mandates-numbers-so-far.

293 *They worked for many employers*: Emma G. Fitzsimmons and Sharon Otterman, "New York City Ends Vaccine Mandate for City Workers," *New York Times*, February 6, 2023; Oriana González, "United Airlines: Employee Deaths Dropped to Zero after Vaccine Mandate," Axios, January 11, 2022; Samira Sadeque, "Nearly All Fox Staffers Vaccinated for Covid Even as Hosts Cast Doubt on Vaccine," *Guardian*, September 15, 2021.

Epilogue

297 *I once covered*: Donald G. McNeil Jr., "In Remote Villages, Surprising New Measures Save Children with Malaria," *New York Times*, December 10, 2018.

297 *My February 2, 2020, story*: Donald G. McNeil Jr., "Wuhan Coronavirus Looks Increasingly Like a Pandemic, Experts Say," *New York Times*, February 2, 2020.

INDEX

ABOUT THE AUTHOR

Donald G. McNeil Jr. spent almost his entire career at *The New York Times*, starting as a copy boy in 1976. For twenty-five years, he was a science correspondent, reporting from more than sixty countries as he covered global health and infectious diseases. His prescient reporting on the Covid epidemic and his insightful appearances on *The Daily* podcast helped the *Times* win the 2021 Pulitzer Prize Gold Medal for Public Service. He also won the 2020 John Chancellor Award for Excellence in Journalism, the 2007 Robert F. Kennedy Journalism Grand Prize, and awards from GLAAD, the National Association of Black Journalists, and the Association of Health Care Journalists. Within the paper itself, he was a union activist and negotiator for the News Guild and a regular at the Alte Kakers table in the cafeteria. Born in San Francisco in 1954, he attended Catholic schools and the University of California at Berkeley.